Policy and Stra

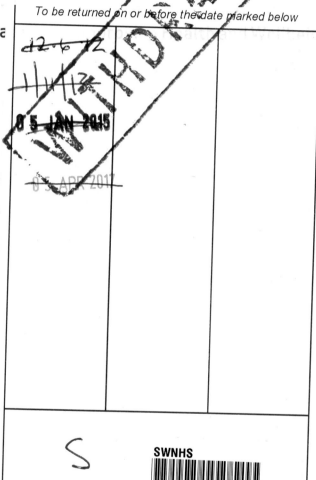

Titles in the Series

Assessing Evidence to Improve Population Health and Wellbeing ISBN 9780857253897
Leadership and Collaborative Working in Public Health ISBN 9780857252906
Measuring Health and Wellbeing ISBN 9780857254337

To order, please contact our distributor: BEBC Distribution, Albion Close, Parkstone, Poole BH12 3LL. Telephone: 0845 230 9000 email: learningmatters@bebc.co.uk. You can also find more information on each of these titles and our other learning resources at www.learningmatters.co.uk.

Policy and Strategy for Improving Health and Wellbeing

Editors: Elizabeth Porter and Lesley Coles

Series Editor:
Vicki Taylor

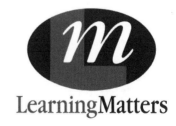

First published in 2011 by Learning Matters Ltd

British Library Cataloguing in Publication Data
A CIP record for this book is available from the British Library.
ISBN 9780857250070

This book is also available in the following ebook formats:
AER ISBN: 978 0 85725 288 3
EPUB ISBN: 978 0 85725 008 7
Kindle ISBN: 978 0 85725 289 0

Cover and text design by Code 5 Design Associates
Project management by Swales & Willis Ltd, Exeter, Devon
Typeset by Swales & Willis Ltd, Exeter, Devon
Printed and bound in Great Britain by Short Run Press Ltd, Exeter, Devon

Learning Matters Ltd
20 Cathedral Yard
Exeter EX1 1HB
Tel: 01392 215560
info@learningmatters.co.uk
www.learningmatters.co.uk

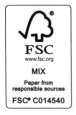

FSC
www.fsc.org
MIX
Paper from
responsible sources
FSC® C014540

Contents

Contents

Foreword from the Series Editor

The publication of the Public Health Skills and Career Framework in April 2008 provided, for the first time, an overall framework for career development in public health in the United Kingdom. Prior to this, the focus had been primarily on the public health specialist workforce. The development of the framework itself was a truly collaborative enterprise involving a large number of organisations and stakeholder groups and was designed to enable individuals at any stage of their career to identify a pathway for skills and career progression.

Within the framework, Public Health is divided into nine areas of work: There are four core areas that anyone working in public health must know about and have certain competences within. There are five non-core or 'defined' areas, representing the contexts within which individuals principally work and develop.

Core Areas	Non-core (defined) areas
Surveillance and assessment of the population's health and well-being	Health improvement
	Health Protection
Assessing the Evidence of Effectiveness of Interventions, Programmes & Services	Public Health Intelligence
Policy & Strategy Development & Implementation	Academic Public Health
Leadership & Collaborative Working	Health & Social Care Quality

This new series, 'Transforming Public Health Practice', has been developed as a direct response to the development of the framework and has a book dedicated to each of the four core areas of public health. Measuring Health and Wellbeing; Assessing Evidence to Improve Population Health and Wellbeing; Policy and Strategy for Improving Health and Wellbeing; and Leadership and Collaborative Working for Health and Wellbeing are all featured.

The framework defines nine levels of competence and knowledge: Level 1 will have little previous knowledge, skills or experience in public health, while those at level 9 will be setting strategic priorities and direction and providing leadership to improve population health and wellbeing. This series is aimed at those who want to develop their skills and knowledge in public health at levels 7–9 (which broadly equates to master's level) although the series will be relevant to a wider group with the publication of the Public Health Practitioner standards (UKPHR) and opening of the Public Health Practitioner Register (UKPHR). This will include those interested in acquiring or developing their public health competences and knowledge and, in particular, those who are seeking to demonstrate their public health skills and knowledge (and may be considering putting together a portfolio to demonstrate this, at specialist or practitioner level).

This series will also be useful for anyone whose work involves improving people's health and wellbeing, or has a direct impact on the health and wellbeing of communities and populations – this encompasses a wide range of work areas and of organisations and agencies.

Individual books in the series outline the key knowledge and skills in the core area and take these further through case studies and scenarios in order to show how these competences can be used in practice. Activities and self-assessment tools are provided throughout the book to help the reader to hone their critical thinking and reflection skills.

Chapters in each of the books follow a standard format. At the beginning a box highlights links to relevant competences. This sets the scene and enables the reader to see exactly what will be covered. This is extended by a chapter overview, which sets out the key topics and what the reader should expect to have learnt by the end of the chapter.

There is usually at least one case study in each chapter, which considers public health skills and knowledge in practice. Activities such as practical tasks with learning points, critical thinking and reflective practice are included. At the end of each chapter a chapter summary provides a reminder of what has been covered.

All chapters are evidence based in that they set out theory or evidence that underpins practice. A list of additional readings is set out under the 'Going further' section, with all references collated at the end of the book.

In summary, this series will provide invaluable support to anyone studying or practising in the field of public health, in a range of different settings.

Vicki Taylor,
Independent Public Health Consultant & Director,
The Roundhouse Consultancy, MK Ltd.
Associate Lecturer, The Open University.
Previously Senior Lecturer, London Southbank University,
Senior Lecturer, Kings College, London.

Foreword from Professor Vari Drennan

Improving the health and wellbeing of populations would seem an objective every citizen could sign up to and thus a goal of all governments. Sixty plus years of a 'welfare state' in the UK have demonstrated that, in reality, these are not easily agreed objectives, nor is there consensus as to the extent and role of government and the public sector. In 2011, as this book is published, the change in political leadership of the UK and specifically England demonstrates the influence of values and beliefs with a raft of new legislation, altering the nature and extent of public policy. Public health practitioners more than ever need to understand how public policy is developed, the factors that influence policy decisions at the macro and micro levels of society and the consequences in local implementation amongst the communities they work within. Contemporary definitions of public health encompass the promotion of health and wellbeing as well as the prevention of disease in populations as part of an organised societal enterprise. Public health practitioners need to understand the ways and means they can contribute to that collective effort in an often changing organisational and political landscape. This text provides the student and novice public health practitioners with a wealth of resources to build their knowledge and skills from. The early chapters examine frameworks for understanding policy processes and the mechanisms for influencing them. The chapters with analyses of the four countries of the UK offer plentiful opportunity to compare and contrast, identifying how different forces can shape local level services and preoccupations. The detailed descriptions and analysis of public policy in housing, child poverty, children and young people, obesity, drug misuse and tackling inequalities give penetrating insights into the extent to which national policies address public health problems as well as the unintended consequences of implementation and implementation gaps. Implementation tools and techniques are defined and range from those of the business and management worlds such as industry standards on project management through to those of whose origins lie in emancipatory politics such as community development.

I commend this text to all public health practitioners for both its breadth and depth for, while it is tailored to the learner and novice through the structured activities, there is much for others to absorb and learn from. While I think all those concerned with public health have always worked in '*challenging*' times and situations, it seems to me the widespread fiscal crisis and its consequences means public health practitioners will need to draw deeply in the coming years on the type of knowledge that this book so competently offers.

Vari Drennan, PhD., MSc. BSc., RN, RHV. Fellow of the Queen Nursing Institute
Professor of Health Policy & Service Delivery
Kingston University & St. George's University of London
February 2011

Author Information

Editor: Elizabeth Porter

Elizabeth Porter is a Senior Lecturer at the University of Southampton, Faculty of Health Sciences. She developed the first MSc in Public Health Practice at the University of Southampton in 2002 for public health practitioners and was programme leader for the MSc Public Health Practice at the University of Southampton 2003–10. The particular focus of her work for the last 23 years has been curriculum development, leadership, management and delivery of public health education for specialist community public health nurses and public health practitioners.

Editor: Lesley Coles

Lesley Coles is a retired Lecturer from the University of Southampton. Following a career in district nursing, Macmillan nursing and health visiting, she entered education and developed some of the first non-medical prescribing programmes for nurses. This later progressed into the development of multidisciplinary programmes for pharmacists, physiotherapists and occupational therapists. During the latter stages of her career she returned to pre-qualification curriculum development in order to enhance and develop public health and medicines management. Her last major role was as Award Leader for the Pre-qualifying Diploma with Advanced Studies in Nursing, with a portfolio focusing on curriculum review, development, re-approval and implementation of new programmes across all branches and academic awards.

David Adams

David Adams is a Lecturer in Health Studies at the Robert Gordon University's School of Nursing and Midwifery. With over 20 years' experience in nurse education, he currently teaches aspects of health policy, at both pre- and post-registration level, to both degree and diploma students. He has previously developed modules in health policy, and has a particular interest in the effects of devolution on the policy process.

Peter Ambrose

Peter Ambrose went to university following periods spent working in a bank and flying in the RAF. He holds degrees from London, McGill and Sussex Universities, and taught at the last of these for 35 years until his retirement in 1998, since when he has been a Visiting Professor in Housing Studies at Brighton University. His current research interests centre on the effect of poor housing on health, welfare and education, and working to assess the public costs of bad housing. He has produced seven books and about 160 other publications.

Heather Bain

Heather Bain is the course leader for BN (Hons) Community Health at Robert Gordon University, Aberdeen. She also leads the Non Medical Prescribing module and the Practice Teacher preparation module. Heather is currently undertaking a Doctorate in Education at Stirling University and is exploring the extent to which experience and education have contributed to community nursing practice. She is also the current chair of the Association of District Nurse Educators.

Jean Cowie

Jean Cowie is the pathway lead for the Specialist Community Public Health Nursing course (Health Visitor/School Nurse), and also the Professional Advisor for Public Health within the School of

Nursing and Midwifery at the Robert Gordon University, Aberdeen. She is also involved with the Erasmus Lifelong Learning Programme and, in her role as European Link Teacher, has taught in universities in Finland and Spain. She also has an interest in advanced practice and A&E nursing.

Marianne Cowpe

Marianne Cowpe is a Principal Lecturer and Divisional Head for Policy Leadership and Clinical Governance at the University of Glamorgan. She has worked as a health visitor and school nurse in both rural and inner-city areas. She has undertaken a Post Graduate Certificate in Education and a master's degree in Public Health. She is award leader for the BSc and the PG Certificate in Clinical Leadership, and has recently published articles on higher-level work-based learning

Yvette Cox

Yvette Cox is an experienced lecturer in leadership and management at the University of Southampton's Faculty of Health Sciences. She co-ordinates and teaches on all leadership and management modules, and is the module leader for Strategic Leadership and Management for Health and Wellbeing within the MSc Public Health Practice. Before joining the Faculty, Yvette worked on secondment with the Department of Health and held managerial positions within the NHS.

Samantha Greene

Sam Greene is a final-year medical student at the University of Southampton. She was awarded a distinction in her master's degree in Public Health Nutrition in 2011. Her dissertation was a review of the evolution of the obesity policy in England and is the basis of her chapter in this book.

Jenny Hacker

Jenny Hacker is a public health specialist and currently works as Consultant in Public Health Intelligence at Croydon Primary Care Trust. She began her career in local government, working for Manchester City Council housing directorate for ten years, before entering the world of health services research. She retained a keen interest in housing and health issues, establishing the Housing and Health Special Interest Group of the UK Public Health Association, which she chaired until recently.

Deirdre Heenan

Deirdre Heenan is Professor and Dean of Academic Development at the Magee Campus of the University of Ulster. She is a National Teaching Fellow and has extensive experience of teaching at both undergraduate and postgraduate levels. She has published widely on ageing, disability and social exclusion.

Marcus Longley

Marcus Longley is Professor of Applied Health Policy, and Director of the Welsh Institute for Health and Social Care, University of Glamorgan. He was educated at the Universities of Oxford, Cardiff and Bristol, and worked in a managerial and planning post in the NHS until he joined the University of Glamorgan in 1995. He is particularly interested in the relationship between policy and service delivery, in how to get patients, professionals and healthcare organisations to work together in partnership, and in the future sustainability of the NHS.

Lisa Luger

Lisa Luger is Principal Lecturer and Programme Leader for Substance Use and Misuse Studies at Thames Valley University. She is a social scientist and educationalist working in learning, development and research. Her expertise involves a range of subjects, such as substance misuse, sexual health, HIV/AIDS and cultural competence.

Linda Mages

Linda Mages is Subject Lead for Public Health at the University of Glamorgan. In this role she is Programme Leader for a newly validated MSc in Public Health and, with her background in public health nursing, leads the Specialist Community Public Health Nursing Programme, too. She is also involved in developing inter-professional education on domestic violence and sexual abuse. Her research interests include exploring perspectives held by children and young people, and developing child and youth-centred methodologies.

Penelope Nestel

Penny Nestel has a background in international nutrition and tropical agricultural development, and is currently the Programme Director for the Master's in Public Health Nutrition at the University of Southampton. She has experience in managing operations research and policy programme development and implementation, with a focus on micronutrient malnutrition.

David Ormandy

David Ormandy is head of the WHO Collaborating Centre for Housing Standards and Health at the Institute of Health, University of Warwick. He specialises in the relationship between the housing environment and health. His particular interests include carbon monoxide poisoning, domestic energy precariousness and children's unintentional injuries. He was involved in the development of health-based housing assessment tools for the UK government, the US Department for Housing and Urban Development, and others, and has written papers and co-authored and edited books on housing and health.

Susie Sykes

Susie Sykes is currently a Senior Lecturer at London South Bank University where she teaches on the MSc programme in Public Health and Health Promotion. With a background in health promotion and public health, she has experience of working in both the voluntary and public sectors. Her areas of particular interest are community development, policy making and health literacy.

Steve Tee

Steve Tee is currently Associate Director of Education in the Faculty of Health Sciences at the University of Southampton. Since qualifying in nursing in 1988 he has worked in a number of clinical, managerial and educational leadership roles within healthcare provider organisations and higher education institutions. He has a particular interest in participatory approaches to healthcare practice, education and health promotion. He completed a doctorate in 2005, focusing on service user involvement in clinical decision making.

Sue Toward

Sue Toward is a Lecturer in the Faculty of Health Sciences, University of Southampton. She began her career in NHS general management, but has worked in academic health policy since 1988 when she was appointed as a research fellow at the Institute for Health Policy Studies, University of Southampton. Sue has extensive experience of teaching policy, leadership, and managing for innovation and improvement at undergraduate and postgraduate level.

Introduction
Elizabeth Porter and Lesley Coles

This book explores the knowledge and skills of policy development and implementation for the improvement of health and wellbeing. As public health policy at a national level has an ever increasing impact on local health services, it is essential that practitioners understand how the development and implementation of policy provides an enduring framework for quality and service improvement in the delivery of a public health system designed to improve the health and wellbeing of populations, communities, families and individuals. The debate is therefore about priorities and progress in health improvement for all.

For practitioners this translates as having more autonomy, accountability and democratic legitimacy. This means understanding what policy is, and combining knowledge of policy development (strategy) with policy implementation (operationalisation) in different ways. The changing nature of these elements and the opportunity to improve health outcomes while working in partnership with clients and patients should become the norm: *no decision about me without me* (Department of Health (DoH), 2010a, p3). This demands that practitioners are more innovative in their practice and services more integrated in their approach, and consequently delivered in a more proactive manner.

Is this book for me?

This book is one of a series of four textbooks aimed at addressing the core standards for public health practice. It provides a strategic approach to understanding policy and its development, and aims to familiarise you with the strategic context of policy, its development, implementation and impact on national and local services.

Through the use of case studies and activities, linked directly to policy development and implementation, the book takes a national perspective and covers a range of practice settings across the United Kingdom (UK) of Great Britain and Northern Ireland. Drawing on expertise from across the UK, this approach gives the reader an opportunity to examine ways of contributing to policy development and implementation, not only locally but from a national viewpoint.

How the book works

The book is divided into two parts. The first (Chapters 1–5) provides a strategic overview and explores the development of national policies; this provides the foundation for the development and implementation of policy at local level. The second (Chapters 6–12) explores the specific development and implementation of policy from across the United Kingdom of Great Britain and Northern Ireland, with examples to support the thinking of part one. The chapters in part two focus on public health initiatives, and critique the importance and impact of public health policy and legislation on health and wellbeing at local level.

How to use this book

Once you know the focus of your studies for the day, whether (for example) it is determining how policy is made or its implementation, look at the table below, which gives you a quick guide to the chapter titles and specific occupational public health practice (PHP) or public health specialist (PHS) standard, the Career Framework academic standard (knowledge) and career academic standard (competence) covered within the chapter. A chapter overview, at the beginning of each chapter, augments this information and sets you in the right direction.

Chapters, occupational standards and Career Framework academic standards (Public Health Resource Unit (PHRU) and Skills for Health, 2008)

Chapter	Occupational standard	Career Framework academic standards – knowledge	Career Framework academic standards – competences
1 Policy: What is It? How is It Made?	PHP35: Advise on how improvement can be promoted in policy development PHP36: Contribute to the formulation of policy specifically focused on improving health and wellbeing	Level 5b: Awareness of the complexity of the policy context and how policy is made Level 7b: Knowledge of the policy setting context and the process of policy development Level 7e: Understanding the concepts of power interests and ideology in policy development Level 8b: Understanding of the strategic context of policy development	
2 Political and Ideological Context of Policy	PHP39: Present information and arguments to others on	Level 6b: Knowledge of major government policies relevant to	

	how policies affect health and wellbeing DA AB 3: Contribute to the development of organisational policy and practice	health and wellbeing Level 6d: Knowledge of public service organisation and delivery Level 7b: Knowledge of the policy setting context and the process of policy development Level 7e: Understanding of the concepts of power, interests and ideology in policy Level 8c: Understanding of the political environment in which own organisation is set and how this affects policy	
3 Strategic Context of Policy: A Look at UK Policy for the Four Nations	PHP38: Monitor trends and developments in policies for their impact on health and wellbeing PHP39: Present information and arguments to others on how policies affect health and wellbeing PHP40: Evaluate and recommend changes to policies to improve health and wellbeing	Level 6a: Understanding of the policies and strategies that affect own area of work	Level 7.1: Interpret and communicate local, regional and national policies and strategies within own area of work Level 7.5: Assess the actual or potential impact of policies and strategies on health and wellbeing
4 Communicating and Implementing Policy and Strategy to Improve Health and Wellbeing	PHP39: Present information and arguments to others on how policies affect health and wellbeing	Level 5a: Knowledge of the policies and strategies that affect the overall area in which one works Level 5b: Awareness of the complexity of the policy context and how policy is made	Level 7.1: Interpret and communicate local, regional and national policies and strategies within own area of work Level 8.1 Interpret and apply local, regional and national policies and strategies

		Level 7f: Understanding of how to communicate and implement policy and strategy to improve the population's health and wellbeing	
5 Developing a Strategy for Implementation of Policy	PHS 15: Implement strategies for putting policies to improve health and wellbeing into effect PHP39: Present information and arguments to others on how policies affect health and wellbeing	Level 6e: Knowledge of tools used in strategic decision-making and planning Level 7a: Understanding of various methods to assess the impact of policies on health and wellbeing Level 7c: Understanding of the variety of tools that can be used to aid strategic decision-making and planning Level 8b: Understanding of the strategic context of policy development	Level 5.3: Contribute to development of specific policies and strategies Level 6.3: Appraise draft policies and strategies and recommend changes to improve their development
6 Tackling Health and Social Inequalities	PHP30: Work in partnership with others to plan how to put strategies for improving health and wellbeing into effect PHP31: Work in partnership with others to implement strategies for improving health and wellbeing PHP33: Work in partnership with others to make a preliminary assessment of the		Level 6.2: Implement relevant aspects of policies and strategies in own area of work Level 6.3: Appraise draft policies and strategies and recommend changes to improve their development Level 6.4: Contribute to assessing the potential or actual impact of policies and strategies on health and wellbeing in own area of work

	impact of policies and strategies on health and wellbeing PHP35: Advise how health improvement can be promoted in policy PHP39: Present information and arguments to others on how policies affect health and wellbeing PHP40: Evaluate and recommend changes to policies to improve health and wellbeing DA AB 3: Contribute to the development of organisational policy and practice		Level 7.1: Interpret and communicate local, regional and national policies and strategies Level 7.5: Assess the actual or potential impact of policies and strategies on health and wellbeing Level 7.6: Provide specialist input to policies and strategies that are under development Level 7.7: Alert the relevant people to issues and gaps in policies and strategies that are affecting health and wellbeing Level 8.1: Interpret and apply local, regional and national policies and strategies Level 8.2: Influence the development of policies and strategies at other levels and/or in own area of work Level 8.3: Develop and implement policies and strategies in own area of work Level 8.4: Identify opportunities for policy development that will improve health and wellbeing and reduce health inequalities Level 9.1: Identify where new policies and strategies are needed to improve the population's health and wellbeing
7 Determinants of Health – Housing: A UK Perspective	PHS 14: Assess the impact of policies, and shape and influence them to improve health and	Level 6d: Knowledge of public service organisation and delivery	Level 6.4: Contribute to assessing the potential or actual impact of policies and strategies

	wellbeing and reduce inequalities PHS 15: Implement strategies for putting policies to improve health and wellbeing into effect	Level 7d: Understanding of public service organisation and delivery Level 8c: Understanding of the political environment in which own organisation is set, and how this affects its policy and strategy	on health and wellbeing in own area of work Level 8.3: Develop and implement policies and strategies in own area of work
8 Social Determinants of Health – Child Poverty: A Northern Ireland Perspective	PHP35: Advise how health improvement can be promoted in policy PHP37: Evaluate and review the effects of policies on health improvement PHP39: Present information and arguments to others on how policies affect health and wellbeing PHP40: Evaluate and recommend changes to policies to improve health and wellbeing		Level 7.1: Interpret and communicate local, regional and national policies and strategies within own area of work Level 7.5: Assess the actual or potential impact of policies and strategies on health and wellbeing Level 8.4: Identify opportunities for policy development that will improve health and wellbeing and reduce inequalities Level 8.2: Influence the development of policies and strategies at other levels and/or within own area of work Level 9.1: Identify where new policies and strategies are needed to improve the population's health and wellbeing
9 Development and Implementation of Policy –	PHP30: Work in partnership with others to plan how to put strategies for improving		Level 6.1: Contribute to the interpretation and application of policies and strategies in own

Children and Young People: A Welsh Perspective	health and wellbeing into effect PHP34: Work in partnership with others to undertake a full assessment of the impact of policies and strategies on health and wellbeing PHP38: Monitor trends and developments in policies for their impact on health and wellbeing PHP39: Present information and arguments to others on how policies affect health and wellbeing PHP40: Evaluate and recommend changes to policies to improve health and wellbeing	area of work Level 6.3: Appraise draft policies and strategies, and recommend changes to improve their development Level 6.4: Contribute to assessing the potential or actual impact of policies and strategies on health and wellbeing in own area of work
10 Communities and Health: A Scottish Perspective	PHP31: Work in partnership with others to implement strategies for improving health and wellbeing PHP34: Work in partnership with others to undertake a full assessment of the impact of policies and strategies on health and wellbeing PHP35: Advise how health improvement can be promoted in policy PHP37: Evaluate and review the effects of policies on health improvement	Level 6.4: Contribute to assessing the potential or actual impact of policies and strategies on health and wellbeing in own area of work Level 7.1: Interpret and communicate local, regional and national policies and strategies within own area of work Level 7.2: Work with a range of people and agencies to implement policies and strategies in interventions, programmes and services Level 7.3: Contribute to the development of policies and strategies beyond own area of work

		Level 7.5: Assess the actual or potential impact of policies and strategies on health and wellbeing
		Level 7.7: Alert the relevant people to issues and gaps in policies and strategies that are affecting health and wellbeing
11 Lifestyle Factors – Nutrition: An English Perspective	PHP29: Work in partnership with others to develop and agree priorities and targets for improving health and wellbeing PHP32: Work in partnership with others to monitor and review strategies for improving health and wellbeing PHP34: Work in partnership with others to undertake a full assessment of the impact of policies and strategies on health and wellbeing PHS 14: Assess the impact of policies, and shape and influence them to improve health and wellbeing and reduce inequalities	Level 7.1: Work with a range of people and agencies to implement policies and strategies in interventions, programmes and services Level 7.6: Provide specialist input to policies and strategies that are under development Level 8.1: Interpret and apply local, regional and national policies and strategies Level 9.2: Lead on the development and implementation of policy and strategy to improve the population's health and wellbeing Level 9.3: Lead on assessing the impact of policies and strategies on the population's health and wellbeing
12 Lifestyle Factors – Substance Use and Misuse: A UK Perspective	PHS 14: Assess the impact of policies, and shape and influence them to improve health and wellbeing and reduce	Level 6.1: Contribute to the interpretation and application of policies and strategies in own area of work.

inequalities	Level 7.4: Contribute to the development of policies and strategies within own area of work
PHP29: Work in partnership with others to develop and agree priorities and targets for improving health and wellbeing	
	Level 7.5: Assess the actual or potential impact of policies and strategies on health and wellbeing
PHP35: Advise how health improvement can be promoted in policy	
PHP39: Present information and arguments to others on how policies affect health and wellbeing	Level 9.1: Identify where new policies and strategies are needed to improve the population's health and wellbeing
DA AB 3: Contribute to the development of organisational policy and practice	Level 9.4: Influence the development of policies and strategies to improve the population's health and wellbeing

Abbreviations: PHP= public health practice; PHS = public health specialists; DA = drugs and alcohol

chapter 1

Policy: What Is It? How Is It Made?

Susie Sykes

Meeting the Public Health Competences

Core area 3: Policy and strategy development and implementation to improve population health and wellbeing

This chapter will help you to evidence the following competences for public health (Public Health Skills and Career Framework):

- Level 5(b): Awareness of the complexity of the policy context and how policy is made;
- Level 7(b): Knowledge of the policy setting context and the process of policy development;
- Level 7(e): Understanding of the concepts of power, interests and ideology in policy development;
- Level 8(b): Understanding of the strategic context of policy development.

This chapter will also assist you in demonstrating the following National Occupational Standard(s) for public health:

- PHP35: Advise on how improvement can be promoted in policy development;
- PHP36: Contribute to the formulation of policy specifically focused on improving health and wellbeing.

This chapter should also be useful in demonstrating Standard 10 of the Public Health Practitioner Standards:

Standard 10: Support the implementation of policies and strategies to improve health and wellbeing outcomes – demonstrating:

a. knowledge of the main public health policies and strategies relevant to own area of work and the organisations that are responsible for them;
b. how different policies, strategies and priorities affect own specific work and how to influence their development or implementation in own area of work;
c. critical reflection and constructive suggestions for how policies, strategies and priorities could be improved in terms of improving health and wellbeing and reducing health inequalities in own area of work.

Overview

This chapter will help you to consider what is meant by the term policy – and, in particular, health policy – and examine the importance of it and the role it plays in public health. It will explore the different approaches to policy making and the various stages involved in the policy-making process. It will help you to consider the key drivers of policy, and will look at the role of political and ideological factors, research and evidence, stakeholders and actors, and contextual issues in getting public health issues on to the policy agenda and in influencing the shape of policies.

Introduction

Public health practitioners are continually called on to implement organisational, local or national policy directives. A clearer understanding of how these policies have been formed, and why they have taken the shape they have, enables the practitioner to assess them more critically, gauge their potential effectiveness and implement them more successfully. Understanding the policy development process also enables the public health practitioner to recognise the opportunities that exist to influence the policy-making process and to see themselves as part of the political process that underpins public health.

What is 'policy'?

The term policy is one that enters the dialogue of public health practitioners on an almost daily basis. Policy governs and informs the planning and implementation of both strategies and projects, and provides a framework for the professional development of the workforce. This creates an understanding of the term that Jenkins has described as a tacit, *practical working consensus* (Jenkins, 2002, cited in Hodgson and Irving, 2007, p23), and for many operating within this working consensus the defining element of a policy is that it is embodied within a single written document (Green, 1995). However, on closer scrutiny, it is clear that it is not an exact or clearly defined term, and very often cannot be traced to one written source or document. Rather, policy takes on different forms, operates within different parameters, is arrived at following different processes, and is represented and communicated in many different ways.

ACTIVITY 1.1

Consider how you would define the term 'policy'? What key features distinguish something as a policy?

Numerous definitions of the term have been offered in the literature, many of which emphasise two aspects: 'decision' and 'action'. For many, the fundamental definition of a policy is that it is a set of decisions made by those with responsibility for an area of public life (Buse *et al.*, 2005). Hill (2005) makes the link between decisions and action, describing how a complex decision network may be involved in producing action. Thus policy is not static but a shifting phenomenon that may evolve with time as it is implemented and reviewed. Hill (2005) goes on to describe how policy is not necessarily expressed as a single decision, or indeed within a single document, but is often represented in a collection of decisions that relate to previous and existing policies. Indeed, policy decisions may not be explicit, but may remain implicit and simply understood as being the agreed position on an issue. 'Non decision making', or maintaining the status quo, may be as important in establishing a policy position as action-based decisions (Crinson, 2009). As Walt (1994) highlights, policy should be seen as something that governments say they will do, what they actually do and what they decide not to do.

For many, though, policy is about change and addressing an identified problem or achieving a specific goal. Titmuss's often quoted definition embodies this when he describes policy as *the principles that govern action directed towards given goals. The concept denotes action about means as well as ends and it, therefore, implies change: changing situations, systems, practices, behaviour* (Titmuss, 1974, p23). Indeed, for Torjman (2005), the selection of a destination or desired goal is the core of policy development. This perspective was represented in New Labour's view of policy as part of its modernisation of government: *Policy Making is the process by which governments translate their political vision into programmes and actions to deliver 'outcomes' – desired changes in the real world* (Cabinet Office, 1999, para. 2.1).

Decision making requires some form of legitimacy and Colebatch's definition emphasises policy as the maintenance of order in society through legitimate authority that is informed by relevant expertise (Colebatch, 2002). It is clear that policy can be dictated at an international, national, regional, local and organisational level, but that the decision makers must have the appropriate authority to do so. As such, these decisions will be influenced by the values of those decision makers, leading Easton (1953) to describe policy as the *authoritative allocation of values*. This is not to say that policy is defined only by decisions made by what Buse *et al.* (2005) term the *policy elite*. Policy is also the result of the actions taken by professionals during the implementation stages of policy making (Barrett and Fudge, 1981). The issue of influencing policy through implementation will be looked at in more detail later.

It is helpful to see policy as an umbrella term embodying other terms, such as public policy or the general actions and regulations put in place by government, health policy – or those regulations that relate specifically to the health of the population, whether this is the allocation of resources, development and management of services or measures to reduce inequalities in health and social policy – or the actions and regulations designed to protect and improve the social welfare of a population. It is important to add to these types of policies the term healthy public policy. This is the positioning of *health on the agenda of policy makers in all sectors and at all levels, directing them to be aware of the health consequences of their decisions and to accept their responsibilities for health* (World Health Organization (WHO), 1986, p2). Thus, healthy public policy is more than policy put in place to govern healthcare – it is concerned with the role of all government departments in creating conditions that support and promote health, and ultimately reduce inequalities in health.

Characteristics of policy

Jenkins (2002), in his analysis of definitions of the term policy, identifies a number of core propositions that underpin them.

- Policy is an attempt to define, shape and steer orderly courses of action, not least in situations of complexity and uncertainty.

- Policy involves the specification and prioritisation of ends and means, and the relationships between competing ends and means.
- Policy is best regarded as a process, and as such it is ongoing and open ended.
- The policy process is, by definition, an organisational practice.
- The policy process is embedded in and is not distinct from other aspects of organisational life.
- Policy appeals to, and is intended to foster, organisational trust – that is, external trust of organisations, and trust within organisations – based upon knowledge claims and expertise.
- Policy appeals to, and is intended to foster, organisational trust based on legitimate authority.
- Policy is about absences as well as presences, about what is said as much as what is not said.
- Policy may be implicit as well as explicit.

ACTIVITY 1.2

Consider what the difference is between:

- policy;
- strategy;
- programme;
- guidelines.

Comment

While a policy represents the decision makers' position on a particular issue, a strategy represents the high-level plan or course of action that will be taken to bring about change. A programme can be defined as an intervention or series of interventions that have been developed to achieve particular aims and objectives. Guidelines offer the practitioner an outline of how to operate based on best practice when undertaking a particular activity.

Despite the difficulties in agreeing a definition of the term, it is clear that policy plays a crucial role in managing both the health service and health inequalities. The complex nature of health and its wide determinants, the size of the health sector and huge cost of the health service, as well as the potentially life-and-death nature of the field mean that strategic decision making and planning are essential. Milio (1986) identifies five key ways in which policy supports health:

1. fiscal/monetary – incomes and incentives;

2. regulation;

3. provision of goods and services;

4. supporting participation;

5. research, development, information and education.

ACTIVITY 1.3

Identify a public health issue that you are involved in addressing. What policy exists to address that issue and underpins the work you do?

Using Milio's framework, consider in what ways this policy supports the issue. Does the existence of a policy on this issue help or hinder you in your work?

As indicated above, policy can be developed at organisational, local, regional, national and even international levels. While it is possible to take different ideological positions regarding the extent to which the state should exert control and make policy on health and social issues, it is clear that its role has expanded in recent decades. Indeed, governments have a duty to ensure that the conditions for health are maintained. However, how far they should go in controlling people's freedom of choice is debatable.

Approaches to policy making

Two main perspectives exist that represent the broad approaches to policy making: the 'rational' and the 'incremental'. Rational models linked to the work of Simon (1957) suggest that having identified a problem and agreeing the goals, values and objectives to address the problem, the policy-making process consists of the systematic gathering and review of all the data relating to alternative possible solutions and their potential outcomes. Having identified the options, the policy makers choose the one that maximises their objectives and values. A number of difficulties associated with this model have been identified. As Hill (2005) points out, the question must be asked as to whose values, objectives and goals should be used. In addition to this the reality of policy making is unlikely to follow such a logical and linear process, and policy issues are rarely discrete issues that can be dealt with in isolation from other areas and past policies. Also, as Beaumont *et al.* (2007) argue, policy makers may be more concerned with finding a politically acceptable solution than they are with finding a rational one. Simon (1957) offered this as an idealised view of decision making and acknowledged some of its limitations. His developed idea of 'bounded rationality' involves reviewing data on a more limited range of possible solutions.

The complexity of the policy-making process is recognised in the incrementalist perspective. This school of thought suggests that, in reality, policy making involves the consideration of a limited number of alternatives that differ only slightly from existing policies so that policies tend to evolve and emerge out of previous policies rather than representing radical and fundamental change. Within this process a good policy will secure the support of a range of stakeholders. If too much opposition exists, an alternative policy closer to the existing position would be adopted. Lindblom (1959) famously describes this process as the *science of muddling through* and describes new policy as being *tried, altered, tried in its altered form, altered again and so forth* (Braybrooke and Lindblom, 1963, p73). Lindblom (1959) states that not only does incrementalism offer a more accurate account of the realities of policy making, but it is the approach the policy makers should aspire to, arguing that it offers a more democratic process and reduces the chance of making mistakes that might occur through the adoption of more radical or untested measures.

Incrementalism also has its critics in both its accurate description of the policy-making process and in its basis as a model of good practice. Not all policies are minor adjustments of previous positions and radical shifts do remain an option for policy makers. Adopting an incrementalist position is essentially confining oneself to a conservative position, and may result in more innovative and ambitious alternatives being overlooked, particularly when stakeholders with more power object.

Mixed scanning approach

Attempts have been made to offer hybrid solutions to the question of how policy is made, including Hancock's (1992) 'goal directed muddling through' and Colebatch's (1998) 'combination model'. In 1967 Etzioni offered a third model, which he claimed was not as utopian in its assumptions as the rationalistic approach and less conservative than the incrementalist approach. In this attempt to combine the positive aspects of both approaches, Etzioni proposes taking a sweeping and general view of the whole problem while focusing in on specific components of the issue for more detailed analysis. Through this process, broad analysis is taken on fundamental issues, while more detailed analysis is undertaken on the minor decisions that may result from a fundamental decision. Criticisms that have been levelled at this approach are that it fails to offer anything significantly new and that the distinction between fundamental and minor decisions is hard to make.

The process of policy making

In order to aid the systematic analysis of policy making, the often complex and multi-tiered process is frequently broken down either using a systems perspective or by setting the process out into different policy stages. Easton's (1965) systems model represents an organic view of politics and describes a series of continual steps. At the beginning of this cyclical process, changes in the social or physical environment produce 'demands' or 'supports' for change (or alternatively for maintaining the current position) and these are represented as inputs towards the political system or the 'black box' of decision making. These demands and supporting interests create an element of competition within the political system known as the conversion process. It is this that then leads on to produce outputs or the decisions and policies of the policy elite. As this new policy interacts with the environment there are ultimate outcomes for the population that may create change in the social and political environment, in turn creating new demands or supports. Thus the process continues.

A stages approach is also concerned with representing the process in a simpler form, and is often represented in four stages: problem identification and issue recognition, policy formulation, policy implementation, and policy evaluation. This model is known as the Stages Heuristic (Sabatier and Jenkins-Smith, 1993); it does not claim to represent the actual process of policy making but seeks to provide a theoretical device that breaks down the process into stages that can more easily be conceptualised and analysed. While these are helpful in understanding the complex set of factors that contribute to policy, neither system nor stages approaches should be seen to represent a linear or chronological process. The different stages do not exist in isolation from each other and there exists a complex interplay of factors. Colebatch (2006) warns us that policy practitioners tend to find that their experiences do not reflect the assumptions that underpin such models and that policy outcomes usually reflect much broader processes.

ACTIVITY 1.4

Consider a public health issue and identify the current policy position on this. Reflect on how this policy position has changed over recent years. Have new policy documents that have been published on this issue over recent years represented a rational or incremental change?

Getting things on the policy agenda

Clearly there are many factors that influence the shape that a policy might take, but it is important to consider the stage before a policy is formulated – that is, to consider why some issues are given priority over others and are raised on to the policy agenda in the first place. The policy agenda has been described by Kingdon as *the list of subjects or problems to which the government officials and people outside of government closely associated with those officials are paying serious attention to at any given time* (Kingdon, 1984, p53).

ACTIVITY 1.5

Consider the debates that were conducted during the 2010 general elections. What issues did the different parties prioritise as part of their policy agendas? How did these vary from party to party, and why did certain issues gain a place on the agendas while others didn't? How did the policy agendas of the Conservative and Liberal Democrat Parties alter once a coalition government was established?

It may often seem obvious why certain issues gain a place on the policy agenda. It may, for example be a response to a particular event, often referred to as a focusing event, or crisis such as an environmental disaster or scandal in the public sector (Birkland, 1997). Parliamentary reform, for example, was raised up the policy agenda following the revelations of misuse of the parliamentary expenses system by MPs. Similarly, it may be an issue that provokes particular public attention or anger, such as hospital waiting times or cancer treatments. However, there are other occasions when issues gain a profile on the policy agenda and it is less clear why a government thinks they are important enough to occupy their time now when previously it, or former administrations, did not. Why, for example, did the New Labour government consider smoking an important enough issue on which to produce a White Paper (DoH, 1999c) when previous governments did not? There is an almost infinite number of issues to which the government could give its attention. With limited time and resources, understanding how things get on to the agenda is key to understanding how things change. There are several useful models that have been developed to help gain an understanding of this.

Kingdon (1984) presents a model that describes how 'policy windows' or opportunities emerge for an issue to gain the attention of a government. These policy windows are created when three different streams – a problem stream, a policy stream and a political stream – converge at one point in time. The coming together of these issues can be exploited by policy entrepreneurs, who identify that the political climate offers a conducive time to push their issue. Policy windows, however, do not just appear by chance, they can be created. Hall *et al.* (1975) also outline the coming together of different factors in order to push an issue on to the agenda. They describe how an issue will gain government attention only when it has high levels of legitimacy, feasibility and support. This suggests that policy makers will assess the degree to which an issue possesses these three factors before deciding to place it on their agenda.

Agenda setting

Kingdon's Theory of Multiple Streams (Kingdon, 1984)

- Problem stream: represents information and perception of a problem as one requiring government action. Issues are more likely to be placed on the agenda if a problem is perceived as being serious and therefore problem recognition is important.

- Policy stream: refers to the knowledge or advice given by researchers and policy advisers that offer a solution or alternative solutions that could be considered by decision makers. As such, the policy stream refers to proposals and these are more likely to hold credibility if they are seen as feasible, compatible with the values of decision makers, reasonable in cost and appealing to the public (Coffman, 2007).
- Political stream: represents the will of the political establishment and key actors to place an issue on the agenda. This may be influenced by public opinion, pressure from interest groups and changes in government.

The Hall Model of Agenda Setting (Hall et al., 1975)

- Legitimacy: issues that governments feel they have either a right or a duty to intervene on.
- Feasibility: issues that the government feels it has the ability to address based on knowledge, skills, resources, infrastructure, technology, etc.
- Support: existence of public support for the issue to be addressed by government.

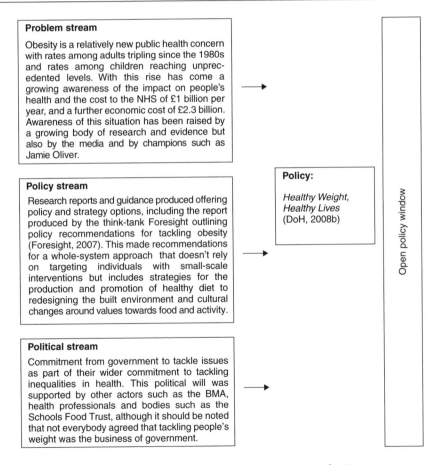

Figure 1.1 Applying Kingdon's Theory of Multiple Streams to obesity

Influencing policy

Having achieved its place on the policy agenda, there are clearly a number of policy responses to public health issues that could be decided upon. The factors that influence how a policy takes shape are a complex matrix of political, ideological, economic and contextual drivers, and the process has been described by John (1998) as the continuing interaction among institutions (the structures and systems that govern how decisions are made), interests (the groups and individuals who will be affected by changes) and ideas. To help unravel these factors, Walt and Gilson (1994) have developed a framework, based on a political economy perspective, for policy analysis, which draws the policy reader's attention to the interaction of content, context, process and actors. While the framework offers a simplicity and logic to the analysis process, it has been lauded for going beyond the consideration of the content of a policy and acknowledging the political dimensions of it (Walt *et al.*, 2008). The framework is represented as a triangle (see Figure 1.2).

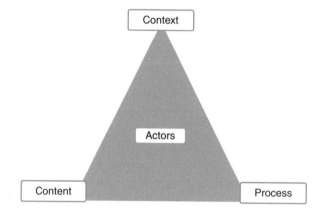

Figure 1.2 The Health Policy Triangle

Source: Walt and Gilson (1994)

Buse *et al.* (2005) warn us that the relationship between these four areas is complex and they should not be considered in isolation from each other. The triangle has been used as a basis for analysing policy internationally and encourages the systematic analysis of the different dimensions affecting the policy-making process.

Dimensions of the Health Policy Triangle (Walt and Gilson, 1994)

- Actors: this is placed at the centre of the triangle and refers to individuals, groups and organisations, or even the government. Actors are those who try and influence the policy process, and may operate at a local, regional, national or international level. They may form interest or professional networks, but the degree of influence they have will depend on the power they hold.

- Context: this is described as the systemic political, economic and social factors that influence the shape a policy takes. Sub-categories of this domain are based on Leichter's (1979) work and are as follows:
  - Situational factors: the temporary events or conditions that have an impact on policy. These may also be described as focusing events.
  - Structural factors: the stable and relatively unchanging systems within a society including the political system, the economic structure, opportunities for democratic participation, demographic features and so on.
  - Cultural factors: the values that underpin a society, including attitudes towards different issues and groups in society and different religious views.
  - International or exogenous factors: the factors that exist externally to the domestic political system, but that influence how issues can be dealt with internally.
- Process: this refers to the stages that were undertaken in the making of a policy. This may include the four stages described above in the Stages Heuristic model (Sabatier and Jenkins-Smith, 1993).
- Content: this refers to what the policy seeks to do, the goals it seeks to achieve, and how it proposes to do this. It is this dimension that many policy analyses focus on.

One of the key elements of the Health Policy Triangle (Figure 1.2) is the inclusion of the political dimension as an underpinning theme. One of the key drivers behind any policy decision is likely to be the ideological perspective of the administration. Policy debates often lay bare ideological differences between parties, particularly around the relationship between individuals and society, how the roles and responsibilities of the state and of individuals should be allocated and, with particular reference to health policy, whether the individual has the autonomy and resources to exercise free choice or whether the state should take a proactive role in protecting its citizens' health. A complex spectrum of positions exist and these ideological perspectives are explored in detail in Chapter 2.

The idea that ideology and its influence in policy making are waning is not a new one. In 1960 Bell wrote *The End of Ideology: On the Exhaustion of Political Ideas in the Fifties*. Although many of his ideas were criticised at the time, the question of the current relevance of ideology remains. In 2003 a report for the Nuffield Trust concluded that

> *Political ideology still informs the values that guide government – such as, in this case, a concern with the health and well-being of the people. We are, however, in an era where an evidence-based rather than an ideological approach seems to be the most appropriate method of policy formulation.*
>
> (Monaghan *et al.*, 2003)

This position represents a movement that grew and gained political acceptance in the 1990s, which called not only for evidence-based practice but for evidence-based policy making.

Moving into an evidence base

While the need for policy decisions to be informed by research and to have a sound evidence base would seem to be logical and self-evident, the relationship between research and evidence in the policy-making process requires closer consideration. Black (2001) provided a useful review of how research has traditionally influenced three different types of health policy: practice policies (use of resources by practitioners), service policies (resource allocation and pattern of services) and governance policies (organisational and financial structures). He argues that the case for practice policies to be based firmly on evidence is well established, although there exists a delay in implementing findings. The relationship between research evidence and service policies is however weaker for reasons such as those listed in the accompanying box, and even weaker still for governance policies.

Factors that may reduce the influence of research and evidence on policy

- Policy makers may be influenced by other political, social or economic factors.
- Research may be dismissed as irrelevant if it comes from a different sector or speciality.
- There may be a lack of consensus about evidence because of its complexity, scientific controversy or different interpretations.
- Policy makers may be influenced by less scientific evidence such as personal experience, local feedback, expert opinion.
- The social environment may not be conducive to change.
- The 'knowledge purveyors' may be inadequate. These are the people who bring the research to the policy makers and are often civil servants. They may not be experts in the policy area.

New Labour used 'Evidence Based Policy Making' as a key element of its modernisation agenda and made a declaration in its 1997 manifesto that *What counts is what works* (Labour Party, 1997), stating in its Modernisation White Paper that *policy decisions should be based on sound evidence* (Cabinet Office, 1999). However, a review by Wells (2007) of the role evidence-based policy making played under New Labour shows that its attitude moved from placing it as an integral part of social and welfare policies to one where it was used in a more selective and focused way. Wells (2007) identified a number of reasons for this, including the fact that, despite the importance of evidence, issues such as power, politics and people remain important, and that evidence-based policy making is a contested term and means different things across the policy domains. He goes on to argue that evaluative research explored with an understanding of political ideas, institutions and contexts provides a richer basis for decision making.

New Labour, during its time in government, made increasing use of the review process, whereby rather than commissioning significant amounts of formal research, it commissioned 'independent reviews' chaired by independent experts such as academics, with support groups consisting of lay and expert opinion from different spheres. The expectation of review bodies is to go beyond presenting social scientific research as evidence, and to look at a broader range of evidence and expert opinion and translate it into policy recommendations.

Case Study: Example of the review process

In November 2008, Professor Sir Michael Marmot was asked by the Secretary of State for Health to chair an independent review to propose the most effective evidence-based strategies for reducing health inequalities in England from 2010. The strategy includes policies and interventions that address the social determinants of health inequalities.

The review had four tasks:

1. identify, for the health inequalities challenge facing England, the evidence most relevant to underpinning future policy and action;
2. show how this evidence could be translated into practice;
3. advise on possible objectives and measures, building on the experience of the current PSA targets on infant mortality and life expectancy;
4. publish a report of the review's work that will contribute to the development of a post-2010 health inequalities strategy.

Fair Society, Healthy Lives: A Strategic Review of Health Inequalities in England Post-2010 was published on 11 February 2010 and called for action on six policy objectives, as follows:

1. Give every child the best start in life.
2. Enable all children, young people and adults to maximise their capabilities and have control over their lives.
3. Create fair employment and good work for all.
4. Ensure a healthy standard of living for all.
5. Create and develop healthy and sustainable places and communities.
6. Strengthen the role and impact of ill-health prevention.

Source: **www.marmotreview.org**

The point raised by Black (2001) that 'knowledge purveyors', or those individuals who bring research findings to policy makers, may not be researchers, academics or even experts in the area, and therefore may not translate the findings effectively, is an important one. Kingdon's (2003) research in the United States showed that in order to have more than a short-term impact on policy making it is not uncommon for researchers and academics to build 'inner-outer' careers in which they move between academia and government positions in order that they might develop routes through which their research can be filtered. Thus, the role of the individual personality or policy actor is highlighted.

Policy actors

The term 'policy actor' is perhaps more usefully seen as an umbrella term to represent all those individuals, groups or organisations that work to influence some stage of the policy-making process. Buse *et al.* (2005) place actors at the core of their Health Policy Triangle (Figure 1.2), demonstrating their central significance. These actors may differ in their make-up, work, the stage of the policy-making process that they may be involved in and the level of their influence.

Policy actors: terms

- Stakeholder: those individuals or organisations who are likely to be affected by a policy. This does not necessarily mean they have been involved in making the policy.
- Policy keeper: the agency that, whether by mandate or through its own initiative, holds a policy and moves it on to the next stage in the policy-making process.
- Interest (or pressure) group: a group that exists outside government and seeks to influence the policy-making process in order to achieve a specific goal or set of objectives. Usually associated with one particular issue.
- Policy champions: individuals, often with an existing high profile, who champion a particular cause or advocate on behalf of a population group, e.g. Joanna Lumley championing the rights of retired Gurkhas in Great Britain, and Jamie Oliver and his campaign on school dinners and healthy eating for children.
- Policy elite: those individuals who hold privileged positions within the policy-making process and who are involved in key decision making.
- Policy communities: network of groups and organisations that operate within a policy area, e.g. within the field of health or education. There is likely to be a sharing of values and interests.
- Issue network: a large and diverse network of organisations that share an interest in a policy area but may have little else in common, often brought together as part of a consultative process.

Clearly, key actors are the members of political parties and, in particular, the members of the government who set out the policy agenda are key policy actors, or the policy elite. However, they are influenced from many quarters. The civil service plays a key role in both policy making and implementation. Top civil servants such as Permanent Secretaries have, as one of their tasks, the advising of ministers on policies relevant to their departments. While some argue that they may carry too much influence for a non-elected position, others argue that new governments bring new and often inexperienced ministers, and civil servants offer consistency and experience to support this.

Actors outside of the government and state bureaucracy include interest groups or pressure groups. Buse *et al.* (2005) identify the key features of interest groups as being their voluntary nature, with people choosing to join them; that they have an aim to achieve a particular goal and want to influence the decision-making process but not to the extent of becoming part of the formal government process. They range in size and may include organisations as large as the Confederation of British Industry (CBI), which represents thousands of businesses across the country, or they may be single-issue local groups. For many, interest groups offer the opportunity for members of civil society to influence or play a part in the political process beyond the exercising of their franchise.

Different types of interest or pressure group

- Sectional pressure groups: those groups that represent the needs and interests of one section of society, such as professional bodies and trades unions.
- Promotional pressure groups: those that advocate a particular cause. Members of these groups may not directly benefit from the outcomes because it is a cause that is at the heart of the work. Examples may include Alcohol Concern or Greenpeace.
- Insider pressure groups: those that have direct links with decision makers and are seen by them to be legitimate, thus giving them increased access and influence.
- Outsider pressure groups: those groups that do not have the direct ear of the policy elite and cannot assume to be consulted upon in the policy-making process.

Interest groups may adopt a number of different strategies to promote their goals and influence the policy-making process, depending on their relationship with the government. Some may be formally included in the consultative stages of policy making and have the opportunity to express views; others may undertake advocacy or lobbying activities in an attempt to influence government. Equally they may run campaigns, try to influence public opinion and the media, or commission their own independent research.

Though the media cannot be justly described as a pressure group, their influence can be considerable. The media may play a role in bringing an issue to public attention, but also in framing an issue and influencing public opinion. Buse *et al.* (2005) argue that the influence of the media in policy making has, in the past, been underestimated and that they serve a range of functions:

- sources of information;

- propaganda mechanisms;

- agents of socialisation – transmitting a society's culture and instructing people in the values and norms of society;

- agents of legitimacy – generating acceptance of dominant institutions such as democracy or capitalism;

- critics of the way society and government operates.

Case Study: Example of pressure groups' work (Harkins, 2010)

The Portman Group has as its stated aim the promotion of social responsibility in the alcohol industry and, in particular, of responsible marketing. While it claims not to lobby on behalf of the industry, evidence has been presented that it is involved in policy consultations and has shown at times some considerable influence in determining alcohol policy. The group has attacked evidence around minimum pricing for alcohol despite the evidence being supported by the Chief Medical Officer for Health, Sir Liam Donaldson. It has also criticised Sir Liam, the British Medical Association (BMA) and Alcohol Concern for their support of a ban on advertising, again despite a rigorous evidence base. The influence of the alcohol industry on alcohol policy under New Labour was criticised in the Parliamentary Health Select Committee's report on alcohol when it said: *We are concerned that government policies are much closer to, and too influenced by, those of drinks industry and supermarkets than those of health professionals* (House of Commons, 2010, p123, in Harkins, 2010).

The ability of any policy actor to influence or to exert any form of control on the policy-making process depends ultimately upon the type and amount of power it holds. Understanding the influence of policy actors therefore requires us to have an understanding of the nature and distribution of power. Understanding and even defining power is complex and contested. Weber (1947) offered an important starting point when he defined power as *the probability that one actor within a social relationship will be in a position to carry out his own will despite resistance* (Weber, 1947, p152), going on to offer a distinction between power that manifests itself on a consensual basis and power that manifests itself despite resistance or through coercion. The eminent political theorist Steven Lukes (2004) identifies *three dimensions of power* – a theory which claims that power is exerted in three ways: power as decision making (a process whereby one party resolves a dilemma in their own favour through a formal process); power as non decision making, which includes the first dimension but also the added element of not allowing something to appear on the agenda in the first place and thus maintaining the status quo; and, finally, ideological power or the power to mould the wishes of a less powerful group through the accepted supremacy of the values, norms and beliefs of the dominant ideology. This third dimension of power may be exercised through the moulding of views through the education system, control of the media and so on, and as a form of power that may be less observable, but has the potential to be highly pervasive.

Not only is it important to recognise and understand differing views on how power can be conceived, it is also important to understand the different theories on how power is distributed through society and through the political system. Distinctions in the spectrum of theories range from those that see the state as holding a neutral position, acting only to enact the will of the people through a democratic process, to those that see the state as acting to maintain the status quo and protect the interests of dominant groups in society (Crinson, 2009).

A pluralist position sees power as being distributed across society with the state acting as a neutral arbitrator to serve the diversity of society. This position acknowledges division and diversity in society but argues that, while elites may exist, they do not dominate the political landscape at all times because the sources of power, such as money, skills, knowledge and so on, are distributed across society and can be accessed in some form by different groups. Thus people are free to exercise their franchise, organise themselves into pressure groups, articulate their wishes and lobby government, so ensuring that their political will is heard and ultimately adopted if they are sufficiently determined and organised.

Critics of the pluralist position argue that this is an unrealistic perspective of how power is distributed (Hill, 1997), that it focuses too much on the visible forms of power and that the British system of government is not open to influence in the way that pluralists claim (Ham, 1999). Alternate theories argue that there will always be those in society that have greater access to the sources of power and that, because of the way the political system is structured, some groups will always have a greater potential to dominate it. Governments will inevitably primarily advocate the interests of themselves and those they represent as a form of ruling elite. Within theories of elites certain pressure groups are better placed to influence policy because of their strategic position within society. Such theories hold particularly resonance in relation to economic policy but commentators such as Cawson (1982) argue that it extends to social policy and in particular health policy because of the dependence on the medical profession for expert opinion and delivery.

Implementation of policy

A shift in the study of policy analysis occurred in the 1970s, from focusing on the process of policy formulation to including a focus on implementation as part of the policy process. This shift represented a recognition that policy continues to be shaped and changed as it is put into practice, and gets exposed to and influenced by a different set of actors and drivers. There is indeed frequently a significant gap between policy objectives and policy outcomes, described as the *implementation deficit* (Crinson, 2009).

Models that have been developed to help us understand the implementation of policy are often represented as two diametrically opposed positions, sometimes described as the 'top-down' approach and the 'bottom-up' approach. The top-down approach draws on the stagist approach and sees policy operating in a sequential way with implementation being the final stage. Implementation is understood as a fairly technical process of carrying out the political stage of policy making with those involved in the political stage owning the policy (Buse *et al.*, 2005). While this offers a tangible framework for understanding how policy reaches the implementation stage, critics argue that it fails to recognise the true complexity of the process and in particular the power and influence of actors operating at the level of implementation to influence the policy process or the impact of professionals operating within multiple policy contexts. Hill (2005) goes on to point out that in some extreme cases policies may be *deliberately made complex, obscure, ambiguous or even meaningless* (Hill, 2005, p179) as forms of 'symbolic' policy that are intended as a political statement rather than to be actioned.

The bottom-up perspective acknowledges the influence of professionals tasked to deliver a policy as part of the policy-making process, and sees the policy process as a continous cycle where actions are affected by a number of variables and represent choices in reponse to particular and sometimes unforeseeable problems. Thus, policy may change during the implementation stage; however, this doesn't represent an implementation deficit but rather the next stage of the policy development process.

Colebatch's model (Figure 1.3) blends the vertical and horizontal dimensions of policy. The vertical strand represents the authoritative elements of decisions being

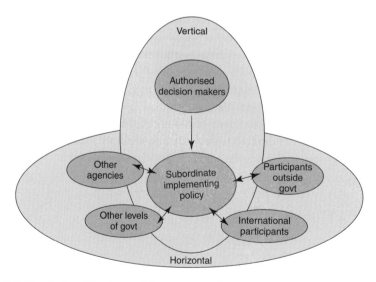

Figure 1.3 Vertical and horizontal dimensions of policy

Source: Colebatch (1998, p38)

transmitted down for implementation while the horizontal dimension represents the role of those outside the legitimate decision makers who are, however, linked together by the issue and influence its implementation according to their own circumstances, agenda and interpretations.

Lipsky (1980) also challenges the view put forward by the proponents of the top-down theories that policy formulation is the political stage and that policy implementation is a technical stage, by arguing that grassroots workers are carrying out a political role in that while they may see themselves as being controlled by the organisations they work for, their clients and researchers often see them as holding a great deal of discretionary freedom and autonomy. Lipsky's description of professionals as *street-level bureaucrats* is based on the idea that these implementers of policy have to cope with a number of pressures and limited resources, and have to constantly make decisions about how to interpret and act on policy within these constraints: *I argue that the decisions of street-level bureaucrats, the routines they establish, and the devices they invent to cope with uncertainties and work pressures, effectively become the policies they carry out* (Lipsky, 1980, pxii). The influence they hold is significant, but is often led by the need to develop coping mechanisms rather than by ideals.

Factors required for successful policy implementation (Hogwood and Gunn, 1984)

Hogwood and Gunn (1984) identify a number of factors that they argue would need to be in place in order for a policy to be successfully implemented with a minimal policy deficit.

- The circumstances external to the implementing agency do not impose crippling constraints.
- Adequate time and sufficient resources are available.
- The required combination of resources is available.
- The policy is based on a valid theory of cause and effect.
- The relationship between cause and effect is direct.
- Dependency relationships are minimal.
- There is understanding of, and agreement on, objectives.
- Tasks are fully specified in correct sequence.
- Communication and co-ordination are perfect.
- Those in authority can demand and obtain perfect compliance.

ACTIVITY 1.6

Consider a policy that underpins an area of your work.
How familiar are you with the detail of the policy?
To what extent have you or your team been able to apply your own interpretation to how you implement that policy?
Could you or your team have made different decisions about how to implement that policy?
What influenced your decisions about how to implement the policy?

Conclusion

Health is an increasingly political issue. Just as a country's political agenda cannot be discussed without reference to health, public health (and in particular the tackling of inequalities) cannot be discussed without reference to politics and policy. An understanding of the key drivers behind policy, the complexity of the policy-making process and the opportunities to influence the development and implementation of policy is fundamental for the public health practitioner at both a delivery and strategic level.

Chapter 1 summary

The models and theories presented in this chapter are an aid to understanding those processes but it is important not to allow their rational representation of the issues to mask the convoluted nature of policy making, which often takes place in what Kickbush (2010, p263) terms an *environment of organised anarchy*.

GOING FURTHER

Baggott, R (2010) *Public Health Policy and Politics* (2nd edn). Oxford: Wiley Blackwell. *This new edition visits the contemporary debate surrounding public health, exploring the many facets of health improvement and promotion within their historical, socioeconomic and political contexts.*

Buse, K, Mays, N and Walt, G (2005) *Making Health Policy*. Berkshire: Open University Press/McGraw-Hill Education. *This book views power and process as integral to understanding policy, and focuses on the three key elements in policy making: the context, the actors and the processes.*

Hill, M (2005) *The Public Policy Process* (4th edn). Essex: Pearson Education. *This book provides core readings about decision making and policy making.*

Global Public Health. An international journal for research, policy and practice. Online at: www.tandf.co.uk/journals/titles/17441692.

chapter 2

Political and Ideological Context of Policy

Sue Toward

Meeting the Public Health Competences

Core area 3: Policy and strategy development and implementation to improve population health and wellbeing

This chapter will help you to evidence the following competences for public health (Public Health Skills and Careers Framework):

- Level 6(b): Knowledge of major government policies relevant to health and well-being and inequalities;
- Level 6(d): Knowledge of public service organisation and delivery;
- Level 7(b): Knowledge of the policy setting context and the process of policy development;
- Level 7(e): Understanding of the concepts of power, interests and ideology in policy development;
- Level 8(c): Understanding of the political environment in which own organisation is set and how this affects policy and strategy.

This chapter will also assist you in demonstrating the following National Occupational Standards for public health:

- PHP39: Present information and arguments to others on how policies affect health and wellbeing;
- DA AB3: Contribute to the development of organisational policy and practice.

This chapter should also be useful in demonstrating Standard 10 of the Public Health Practitioner Standards:

Standard 10: Support the implementation of policies and strategies to improve health and wellbeing outcomes – demonstrating:

a. knowledge of the main public health policies and strategies relevant to own area of work and the organisations that are responsible for them;
b. how different policies, strategies and priorities affect own specific work and how to influence their development or implementation in own area of work;
c. critical reflection and constructive suggestions for how policies, strategies and priorities could be improved in terms of improving health and wellbeing and reducing health inequalities in own area of work.

Overview

This chapter will introduce you to a range of ideas and related terms relevant to an exploration of the political and ideological context of policy. The key concepts we will consider are values, principles, culture and ideology (both political and welfare ideologies). These concepts will then be considered in relation to health policy, with a focus on England.

Introduction

Values, principles, culture and ideology

Abstract concepts such as values, principles, culture and ideology can seem very remote from the *stuff of everyday social policy: health care, housing, social care, social security, poverty* (Lister, 2010, p1) and therefore from the 'real world' inhabited by front-line practitioners delivering services. However, as we shall see, these concepts are of fundamental importance when it comes to understanding policy and its relationship with politics and the political process. For example, policy itself is often defined in terms of values – beliefs and core principles that guide behaviour, activity, decisions and priorities at an individual and collective level. Easton (1953) considers that political activity can be characterised by its concern with the *authoritative allocation of values* in society and that *a policy . . . consists of a web of decisions and actions that allocate . . . values* (quoted in Ham, 2009, p131). Similarly, Colebatch suggests that the term 'policy' can be used to mean a statement of values, and cites the example of the aphorism *honesty is the best policy* (Colebatch, 2009, p7).

The idea of shared values at a collective level leads us on to the term 'culture'. Mannion's perspective on culture focuses on that which is shared between people in organisations – for example:

- Beliefs, values, attitudes and norms of behaviour
- Routines, traditions, ceremonies and rewards
- Meaning, narratives and sense making.

(Mannion, 2010, p20)

Such shared ways of thinking and behaving help define what is acceptable within any given organisation and constitute a type of 'glue' that holds an organisation together.

What we have said so far about values, principles and culture may still seem far removed from the 'real world' of practice and organisations. However, the NHS Constitution, developed for the National Health Service (NHS) in England as part of the NHS Next Stage Review process in 2007/08, is arguably a 'real world embodiment' of principles and values in the sense that these underpin a series of legal rights, pledges and responsibilities affecting patients, the wider public and staff (DoH, 2010b). The Constitution, which the Conservative–Liberal Democrat coalition government elected in May 2010 is committed to upholding, sets out seven principles for guiding the NHS in all it does. The principles are based on six core NHS values derived from extensive discussions with staff, patients and the public (see the accompanying boxes).

Principles that guide the NHS

1. The NHS provides a comprehensive service, available to all.
2. Access to NHS services is based on clinical need, not an individual's ability to pay.
3. The NHS aspires to the highest standards of excellence and professionalism.
4. NHS services must reflect the needs and preferences of patients, their families and their carers.
5. The NHS works across organisational boundaries and in partnership with other organisations in the interest of patients, local communities and the wider population.
6. The NHS is committed to providing best value for taxpayers' money, and the most effective, fair and sustainable use of finite resources.
7. The NHS is accountable to the public, communities and patients that it serves.

Source: Department of Health (2010b, pp3–4)

NHS values

1. Respect and dignity
2. Commitment to quality of care
3. Compassion
4. Improving lives
5. Working together for patients
6. Everyone counts

Source: Department of Health (2010b, p12; online at
www.dh.gov.uk/en/Publicationsandstatistics/Publications/
PublicationsPolicyAndGuidance/DH_113613)

ACTIVITY 2.1

Read through the NHS Constitution and think about the ways in which the principles and values it sets out have shaped the rights, pledges and responsibilities for patients, the public and staff. Has the Constitution succeeded in translating abstract concepts into the *stuff of everyday social policy* – in this case healthcare (Lister, 2010, p1)?

While it does not refer explicitly to culture, several statements in the NHS Constitution imply that shared values are an important ingredient in the 'glue' of a national institution such as the NHS. For example, we read that *the NHS is founded on a common set of principles and values that bind together the communities and people it serves – patients and the public – and the staff who work for it* (DoH, 2010b, p2). A little further on, the NHS is described as an *integrated system of organisations and services* (Department of Health, 2010b, p4), consisting not only of NHS bodies but also private and third-sector providers supplying NHS services. The NHS *and* its extended family are considered to be bound together in a cultural sense by NHS Constitution principles and values. In addition they share a legal obligation to take account of the Constitution in their decisions and actions.

The NHS Constitution sets out a range of traditional – or founding – and modern principles and values. This is an idea we shall return to when we consider the impact of ideology on health policy development. For now, it is worth noting the strength of commitment on the part of patients, staff, the wider public and politicians to certain 'ends' or overarching goals in the NHS. These can be framed in terms of NHS traditional values – comprehensive, available to all, based on need not individual ability to pay – and newer values – excellence, patient-centredness, partnership, efficiency, effectiveness and accountability. There may not be the same degree of consensus, however, on the means or the best way of delivering the overarching goals. Debates about means tend to focus on the funding, organisation, structure and ownership of health services. The policy positions reached by different political parties on these contested areas reflect a range of ideological perspectives. Ideology is a concept we now turn to in more detail.

Ideology

Ideology has been defined by George and Wilding as *a set of values and beliefs held by individuals, groups and societies that influence their conduct* (1994, pp4–5). So ideology has a bearing on decisions and actions; in the political realm it has policy consequences. For example, in the area of health policy, the ideological position of politicians in power influences decisions, actions and priorities set for both healthcare policy and policy for health or public health policy (Hunter, 2003). Healthcare policy is mainly concerned with the 'means' of service delivery we referred to above. In recent years it has been dominated by debate about the extent to which market mechanisms such as choice, competition between diverse providers and contracting should be used to drive efficiency and quality improvements in the NHS. The very different perspective of public health policy is suggested by the Acheson Report's definition of public health as *the science and art of preventing disease, prolonging life and promoting health through the organised efforts of society* (Cm 289, 1988). Key strands of public health policy include individual and population health improvement (people's lifestyles, health inequalities and the wider social influences of health) and health protection (infectious diseases, environmental hazards and emergency preparedness) (Griffiths *et al.*, 2005).

As Lister argues, all governments draw implicitly or explicitly on theoretical perspectives and concepts derived from political and welfare ideology (Lister, 2010). She also suggests that welfare ideologies as they operate in the political realm go beyond George and Wilding's definition of ideology quoted above. For example, one key feature of welfare ideologies is that they provide a *'view of the world', especially of human nature and of the relationship between state and society* (George and Wilding, 1994, p6; also cited in Lister, 2010, p5).

Both political and welfare ideologies are suffused by particular beliefs about the individual in terms of human motivation and behaviour, the state and society. These important concepts also highlight what Lister describes as *the critical issue* (Lister, 2010, p18) at the heart of much ideological debate in social policy – the proper role of the state. It is this critical issue, and related questions about where the boundaries between state, individual and societal responsibility for welfare provision should lie, that largely delineate the ideological perspectives we go on to explore in relation to health policy.

Ideology and health policy

One of the conceptual frameworks for analysing policy that Baggott sets out in his book *Understanding Health Policy* (2007) is policy, ideology and political parties. The relevance of this framework for considering health policy is apparent if we consider particular phases of policy development and the political ideologies that shaped them. The three main western political traditions of the post-war period are socialism, conservatism and liberalism (Baggott, 2007), although, as Lister has pointed out, each tradition has spawned many sub-strands (see Figure 2.1).

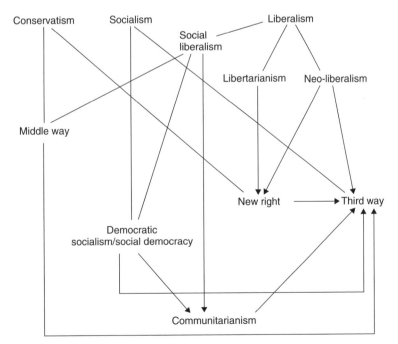

Figure 2.1 Traditions of western political thought

Source: Lister (2010, p33). Reproduced with permission.

The sub-strands we are going to focus on in our exploration of key phases of health policy development are democratic socialism/social democracy, middle way, neo-liberalism and third way. The direction of health policy since the election in 2010 of the Conservative–Liberal Democrat coalition government will also be considered.

Socialism and collectivism

The political tradition of socialism is associated with left-of-centre politics and its key channel of influence in the UK's party political system is through the Labour Party. While socialism is a very broad philosophy, its motivating principle is social equality. Stemming from this is a root-and-branch critique of capitalism and the *inequality, exploitation, social class divisions, competitive individualism and materialist values that it generates* (Lister, 2010, p30). The state is assigned a key role in bringing about a more equal, socially just society through the redistribution of wealth, the common ownership of the means of production and distribution, and the regulation of capitalist enterprise (Baggott, 2007). Other important values underpinning the socialist political tradition are societal responsibility and social solidarity. The interdependence of members of a society means that collective approaches to meeting need, with the state playing a key role, should be sought. This will result in strengthened social solidarity or, to use more modern parlance, social cohesion.

The sub-strands of socialism that shaped the political philosophy of the Labour Party for most of the twentieth century are democratic socialism and social democracy, terms that, despite the subtle difference of emphasis between them, are often used interchangeably (Lister, 2010). However, if we consider the welfare legislation enacted under the 1945–51 Labour government, it is the ideals of democratic socialism – equality, liberty and fraternity or solidarity – that *translated into a commitment to universal welfare services and benefits on the grounds that they foster integration and altruism* (Lister, 2010, p40). The creation in 1948 of the NHS is widely seen not only as a defining moment in UK health policy but also as the crowning achievement of democratic socialism.

In her analysis of the creation of the NHS, Allsop identifies five principles infusing the 1946 NHS Act, which established a remarkably enduring pattern of healthcare in Britain (Allsop, 1995). The five principles are collective responsibility, comprehensiveness, universalism, egalitarianism and professional autonomy. As we have already seen, the founding principles or traditional values of comprehensive services, available to all, based on need not individual ability to pay, have been largely restated in the NHS Constitution (DoH, 2010b). However, a central aim of the 1946 Act was that the *state* should provide healthcare free at the point of service for those in need, reflecting the collectivist principle of state responsibility for its citizens. This principle of collectivist state provision of health services has arguably not endured in the same way as other NHS founding principles identified above. As we shall see when we consider neo-liberal, third way and 'Cameronist' political ideologies, ideas about the proper role of the state in welfare provision have been largely reframed since 1948. While the NHS continues to be funded mainly out of general taxation and remains free at the point of use, there is now less emphasis on 'centralised state organisations' providing a service (Allsop, 1995). Growing numbers of NHS patients are being treated and cared for by independent and private-sector providers.

In the 1940s collective state provision was considered to be fundamental to the realisation of the principle of social equality. In 1946, Aneurin Bevan, the Minister of Health of the 1945 Labour government, argued that *we have got to achieve as nearly as possible a uniform standard of service for all – only with a national service can the state ensure that an equally good service is available everywhere* (Bevan, 1946, quoted in Allsop, 1995, p29). While the commitment to egalitarianism has largely endured, the provision of equally good services everywhere is now not necessarily considered to hinge on a monopoly role for the state in direct service provision.

The practical policy consequences of the five principles that infuse the 1946 NHS Act are evident in the NHS's tripartite administrative structure and decision-making processes – designed to ensure uniformity, equality and professional autonomy – at its inception in 1948. The principle of professional autonomy has proved very enduring; for example, a recent policy iteration of the principle can be found in the 2010 coalition government White Paper *Equity and Excellence: Liberating the NHS* (Cm 7881, 2010) for the English NHS. This states a commitment to increased autonomy on the front line by 'liberating' professionals from stifling bureaucracy and interfering managers and government. GPs' liberation is to be achieved through the development of GP commissioning consortia and the abolition, by 2013, of Primary Care Trusts.

Turning now to consider socialist and collectivist ideology in relation to public health policy, Hunter's second meaning of the term health policy (Hunter, 2003), the history of public health policy provides many examples – clean air and water, sanitation, mandatory vaccination, the protection of children and workers through specific legislation – of state intervention (Nuffield Council on Bioethics, 2007) and of the state being closely identified with public health. As Baggott points out, the beneficial role of the state and of other collective arrangements, for example mutual societies, is much emphasised by socialists and collectivists (Baggott, 2010). Unfettered individualism and capitalism are detrimental to health, and the state has a responsibility to intervene to address their health-damaging consequences and to tackle the underlying socioeconomic causes of ill health. Equity in health is an important element of social justice and reflects a key socialist principle. Priority should be given to promoting everyone's health, regardless of their social and economic circumstances, age, gender and ethnic background (Baggott, 2010).

The extent to which it is acceptable for the state to intervene to influence population health, and the question of where the line should be drawn between government and individual responsibility for health, persist as central issues in public health. A useful concept for exploring them is that of stewardship (Jochelson, 2005; Nuffield Council on Bioethics, 2007). The stewardship model of the state recognises that states are stewards both to individual people and to the population as a whole – that is, they have a responsibility to look after the needs of people individually and collectively. The model emphasises the obligation of states to provide conditions that allow people to be healthy and, in particular, to take measures to tackle health inequalities. The state should protect its citizens from harm caused by others, and safeguard the health of vulnerable groups such as children. At the same time, states should not coerce people or restrict their freedoms unnecessarily (Nuffield Council on Bioethics, 2007).

Stewardship-guided states carry out public health programmes with certain core characteristics (Nuffield Council on Bioethics, 2007) and intervene using a variety of actions. The ladder of interventions, also developed by the Nuffield Council on Bioethics (2007) ranks interventions according to how intrusive they are, from least intrusive – do nothing or monitor – on the bottom rung, to most intrusive – the restriction and elimination of choice – on the top two rungs of the ladder (see Figure 2.2). The more intrusive or interventionist an action, the stronger the justification has to be. The most intrusive or authoritarian measures, including coercion, can be justified if the collective interest outweighs the individual.

The stewardship model bears the imprint of important ideological debates about the freedom of the individual, the authority of the state, and the balance to be struck between individual and collective responsibility. Baggott's exploration of the stewardship model (2010) links it to collectivism and socialism on the basis that the concept of stewardship implies a state that has an active and positive role in promoting the health of the public and in addressing health inequalities (Reeves, 2010).

Eliminate choice. Regulate in such a way as to entirely eliminate choice, for example through compulsory isolation of patients with infectious diseases
Restrict choice. Regulate in such a way as to restrict the options available to people with aim of protecting them, for example removing unhealthy ingredients from foods, or unhealthy foods from shops or restaurants
Guide choice through disincentives. Fiscal and other disincentives can be put in place to influence people not to pursue certain activities, for example through taxes on cigarettes, or by discouraging the use of cars in inner cities through charging schemes or limitations of parking spaces
Guide choice through incentives. Regulations can be offered that guide choices by fiscal and other incentives, for example offering tax breaks for the purchase of bicycles that are used as a means of travelling to work
Guide choices through changing the default policy. For example, in a restaurant, instead of providing chips as a standard side dish (with healthier options available), menus could be changed to provide a more healthy option as standard (with chips as an option available)
Enable choice. Enable individuals to change their behaviour, for example by offering participation in a NHS 'stop smoking' programme, building cycle lanes, or providing free fruit in schools
Provide information. Inform and educate the public, for example as part of campaigns to encourage people to walk more or eat five portions of fruit and vegetables per day
Do nothing or simply monitor the current situation

Figure 2.2 The intervention ladder

Source: Nuffield Council on Bioethics (2007, pxix). Reproduced with permission.

Our exploration of the impact of socialism and collectivism on health policy started with a discussion of the extent to which democratic socialist values and principles shaped the NHS at its inception in 1948. We now turn to the political tradition of conservatism and consider what sort of health service might have been developed if a right-of-centre government had been in power between 1945 and 1951. Our discussion will consider the key values associated with conservatism and the implications for welfare ideology.

Conservatism, the creation of the NHS and welfare state consensus

Conservatism is the tradition of western political thought that has shaped the philosophies and policies of right-of-centre governments. However, one thing conservatism has in common with socialism is that it also has a number of sub-strands, as Figure 2.1 illustrates. According to Baggott (2007), conservatism emphasises the importance of tradition, hierarchy, private property, paternalism and social order. In the British Conservative Party, there has been a long-standing emphasis on the principles of individual responsibility, private property and enterprise, along with a scepticism about the state and a dislike of public spending and taxation.

As we have already seen, the 1946 NHS Act was a major political achievement for a Labour government. However, by 1945 there was a broad, cross-party consensus about the need for a comprehensive health service. This consensus is generally attributed to the social solidarity that had developed from the nation's shared experience of war. The idea of 'nation' – a central theme in the development of welfare provision – is also relevant here. The welfare state with the NHS as a key pillar is argued to have made a vital contribution to *nation-building through helping to create a sense of collective national identity and citizenship* (Lister, 2010, p19).

While the Conservative Party acknowledged the need for a comprehensive system of care and a role for the state in delivering this, it was opposed to Labour plans for the nationalisation – state or public ownership – of pre-NHS facilities such as voluntary and local authority hospitals. Instead the Conservatives emphasised the importance of choice and individual enterprise, and argued for the retention of the voluntary hospital sector, working in partnership with local authority hospitals (Baggott, 2007). However, Baggott also points out that the Conservative governments in power between 1951 and 1964 and 1970 and 1974 *reached an accommodation with the NHS largely for pragmatic reasons* (Baggott, 2007, p7), chief among which was the popularity of the service. Indeed, Conservative governments of this period accepted the need for state intervention in the economy and social welfare despite their ideological principles of individual responsibility, private ownership and markets.

The Conservative Party's post-war accommodation with the NHS can be linked to a particular sub-strand in conservatism identified in Figure 2.1 as 'middle way' and elsewhere as 'One Nation' conservatism. With its emphasis on paternalism, social responsibility, civic values and the protection of the weak and vulnerable (Baggott, 2007), middle way or One Nation conservatism arguably tempers certain tenets associated with more right-wing elements of the British Conservative Party. The origins of the term 'middle way' can be traced back to the 1930s when Harold Macmillan, who went on to become a Conservative Prime Minister in the 1950s, coined the expression. Macmillan's version of conservatism *charted a path between classical liberalism and socialism* (Lister, 2010, p33) and has been described by Pinker as a *classic exposition of the case for Tory collectivism* (Pinker, 2008, p71). This idea of a sub-strand emerging from the process of charting a path between two political traditions is one we shall return to when we consider the 'third way', a political ideology associated with the Labour government elected in 1997.

Neo-liberalism, to which we next turn our attention, arguably provided a fresh ideological departure or, as Baggott puts it, *a blueprint for political action to reverse the tide of paternalism and collectivism* (Baggott, 2010, p9). Paternalism, as we have seen, is particularly associated with middle way or One Nation conservatism in the 1950s. If we come forward 50 years, some commentators suggest that this sub-strand of conservatism has undergone a quiet revival since the election of David Cameron as Conservative Party leader in 2005. This is a question we shall return to when we consider 'Cameronism' as a political ideology. For now, however, it is sufficient to note that a political party is a broad church in the sense that it represents a range of standpoints or ideological positions. These evolve over time and tend to be linked with different wings of a party.

Neo-liberalism, markets and the state

The middle way 'brand' of conservatism was dominant in the Conservative Party for most of the post-war period until 1979 when the first Conservative government led by Margaret Thatcher came to power. The new right sub-strand of conservatism we associate with Thatcherism rejected the broad consensus forged between the middle way and democratic socialism (Lister, 2010). As Figure 2.1 indicates, the sub-strand has its origins in neo-liberal political and economic philosophy.

Adherents of neo-liberalism believe in a smaller state bureaucracy, less government intervention, and a bigger role for the private sector and market forces in the allocation of resources (Green, 1987). The market is considered to be a more efficient producer and allocator of goods and services than state bureaucracies (Lister, 2010), delivering superior quality, value and choice. Core values of neo-liberalism are individual liberty, autonomy, choice, self-reliance and personal responsibility. The state's role should be limited to protecting the liberty and security of the individual and establishing a regulatory framework for the market so that it can operate efficiently (Lister, 2010).

The impact of new right ideas on the public sector during Margaret Thatcher's years in government was profound. The government's aim to reduce the size of the state led to cuts in public expenditure and taxes, and a period of financial restraint across public services, including the NHS. A range of private-sector management ideas and practices – intended to make the NHS more efficient and businesslike – were introduced. These included a system of general management at every level of the NHS (Griffiths Report, 1983), and compulsory market testing of laundry, catering and domestic services. However the most radical changes to healthcare policy of the Thatcher years did not get under way until 1989, following the Conservatives' third consecutive election victory in 1987. The White Paper *Working for Patients* (Secretary of State for Health, 1989) set out far-reaching reforms to the delivery of health services based on the introduction of an internal market. This was intended to create the conditions for competition between hospitals and other service providers through the separation of purchaser/commissioner and provider responsibilities, and the development of autonomous self-governing NHS Trusts and budget-holding GPs (fund holders). Resources would be allocated on the basis of contracts between purchasers and providers and hospitals that failed to secure contracts, and hence income could, in theory, go out of business. However, the fact that no hospital was allowed to 'go to the wall' suggests that the internal market was a managed market that fell short of the neo-liberal purist 'market ideal'.

Our earlier discussion of values and principles drew attention to the traditional – or founding – and modern principles and values set out in the NHS Constitution. It has already been suggested that there is widespread consensus about the 'policy ends' or overarching goals represented by these values and principles. However, there is rather less agreement on the most appropriate means and mechanisms for delivering these ends. The architects of the internal market believed that the newer values – excellence, patient-centredness/choice, efficiency, effectiveness and account-ability – were more likely to be delivered by market forces and mechanisms. At the same time, however, the 1989 *Working for Patients* White Paper (Secretary of State for Health, 1989) stated the government's commitment to preserving the basic principles on which the NHS was founded. General taxation would continue to provide the lion's share of funding, and access to the NHS would be according to need and not ability to pay (Ham, 2009). For all her reforming instincts, Margaret Thatcher, like several of her Conservative prime ministerial predecessors, recognised the popularity of the NHS and did not want to lose votes over it. While she made it clear that she wanted to see a flourishing private sector of healthcare, the NHS and its basic principles was *always a 'fixed point' in her policies* (Baggott, 2007, p26).

Taking responsibility for health

Turning now to public health policy, the neo-liberal ideological perspective asserts that individuals should take responsibility for their health, make their own choices and not be told what to do by an interfering 'nanny state'. The demarcation between individual and state responsibility is different from that associated with the steward-ship model of the state explored in the earlier discussion of socialism and collectiv-ism. The contrast is apparent if we consider policy on prevention and health pursued by Conservative governments in the 1980s. Policy was predicated on notions of per-sonal responsibility and on persuading individuals to change their behaviour. There was a non-interventionist approach to industry also, with the government favour-ing self-regulation (for example, by the tobacco and alcohol industries) over more coercive approaches such as legislation to restrict or ban practices running counter to public health improvement (see Figure 2.2). Although the 1980 Black Report (Department of Health and Social Security (DHSS), 1980) had produced powerful evidence of the link between socioeconomic inequalities and poor health, health inequalities were not on the Conservatives' agenda. Social and environmental determinants of health were downplayed or ignored, and the Black Report's conclusion that widening health inequalities could be attributed primarily to material inequalities rejected. As Baggott (2010) highlights, the Thatcher government favoured alternative explanations – also explored in the Black Report – based on statistical artefact, social mobility, and individual behaviour or lifestyle. Baggott's contention is that the failure to concede the relationship between socioeconomic factors and health inequalities was political (Baggott, 2010).

John Major, who succeeded Margaret Thatcher as Conservative Party leader in 1990, did not entirely share the ideological stance of his predecessor and was considered to be more of a pragmatist than an ideologue. While the Thatcher governments had resisted the development of a national strategy for health, this was subsequently introduced by the Major government in the form of the 1992 *Health of the Nation* strategy (Cm 1986, 1992). Its stated aim was to secure continuing improvement in the health of the population by adding 'years to life' – increasing life expectancy and reducing premature death – and 'life to years' – improving the quality of life and reducing illness. Five priority areas for action – cancer, heart disease/stroke, mental illness, HIV/AIDs and sexual health, and accidents – were identified and two types of target set for each.

Dominance of the medical approach

While opposition parties welcomed the *Health of the Nation* strategy, there was criticism of the dominance of disease-based targets and of the extent to which these reflected a narrow medical perspective that disregarded the broader social context of people's decisions and behaviour. Health inequalities were not targeted and the wider causes of ill health were neglected. However, the Major government did acknowledge the existence of differences in health status between different socioeconomic groups, but chose to refer to these as 'variations', thus avoiding the more toxic and politically charged language of 'health inequalities' (Baggott, 2010). While variations were attributed to *a complex interplay of genetic, biological, social, environmental, cultural and behavioural factors* (Cm 1986, 1992, p122), the policy recommendations for tackling them set out in the 1995 review *Variations in Health* (DoH, 1995b) were narrowly drawn, and based on what the Department of Health and the NHS could do. The narrow medical perspective of the *Health of the Nation* (Cm 1986, 1992) persisted.

It is important not to underestimate the impact of neo-liberal political and welfare ideology on health policy in the 1980s and 1990s, particularly during the Thatcher years. However, while the strong *swing of the political pendulum* (Baggott, 2007, p6) in 1979 gave the Conservative Party great scope to bring its ideology to bear on policy, our analysis of healthcare policy has indicated that a governing party is constrained by a number of factors. Among those identified by Baggott (2007) are practical constraints – for example, it is not possible to reverse at a stroke a previous government's entire programme – and political realities. In the case of healthcare policy, the NHS has proved to be a remarkably popular institution. Margaret

Thatcher was only too aware that politicians who are seen to be tampering with it tend to lose rather than gain votes.

Instead of wholesale changes in policy and ideological direction following the replacement of one political party in office by another, we are more likely to see a degree of continuity with what has gone before. Baggott has described this as a *moving consensus* (Baggott, 2007, p8). This is an idea we shall now explore in relation to the policy and ideology of the Labour government elected in 1997.

Third way: neither capitalism nor socialism but 'what works'

In our exploration of conservatism we touched on the idea of an ideological sub-strand emerging from the process of charting a path between two political traditions. 'Third way', the ideological label that Labour used to describe itself on being elected in 1997, can be understood in a similar way. Baggott (2007) argues that third way incorporates elements of both neo-liberalism and socialism, while Lister refers to a *political philosophy which underlines the distance between New and 'old' Labour as well as providing an alternative to the creed of Thatcherism* (Lister, 2010, p46). So third way is neither 'old left' (democratic socialism) nor new right, and thus transcends the old left–right divide. Third way is pro-market but ambivalent about the state, and it maintains that equality of opportunity is more important than equality of outcome. Third way also endorses an inclusive society where citizens have both rights and responsibilities.

Figure 2.1 highlights the complex set of influences, including communitarianism, that have shaped third-way thinking. Communitarianism emphasises the importance of balancing community values with individual responsibilities and of promoting partnerships with the voluntary and private sectors to pursue the collective good. As far as government is concerned, the imperative is modernisation, with the state's role needing to be recast to enable it to act more entrepreneurially – for example, seeking out new opportunities for wealth creation and for tackling social problems. Another important emphasis in third-way thinking is the need to bring together choice and enterprise with notions of social justice (Baggott, 2007).

Health policy 1997–2010

Turning now to consider health policy between 1997 and 2010, it is clear that the key developments of this period bear the imprint of the complex set of influences we have just described. For example, while in opposition New Labour was very critical of Conservative health policy and pledged to discontinue the divisive internal market. On coming to power in 1997, Labour set about dismantling GP fundholding, but extended the principles of fundholding to all family doctors and community nurses through a network of Primary Care Groups (PCGs). This amounted to a pragmatic retention of the main mechanism for introducing an internal market into the NHS: the purchaser–provider split. However, the government purged all mention of markets and competition from the language it used to set out its reforms, as illustrated by the commitment in the 1997 White Paper to retain *the separation between the planning of hospital care and its provision* (Cm 3807, 1997, p12). The same White Paper also signalled the end of the annual contracting round with its high transaction costs (paperwork and bureaucracy) and a transition to longer-term and more comprehensive service agreements.

Overall the Labour government elected in 1997 reformed rather than abolished the internal market. Labour was not afraid to adopt policy ideas from the right and was prepared to develop its own approach to making greater use of market forces in the delivery of health services. Policies on payment by results, Foundation Trusts, patient choice and consumerism, and practice-based commissioning can be seen in this context. Furthermore, Labour embraced and built on a raft of other Conservative policies – for example, the Private Finance Initiative and contracting with private-sector providers to supply care for NHS patients. However, while Labour stuck initially to the previous government's parsimonious spending plans, the NHS Plan (Cm 4818, 2000) marked a departure from neo-liberal financial restraint and led to a period of unprecedented real-term growth in NHS funding of 7.4 per cent (between 2002/03 and 2007/08) and 4.4 per cent (between 2007/08 and 2010/11) (Appleby *et al.*, 2009).

Ham has described the Labour government's approach to healthcare policy as eclectic as well as pragmatic (Ham, 2009). While the Thatcher government's reforms relied on a core belief in the potential of market forces and mechanisms to drive improvements in NHS performance, Labour used a much wider range of mechanisms to improve efficiency and quality. For example, under Labour, variations in performance were also tackled through national service frameworks and the creation of agencies like the National Institute for Clinical Excellence (NICE) and the Commission for Health Improvement (CHI).

In summary, the argument that third way is simply a continuation of the neo-liberal philosophy of the New Right – the *wolf of neo-Thatcherism in social democratic clothing* (Lister, 2010, p47) – seems to be overly simplistic in relation to healthcare policy. But to what extent did New Labour forge a third way in public health policy and succeed in breaking away from the emphasis on individualism, personal responsibility and non-intervention associated with neo-liberalism? These are questions to which we now turn.

Forging a Third Way in public health policy

During its period in office between 1997 and 2010, Labour published two papers on public health. These were *Saving Lives* (Cm 4386, 1999) and *Choosing Health* (Cm 6374, 2004). Baggott's analysis of these two White Papers (Baggott, 2010) highlights the way in which third-way principles influenced their underpinning philosophy. For example, as far as responsibility for health is concerned, the *Choosing Health* White Paper (Cm 6374, 2004) plots a middle course. On the one hand, it acknowledges that the state has a legitimate role in shaping the environment or creating the conditions that facilitate healthy individual choices, deploying a range of strategies including *regulation, provision of services and information about health risks* (Baggott, 2010, p13). On the other hand, individuals are seen as having a crucial role in taking responsibility for their own health and making healthy choices within the framework provided. Klein's verdict on the overall philosophy of *Choosing Health* is along similar lines. He describes this philosophy as *a sophisticated attempt to balance the spheres of state action (the nanny state) and individual responsibility, avoiding both social determinism and atomistic individualism* (Klein, 2005, p65). Another important third-way principle evident in the *Choosing Health* White Paper is that of partnership, between public-sector organisations such as the NHS and local government and between statutory, voluntary and private-sector bodies. Responsibility for public health improvement does not rest with the government alone, nor does the NHS have a monopoly over the levers of public health improvement.

The *Choosing Health* White Paper (Cm 6374, 2004) is relatively silent on the issue of health inequalities. This is out of step with other policy developments from 1997 onwards (Baggott, 2010) and may reflect an acknowledgement on the part of the government that policy interventions across the whole gamut of social and economic policy have greater potential than those associated with narrower health policy to unlock real progress in tackling health inequalities. In explicitly acknowledging the causal relationship between socioeconomic and health inequalities, the Labour government made a decisive break from the neo-liberal perspective of the previous Conservative government. The Blair government's response to the 39 recommendations made by the independent inquiry into inequalities in health chaired by Sir Donald Acheson (Independent Inquiry into Inequalities in Health, 1998) was positive, and was followed by a commitment to improve the health of the worst off in society, and to narrow the health gap between rich and poor. The Acheson Inquiry's recommendations were wide ranging and addressed key socioeconomic factors affecting health and health inequalities. Many were taken up in subsequent government policy and developed into a range of measures for reducing poverty and social exclusion, regenerating deprived areas and improving housing and the education and welfare of children (Baggott, 2010). This amounted to a cross-government, co-ordinated approach aimed at tackling the social and economic root causes of ill health and health inequalities.

Despite sustained policy activism in relation to health inequalities under Labour, inequalities persisted and, by some measures, widened during the Labour years (DoH, 2009). Baggott identifies several reasons for this, two of which are of particular relevance to the analysis at this point. First, the initial emphasis in government policy on the structural and material causes of health inequalities *gave way to the Choosing Health agenda, which placed more emphasis on individual lifestyles* (Baggott, 2010, p388). Second, by adhering to Conservative neo-liberal economic policies, with their emphasis on markets, privatisation and protecting the interests of the rich, Labour was bound to fail in its efforts to tackle the underlying socioeconomic inequalities that are the main cause of health inequalities (Baggott, 2010).

Continuity and change

Our exploration of key health policy developments under the Conservatives (1979–97) and then under Labour (1997–2010) has suggested both continuity and change in the political and ideological context of policy during the last three decades. In concluding the discussion of the impact of third-way thinking – neither capitalism nor socialism but 'what works' – it is important to acknowledge third way's essential pragmatism.

The synthesis of left and right with a commitment to build on what had worked (under the previous government) helps to explain the emphasis on evidence-based policy during the Labour years. Evidence-based policy not only helped Labour to reposition itself on the centre ground, but also provided a *kind of non-ideological ideology of pragmatism with which nobody can reasonably disagree* (Grayson and Gomersall, 2003, p3). However, the existence of good evidence for policy making should not be taken to imply that ideology can and should be banished from the policy-making process. It is notable that the Marmot Review team was glad to accept the charge that its *Fair Society, Healthy Lives* report on health inequalities could be labelled *ideology with evidence* (Marmot Review, 2010, p4). Its passionate belief that avoidable health inequalities are unfair and that addressing them is a matter of social justice is both striking and challenging.

The next section of this chapter considers the set of values and beliefs associated with David Cameron's Conservative Party: 'Cameronism'. It will also explore the impact on health policy of Cameronism and of the election of a Conservative–Liberal Democrat government in May 2010. The focus will be on public health policy developments heralded by the 2010 White Paper *Healthy Lives, Healthy People: Our Strategy for Public Health in England* (Cm 7985, 2010).

Beyond the third way? Cameronism

At the time of writing, 'Cameronism' is an ideology 'under construction', which is arguably being reshaped following the election of a Conservative–Liberal Democrat coalition government in 2010. However, in terms of its broad political and ideological contours, Cameronism has sought to distance itself from the New Right legacy of Thatcherism, while at the same time *forging the Conservatives' own 'third way' as it trespasses on to political territory which once belonged to Labour* (Lister, 2010, p53). This political territory is the centre ground where the earlier middle-way strand of conservatism could also be located. Lister characterises Cameron's brand of conservatism as modern, liberal and progressive, and based on the core liberal conservative value of social responsibility. While Cameronism is pro-market, it acknowledges that unfettered markets can render people vulnerable. Governments have a duty to respond with compassion. However, Cameronism places more faith in the 'big society' – in particular the private, charitable and informal sectors – than the state to address social problems and drive social progress. Overall the big society vision emphasises individual responsibility and a reduced role for the state, with power being pushed out from the centre and a more devolved system of governance.

Critics of the coalition government elected in 2010 argue that the refashioning of the state implied by the big society vision is far from benign. They argue that social progress will be put into reverse by the deep cuts in public expenditure being implemented by the government, and interpret the cuts in terms of an ideological assault on big government (Lister, 2010). In this analysis, the economic crisis triggered by the 2008 credit crunch is being used as a Trojan horse for the government's unstated mission to shrink the state and recast its role.

Turning now to specific policy, two White Papers on health policy were published during the coalition government's first six months in office. The first of these, *Equity and Excellence: Liberating the NHS* (Cm 7881, 2010), published in July 2010, sets out the government's plans mainly for healthcare policy. The focus of the second White Paper, *Healthy Lives, Healthy People: Our Strategy for Public Health in England* (Cm 7985, 2010), released in November 2010, is public health policy. The first White Paper is the subject of Activity 2.2, while the second is explored in more detail below that.

ACTIVITY 2.2

Read through the *Equity and Excellence: Liberating the NHS* White Paper (Cm 7881, 2010) at **www.official-documents.gov.uk/document/cm78/7881/7881.pdf** and make notes on it in response to the following questions.

1. Describe the values, vision and overarching goals for health policy set out in the White Paper. To what extent are they consistent with 'Cameronism'?
2. Identify the key reforms and policy changes in the White Paper. How will they impact on your work and organisation?

As we have already seen, the focus of the second health White Paper published by the coalition government in 2010 – *Healthy Lives, Healthy People: Our Strategy for Public Health in England* (Cm 7985, 2010) – is public health policy. Our exploration of this White Paper will again draw on George and Wilding's idea that welfare ideologies provide a *'view of the world', especially of human nature and of the relationship between state and society* (George and Wilding, 1994, p6; also cited in Lister, 2010, p5).

Public health policy analysis: Healthy Lives, Healthy People

The analysis will consider the role of individuals, the state and society envisaged by the White Paper in the three domains of public health identified by Griffiths *et al.* (2005): health improvement, health protection and health services (including service planning, efficiency, audit and evaluation).

The *Healthy Lives, Healthy People* White Paper signals the government's commitment to give higher priority to public health, supported by dedicated resources, and sets out a series of measures that relate to all three domains of public health (Griffiths *et al.*, 2005). For example, on health improvement, the White Paper acknowledges that the 'health gap' between rich and poor is increasing and that wider factors determine health, wellbeing and health inequalities. The government's adoption of the life course framework for tackling the wider social determinants of health from *Fair Society, Healthy Lives* (Marmot Review, 2010) highlights the way in which the government's thinking about health improvement has been influenced by some of the Review team's recommendations.

The approach to public health revealed in the White Paper is specific about the role of the state, individuals, the wider community and society in promoting health, preventing ill health and prolonging life. The state should adopt the least intrusive approach possible, avoiding *Whitehall diktat and nannying* (Cm 7985, 2010, p2) or lecturing and hectoring people about the way they should live. While the state should steer clear of intrusive, top-down intervention, it should also avoid a completely hands-off approach. Its proper role should be to establish a framework for empowering local communities, led by local government, to improve public health and to shape an environment that supports people in making healthy choices. Freedom of choice is preserved, but a range of public and private institutions are authorised to steer people in directions that promote their welfare (Reeves, 2010). Overall this implies widely dispersed responsibility for public health improvement, with the efforts *of individuals, families, local and national government and the private, voluntary and community sectors* being harnessed across society (Cm 7985, 2010, p22). However, the emphasis is firmly on local action or localism, a key tenet of Liberal Democrat ideology.

The extent to which the role for the state implied by the White Paper is consistent with the stewardship model of an active, positive state (see the section above on 'Socialism and collectivism') is a question that warrants further consideration. Maryon-Davis and Jolley (2010) highlight a key element of the 'stewardship role': providing a *framework of rules and regulations to help individuals, families and communities make healthier or safe choices in the way they live, work, grow and play* (Maryon-Davis and Jolley, 2010, p4). This could entail setting standards, legislating to ban or circumscribe certain activities, and regulating commercial interests. However, the 2010 public health White Paper signals a shift away from legislative and regulatory approaches, and thus arguably a retreat from the stewardship model. For example, the Public Health Responsibility Deals to be developed will be voluntary agreements, implying a less active, interventionist state. The Deals – focusing on food, alcohol, physical activity, health at work and behaviour change – will be reached collaboratively. Businesses will be expected to take more responsibility for the impact on health and wellbeing of their practices, for example branding and product formulation. Neither businesses nor individuals should be hectored or harangued by government. However, the White Paper also makes clear that if businesses do not become more socially responsible and voluntary approaches fail, the government will, as a last resort, consider more intrusive approaches such as regulation. This would involve stepping up to higher rungs in the intervention ladder shown in Figure 2.2.

The less active, less interventionist state we read about in the White Paper is more appropriately described as a 'nudge state', a term the government itself uses. This type of state 'nudges' behaviour (in the right direction) by making it easier for people to make healthy choices, for example by providing more and better information, by introducing plain packaging of tobacco products, and also by asking non-state organisations to improve their community's health. The 'nudge approach' is based on influencing the 'choice architecture' (Reeves, 2010) and is considered preferable to outright bans that reduce or remove people's choices and infringe their freedom.

A nudge approach

The idea of a nudge state and its accompanying ideology of libertarian paternalism was originally developed by University of Chicago Professors Thaler and Sunstein (2008). However, it has been explored in a UK public health context by the Nuffield

Council on Bioethics (2007) and Reeves (2010). Critics of 'nudge' tend to focus on its aversion to regulation, claiming that non-regulatory approaches are difficult to justify when the greatest advances in public health have come from government action in the form of legislation – for example, on the compulsory wearing of seatbelts or the drink-drive laws. While these types of measure could be argued to have restricted individual freedom, they have undoubtedly saved lives. The public health gains that have followed the ban on smoking in public places in the four countries of the UK are incontrovertible (Maryon-Davis and Jolley, 2010).

What's the evidence?

This activity invites you to consider some of the evidence on the impact of state intervention in public health. Case studies that review historical and contemporary evidence on the impact of state intervention on public health can be found in:

- Jochelson, K (2005) *Nanny or Steward? The Role of Government in Public Health.* London: King's Fund. Online at **www.kingsfund.org.uk/document. rm?id=5792**
- Nuffield Council on Bioethics (2007) *Public Health: The Ethical Issues.* Cambridge: Nuffield Council on Bioethics. Online at **www.nuffieldbioethics.org/ public-health/public-health-what-public-health**.

Obtain one of these papers, and then select and read through a case study that is relevant to you. What options for intervention are described, and what are the implications for your work, your organisation and for government policy makers?

A further criticism levelled at the nudge approach is that it places too much faith in the power of personal responsibility. Appealing to people's sense of personal or social responsibility (to behave better, make lifestyle changes or to play their part in the 'big society') only works up to a point. Opportunities to make healthier choices are not evenly distributed among different population groups, with some people facing more barriers – arising from their personal, social or economic circumstances – than others.

What role central government?

So what public health role should central government discharge, according to the 2010 *Healthy Lives, Healthy People* White Paper (Cm 7985, 2010)? We have already seen that the role is mainly about establishing a framework to empower local communities, and shaping the environment so that it provides more opportunities for healthier choices. It is local government that is considered to be best placed to develop local solutions to health problems and to lead partnership working across social care, the NHS and public health. Local government also holds more of the levers (than central government or the NHS) to influence the wider factors that affect health and wellbeing and to tackle health inequalities. The decision announced in the White Paper to transfer local health improvement functions from the NHS to local authorities by 2013 underlines the extent to which authorities are expected to develop their public health role. NHS Directors of Public Health will also transfer to, and be employed by, local authorities.

A key area of responsibility for Directors of Public Health working within local authorities will be the oversight of local health protection arrangements, and of emergency preparedness and response. However, health protection will be led by central government, with a *strong system to the front line* – Directors of Public Health and local health protection units (Cm 7985, 2010, p23). The 'central state's' responsibility for this important public health domain will be discharged through a new national public health service, Public Health England. This will be set up as part of the Department of Health, and will incorporate the functions of the Health Protection Agency and the National Treatment Agency for Substance Misuse. In addition to leading on health protection, Public Health England will provide leadership for the wider public health community, and support local action through funding and the provision of evidence.

We have seen that the 'proper role' of the state described in the *Healthy Lives, Healthy People* White Paper (Cm 7985, 2010) aligns more with the idea of a nudge state than a stewardship model state. This is also suggested by what the White Paper says about the evidence base for public health interventions. There is a clear indication that much of the evidence to be drawn on will be from behavioural science, a discipline that is central to 'nudge'. The White Paper refers several times to evidence on innovative approaches to behaviour change; for example, on how to reduce the demand for unhealthy goods, products and lifestyles, or to influence social norms and social networks that profoundly impact on individual behaviour. However the White Paper also makes clear that central government will have a key role in promoting evidence-based public health interventions in general, to be discharged through Public Health England.

The government's commitment to a professionally led, rigorous and evidence-based approach to public health is repeatedly stated in the White Paper. However, there are a number of policy issues that will arguably test the strength of this commitment in the coming years. The first test is how the government responds across the spectrum of social and economic policy to the Marmot Review recommendations for tackling health inequalities (Marmot Review, 2010). These were based on the best available evidence and were framed around six priorities (see below).

Six policy objectives to guide action for reducing health inequalities

1. Give every child a healthy start in life.
2. Enable all children, young people and adults to maximise their capabilities and have control over their lives.
3. Create fair employment and good work for all.
4. Ensure a healthy standard of living for all.
5. Create and develop healthy and sustainable places and communities.
6. Strengthen the role and impact of ill health prevention.

Source: Marmot Review (2010)

A second test of the government's commitment to evidence-based policy will come if the nudge approach – with its faith in the power of personal responsibility and preference for avoiding regulation – fails to bring about significant public health improvement. As we have seen, the ban on smoking in public places introduced in England in 2007 provides a powerful example of the way in which regulation through legislation of the so-called 'choice architecture' can have a dramatic effect on demand and behaviour. The public health community has argued that equally significant strides forward in public health could be made by legislating for a minimum price per unit of alcohol (Chief Medical Officer, 2009). NICE has produced guidance on this topic area, which the government has declined to take up. However, plans to deliver the coalition agreement commitment (HM Government, 2010) to ban the sale of alcohol below cost price – defined as the tax drinkers pay, i.e. duty plus VAT – were announced by the government in January 2011. This measure, which affects both England and Wales, will introduce a minimum price of 21p per unit for beer and 28p per unit for spirits. Critics of the government's plans point to the evidence – for example, NICE guidance – that a minimum cost of at least 50p per unit would be necessary to achieve the desired reduction in consumption among harmful and moderate drinkers. It will be interesting to see if, over time, the government comes to a different view of the evidence base on alcohol pricing if the less active, intervention-ist approach it seems to favour produces insufficient progress in tackling harmful levels and patterns of drinking.

Conclusion

The 2010 *Healthy Lives, Healthy People* White Paper (Cm 7985, 2010) sets out a certain *view of the world*, and in particular, of human nature and of the relationship between state and society (George and Wilding, 1994). This view of the world is very consistent with the values and beliefs associated with Cameronism. For example, adults are considered capable of making healthy choices for themselves and their families, but need to be empowered to do so – a process that will boost their sense of self-esteem and personal responsibility. However, responsibility for improving health and wellbeing and for positively shaping social and environmental determinants of health should be widely shared across society. Central government's key role is to establish a framework for effective local action, involving local government, the NHS, corporate interests and civil society – for example, the voluntary and community sectors. State intrusion and interference in people's lives should be kept to a minimum, while personal, social and corporate responsibility should be strengthened.

The public health policy of the Conservative–Liberal Democrat coalition government elected in 2010 is therefore based on an ideology that stresses personal responsibility and individual freedom. This represents a retreat from the previous Labour government's combined approach of intervention, regulation and exhortation, as exemplified by the 'middle course' plotted by the *Choosing Health* White Paper (Cm 6374, 2004).

Chapter 2 summary

This chapter began with a discussion of a range of abstract concepts that are the building blocks to understanding the political and ideological context of policy. The impact of ideology on health policy development during five key phases was then explored. The phases were linked to the ideologies of socialism and collectivism, middle way conservatism, neo-liberalism, third way and Cameronism. Particular attention was paid to what Lister has identified as *the critical issue* (Lister, 2010, p18) dividing ideological perspectives: the proper role of the state. Two models of the state, stewardship and nudge, and their association with particular political and welfare ideologies, were explored.

The degree of continuity between left and right political parties' health policies – for example, on the dividing line between the state and the market in the delivery of health services – suggests that ideological differences may be more rhetorical than actual. Similarly, it is important to acknowledge the common ground shared by the stewardship and nudge models of the state. While they start from different perspectives, and the stewardship approach tends to advocate a higher degree of intervention than nudge, the models are, as Reeves (2010) argues, closer on the continuum or ladder of possible interventions than some commentators might concede.

The chapter concluded with an analysis of the coalition government's 2010 public health White Paper, *Healthy Lives, Healthy People* (Cm 7985, 2010), identifying some of the challenges it sets for individuals, the state and society as its key proposals for health improvement are implemented.

GOING FURTHER

In the years since devolution, key points of difference in policy, priorities and ideology between England and the other countries of the UK have emerged.

For further information on health policy in Scotland, Wales and Northern Ireland, see:

Baggott, R (2007) *Understanding Health Policy*. Bristol: The Policy Press.
Baggott, R (2010) *Public Health Policy and Politics* (2nd edn). Oxford: Wiley Blackwell.
Ham, C (2009) *Health Policy in Britain* (6th edn). Basingstoke: Palgrave Macmillan.

chapter 3

Strategic Context of Policy: A Look at UK Policy for the Four Nations

Heather Bain and David Adams

Meeting the Public Health Competences

Core area 3: Policy and strategy development and implementation to improve population health and wellbeing

This chapter will help you to evidence the following competences for public health (Public Health Skills and Careers Framework):

- Level 6(a): Understanding of the policies and strategies that affect own area of work;
- Level 7(1): Interpret and communicate local, regional and national policies and strategies within own area of work;
- Level 7(5): Assess the actual or potential impact of policies and strategies on health and wellbeing.

This chapter will also assist you in demonstrating the following National Occupational Standard(s) for public health:

- PHP38: Monitor trends and developments in policies for their impact on health and wellbeing;
- PHP39: Present information and arguments to others on how policies affect health and wellbeing;
- PHP40: Evaluate and recommend changes to policies to improve health and wellbeing.

This chapter should also be useful in demonstrating Standard 10 of the Public Health Practitioner Standards:

Standard 10: Support the implementation of policies and strategies to improve health and wellbeing outcomes – demonstrating:

a. knowledge of the main public health policies and strategies relevant to own area of work and the organisations that are responsible for them;
b. how different policies, strategies and priorities affect own specific work and how to influence their development or implementation in own area of work;
c. critical reflection and constructive suggestions for how policies, strategies and priorities could be improved in terms of improving health and wellbeing and reducing health inequalities in own area of work.

Overview

Policy operates at a number of levels, international, national and local, which are all interrelated. This chapter will examine the strategic context of national health policy within the United Kingdom. First, devolution will be explored, then the major government policies from the four UK countries relevant to health and wellbeing, and inequalities, will be discussed, acknowledging the divergence of policy among the four countries since devolution.

Introduction

The creation of the National Health Service (NHS) in 1948 can be regarded as *the* major public health achievement of the twentieth century (Baggott, 2000). Of all the political changes that have taken place within the UK since, it is perhaps devolution that has had the most potential to result in change and divergence within this institution.

Devolution and its effect on the National Health Service and public health policy

The core principles of the NHS were laid down at its birth in 1948; these were of access to services for all, free at the point of delivery and financed through general taxation (Alcock, 2008). These principles have guided the NHS in England, Scotland, Wales and Northern Ireland – the four countries that comprise the United Kingdom – and, prior to devolution, it could be said that there was a broad similarity in the nature of the health policies the four countries produced (Alvarez-Rosete *et al.*, 2005).

The NHS has of course never been a truly unified system, despite the fact that it is usually referred to as '*the*' NHS, which may give rise to notions of it as one institution responsible for the whole of the UK rather than four separate institutions, with a framework in the form of the devolution concordats. These try to ensure that the appropriate departments in the Westminster government and the devolved administrations *co-operate on matters affecting the NHS, public health, wider health issues and social care, seeking to work in an open and helpful manner, with good communication and early involvement of the other parties when appropriate* (DoH, 2001; 2006a).

Initial differences in health policy between the four countries since the inception of the NHS can be explained by the different administrative structures, through which they were governed by Westminster, prior to devolution (BMA, 2007); however, these differences tended to focus on how centrally derived policy was to be implemented.

The advent of devolution for Scotland, Wales and Northern Ireland was in 1999, when their respective administrations were officially convened, the relevant legislation having been passed the previous year. Not all of the devolved administrations have the same powers – for example, Scotland can increase/decrease income tax by three pence in the pound; Wales lacks primary legislative power – therefore major policy change requires agreement from Westminster government; however, all have now a much greater degree of freedom in relation to the health policies they produce.

Since health is a devolved issue, different departments in devolved administrations of the four countries became responsible for its development, implementation and evaluation. In England the responsibility lies with the Department of Health, (PH England). In Scotland it is with the Scottish Government Health Department. In Wales it lies with the Welsh Assembly Health and Social Care, while in Northern Ireland it is the responsibility of the Northern Ireland Department of Health, Social Services and Public Safety.

Some of those seeing the advantages of devolution had felt that it might allow PH policies and priorities to be more sensitive to local situations and needs (Neave, 1999). Others, however, had expected it to have little actual impact on health and social care (BMA, 2007). This latter expectation was perhaps rather naive, given that policies of any description have always tended to be primarily politically driven (Greer, 2008). In this regard the health service and the health agenda has always been a popular arena for political engagement between the parties (Edwards, 2007), often with a 'quick fix' solution being sought (Hunter, 2003), so any change that affects the political balance will almost inevitably result in health policy change.

From the advent of devolution until 2007 there could be said to have been a fair degree of convergence between the four countries in relation to PH policy. In part this was no doubt due to the fact that some drivers for change in the existing health system were common to all four countries. Reports such as *Securing Our Future Health: Taking a Long-Term View* (Wanless, 2002), which took a UK-wide perspective, *The Review of Health and Social Care in Wales* (Wanless, 2003), and *Building a Health Service Fit for the Future* (Scottish Executive, 2005) in Scotland, all identified ageing populations, inequality and increase in long-term conditions as factors the health services needed to address. Other factors, such as the need to respond to EU regulations, may also have contributed to a degree of convergence, however perhaps the most prominent influence at this time was the Labour Party.

During the period from devolution until 2007, Labour formed the ruling administration in Westminster, and Labour/Liberal Democrat coalitions were in power in Scotland and Wales. The political situation in Northern Ireland, which, between a need for maintenance of the status quo to stabilise the opposing parties and suspension of devolution between 2002 and 2007 (during which time there was direct rule from Westminster), gave no real opportunity for real divergence to emerge there.

Following elections for the devolved governments in 2007, however, while Labour remained in power in Westminster, Nationalist parties came to power in both Scotland and Wales, thus changing the political balance. Both Nationalist parties – the SNP in Scotland and Plaid Cymru in Wales – had included promises of improvement in health services in their pre-devolution manifestoes (Ross and Tomaney, 2001) and now had the opportunity to make good on these.

Devolution, then, had set the scene for differences in PH policy in the four countries to become more apparent; and indeed there was evidence that different paths to achieve their aims were soon adopted by the devolved administrations (Greer, 2004a). Some divergence also started to emerge in relation to policy direction itself (Ham, 2004). After the changes following elections to the devolved administrations in 2007 the stage was now set for divergence to accelerate and some sources since then have noted that the nature and provision of services themselves have changed (Maslin-Prothero *et al.*, 2008; Moore, 2009).

ACTIVITY 3.1

Policy is made as a result of networks of decisions involving a wide range of people and organisations at local, national and international levels. From your earlier reading of Chapters 1 and 2 you may have started to realise that values and beliefs underpin policy and the political process. Policy can have either a negative or positive impact on health. To help you appreciate the ideologies that underpin policy, and how they impact upon health and the politics of promoting health, access a health policy from one of the UK countries and analyse it considering a client group from your area of practice. Does the policy have a positive or negative impact on your selected client group? How does this policy support your role as a public health practitioner?

Comment

Recent change in UK government means that, for first time since the advent of devolved governments in the UK, major political differences now exist between a right-wing, Conservative government in Westminster, and predominantly left-wing devolved governments in Scotland and Wales. Given the traditional differences in approach to public health policy between left- and right-wing political parties, the pace of divergence may be set to increase unless all parties concerned can move more towards to the middle ground and fully embrace the 'third way' of policy development, which lies between state control and free market forces (Alcock, 2008).

The extent of current convergence and divergence will now be examined in relation to some of the major policy documents produced by the four countries since devolution.

Scottish health policy

While, with the passage of time, Scottish health policy can be seen to be diverging from that of the other three countries, there has also been a considerable degree of internal convergence to date in the content of policies produced by the different administrations that have governed Scotland in the devolution era.

Two main themes appear to be constant within this period: that of inequalities as a central issue to be tackled to improve the health of the nation, and partnership as being central to the means of doing so.

The concept of inequalities first entered the Scottish policy agenda in *Towards a Healthier Scotland* (Scottish Office, 1999), the last White Paper on health to bear the mark of the Scottish Office of the Westminster government and published just prior to the establishment of the new Scottish Parliament. This paper introduced inequalities (under the title of 'life circumstances') as one focus of a tripartite approach, along with the more conventional areas of lifestyle issues and specific health problems, to improving the health of the public in Scotland. This was the first time that health had been overtly linked to inequalities in a government policy. Though the document was less clear on how the issue was to be dealt with, partnership working was seen as a necessary prerequisite to tackling inequalities, which, by their nature, would require a multi-faceted approach.

From a political viewpoint, this focus on inequalities could be seen as the Labour Party, traditionally well supported in Scotland, picking up the ball again on regaining power after its defeat of the Conservative government in 1997, allowing it to resume its focus on the issue. It had commissioned the *Report of the Working Group on Inequalities* (the Black Report) in 1977, but the Conservative government to which it reported in 1980 had chosen not to implement the recommendations of that report, largely due to the high level of state intervention called for. *Inequalities in Health* (the Acheson Report), published in 1998, showed little had changed since the Black Report was published and, although an English report, was used to inform the direction of Scottish policy on the issue.

Inequalities remained an area to be addressed within the new Scottish Executives paper, *Improving Health in Scotland: The Challenge* (Scottish Government, 2003a). Now, however, rather than inequalities being addressed as a central issue, it became an integral issue to be addressed within four new focus areas of Early Years, Teenage Transition, the Workplace, and Community-Led. Rather than pushing the issue to one side, this could be seen as inequalities as an issue becoming more central to Scottish health policy, and concomitant to this the importance of partnership in dealing with it was also reinforced.

Inequalities agenda in Scottish policy

Improving Health in Scotland had been published as a framework to support the 2003 White Paper, *Partnership for Care* (Scottish Government, 2003b). This policy was intended to announce a change from basing services on normative needs to one based on the expressed needs of individuals and communities. Health improvement was to become the shared responsibility of all, and not just the remit of the Public Health and Health Promotion departments.

This can be seen as the beginning of a move away from the 'professionalism' model of organising health services in Scotland described by Greer (2004a), where the agenda was decided by a medically led elite, to one in which the general population could also have some influence. This approach was evident within how *Improving Health in Scotland* intended to deal with inequalities, with the development of Joint Health Improvement Plans to target disadvantaged communities in both urban and rural settings.

In 2005 another influential report, this time a Scottish-focused one, *Building a Health Service Fit for the Future* (the Kerr Report), was published (Scottish Government, 2005), and was to provide the main drivers for a range of subsequent policies. Three main drivers for change were identified: an ageing population, an increase in the presentation of long-term conditions and, once again, continued high levels of inequalities.

The government response to this was contained in *Delivering for Health* (Scottish Government, 2005b) in what was to be the Labour/Liberal coalition's last health policy document.

Public health intelligence within the document focused on mortality and lifestyle statistics, indicating that the inequality gap between rich and poor in Scottish society was continuing to widen. However, while concern for the issue was clear, the idea of inequalities being integral to all parts of the health agenda seemed to be somewhat diluted from *Improving Health in Scotland*. Many of the initiatives proposed were focused around a shift in focus towards preventative medicine and additional community-based health services within disadvantaged areas. As commendable a proposition as this might be, it could also be said to indicate a return to treating the symptoms of inequalities, rather than focusing on the underlying causes. Partnership remained as an important approach, but the public role in it appeared to have been played down somewhat, with emphasis instead given to co-operation between different government departments.

The event with the greatest potential to change the Scottish health agenda occurred in 2007 when, following the elections to the Scottish Parliament, the Scottish Nationalist Party formed the first minority government since the advent of devolution. In addition this was the first time the ruling administration in Scotland, though still left of centre, would not be formed by either Labour or a Labour-led coalition. There was therefore interest in what direction the health policies of the new administration would take.

The answers to this emerged with the publication of *Better Health, Better Care*, first as a Discussion Document in August 2007 (Scottish Executive, 2007a) to be followed by the Action Plan in December that year (Scottish Government, 2007b). It was clear that inequalities were set to remain as a central concern of health policy. This was perhaps unsurprising as the SNP, a left-of-centre party, was not too far removed from the political perspective of the previous administration in relation to addressing health needs, and indeed had made this clear in its manifesto and in previous support for much of the content of *Delivering for Health*; in addition, its policy acknowledged the same drivers taken from the Kerr Report.

The *Better Health, Better Care* documents set out a strategy for dealing with inequalities that seemed quite far reaching in its scope, with a ministerial task force to be established to gain the public health intelligence necessary to more effectively direct a range of health promotion initiatives and make appropriate changes to existing services – to be based on the needs of deprived communities. It was also made clear that the new government intended to *focus on tackling health inequalities in everything we do*, thus inequalities seemed to be set to regain their status from *Improving Health in Scotland* as an integral part of all policy action.

Partnership and inequalities

The nature of partnership in dealing with inequalities however, though clear in relation to the need for intergovernmental working, is less clear in relation to the involvement with individuals and communities, where it is made specific it is in relation to the provision of healthcare services, rather than in dealing with the underlying causes of ill health in disadvantaged areas.

Better Health, Better Care did present what it referred to as some 'new' policies within its content, predominant among these perhaps the proposal to abolish prescription charges, and reduce the waiting time between initial GP consultation and treatment to 18 weeks by 2011.

Both these initiatives might be seen as the kind of 'popularist' interventions that any new government might introduce, however despite the title, neither of these was new within a UK context. The Labour government of Harold Wilson had abolished UK-wide prescription charges in 1965, only to restore them two years later on the grounds of cost, and in fact in 2005 a Bill to abolish prescription charges in Scotland had been previously introduced in 2005 by the Scottish Socialist Party, only to be thrown out, again on arguments surrounding cost.

A further driver for the SNP, however, is perhaps its underlying drive towards achieving full independence for Scotland; indeed the change in name from 'Scottish Executive' to 'Scottish Government' by the SNP may be seen as part of its move to achieve this. In this light, the SNP needs to be able to convince the public that all services provided under it are at least on a par with, and preferably better than, those in the rest of the UK. As Wales had already moved to abolish prescription charges, and Northern Ireland was on course to follow, Scotland could not be seen to be falling behind. Likewise with waiting times – as England had been moving to an 18-week total patient journey since 2004 this may well have been a catalyst for the Scottish government to announce that it was moving towards the same goal.

Whether *Better Health, Better Care* manages to achieve all its stated aims is still uncertain – cost may prove the greatest stumbling block to this. Free personal care, which the previous administration had introduced and the SNP had pledged to maintain, although popular with the public is already proving difficult to finance, and it remains to be seen if these more recent initiatives will prove equally as difficult to maintain.

ACTIVITY 3.2

Health policy in Scotland has been traditionally medically led.

- What might the advantages, if any, of this be?
- How might this influence approaches to dealing with issues such as inequality and social inclusion?

Dealing with inequality has been a central feature of Scottish health policy since devolution.

- Can you suggest why this issue might have such an apparent priority status within Scottish policy?
- In what way, if any, does the Scottish approach to dealing with inequalities differ from that of the rest of the UK?

Welsh health policy

It is probably true to say that healthcare and the organisation of health services are an integral part of Welsh politics, more so perhaps than anywhere else in the UK. Few Welsh politicians will have failed to make reference to the Welsh origins of the concept of a National Health Service at some time in their careers – as Michael and Tanner (2007) state, *swearing allegiance to Bevan's legacy is an important political gesture in Wales*, and a Bevan Commission still advises the Welsh Assembly on the development of health services in Wales, trying to ensure, among other things, that the NHS in Wales stays true to Aneurin Bevan's original concepts.

It might be expected, then, that the Welsh Assembly would take a rather conservative approach to health policy. However, while still proud of its historical relationship with the NHS, Welsh health policy has not remained stagnant; indeed in some areas where Wales has led others have followed.

Inequalities agenda in Welsh policy

The issue of inequalities is a theme that has featured high in the Welsh policy agenda since devolution. High levels of inequality had long been a feature of Welsh society, linked to the high incidence of ill health; the result of a combination of decline in traditional industries, economic forces and lifestyle choices. An additional complication was perhaps the existence of a large rural population. With devolution, the opportunity arose for the Labour-led Assembly to try to address these issues.

From the outset the decision was taken to have a strong focus on dealing with the underlying causes of ill health by reducing inequalities. Two documents entitled *Better Health, Better Wales* were produced in 1998, the first a discussion document in May, followed by a strategic framework in December that year. Both these documents had a strong public health agenda, and to achieve their stated aim of sustainable health and wellbeing and reduced levels of inequality for the Welsh population, health improvement was seen to be the key. This was to work not only through health promotion activities, but through a joined-up approach to policy that would involve dealing with social, economic and environmental factors that could affect health in a positive or negative manner; thus enhancing wellbeing was seen as being as important as preventing ill health (Welsh Office, 1998a).

Greer (2008) states that Welsh health policy did two things following devolution. First, it showed a commitment to redirecting resources to meet health needs, rather than focus on delivery of services. It then went on to reorganise the structure of the NHS in Wales to put public health and inequalities in the foreground.

The continued importance placed on health improvement was emphasised by the publication *of Promoting Health and Wellbeing* (Welsh Assembly Government (WAG), 2000), and *Improving Health in Wales* (WAG, 2001a) the following year. These documents underlined the Welsh Assembly's commitment to deal with the underlying causes of ill health, and expressed the need for partnership, not only between other public service organisations in order to achieve this, but with the citizens of Wales themselves. The need to review the role of the existing structure of the health service was also postulated.

This desire for joint working to achieve an improvement in the health of the population was reflected in the adoption of what has been described as a 'localism' approach to the design of health services in Wales (Greer, 2004a). This was not new however: since *Putting Patients First* (Welsh Office, 1998b), the emphasis had been placed on Local Health Groups operating through 22 Health Authorities (one for each of the local government areas in the country) as the key to deciding on what services were required within an area, reflecting the priorities of the local communities they served. The idea was that local problems required a local perspective to deal with them, and involvement of the local population would lead to a greater engagement with, and ownership of, services.

This approach was seen as essential for dealing with the underlying determinants of health, since without the population on side the problem of reducing inequalities would be made that much more difficult. Some determinants, however, were recognised as outwith the ability of individuals or communities to deal with, and so some intervention from government would also be required.

A review commissioned by the Welsh Assembly, and chaired by Professor Peter Townsend, was asked to consider the existing arrangements for allocation of resources for health and health services in the face of continued high levels of inequalities. The report from this review, *Targeting Poor Health* (WAG, 2001b), recommended a dual strategy that would address the socioeconomic underpinnings of inequalities, coupled with a new resource allocation process that would more realistically assess health needs. However, initial plans to implement this were revised as they were felt to ignore issues of the higher cost of providing services to Wales' many rural areas, thus highlighting that finding a formula that would be both politically acceptable, and would adequately institute changes that would deal with inequalities, was not going to be easy. Indeed, in some respects, the search for such a solution still goes on.

Partnership and inequalities

A further restructuring of the NHS in Wales was announced in *Improving Health in Wales: A Plan for the NHS with its Partners* (WAG, 2001a). Emphasis was placed on this being a Welsh plan to suit Welsh needs, with a strong emphasis on partnership.

Well Being in Wales (WAG, 2002) built further on this need for strong partnership, and restated the Welsh Assembly's desire to achieve a joined-up approach to health policy by building health into other policy areas, and pointed out that this approach was endorsed by Professor Townsend's report and would be enhanced by the changes made to the organisation of health services to date. The strong focus on health improvement aiming to provide sustainable health and wellbeing, first expressed in *Better Health, Better Wales* (Welsh Office 1998a), was still in place, but now there was the suggestion of greater need for the general population to increase their role by taking more responsibility for their own health.

The Review of Health and Social Care in Wales (Wanless, 2003) also emphasised the need for this, and highlighted the additional pressures that health and social care services would be brought under in the future by an ageing population in particular. It recommended a greater emphasis on the prevention of ill health and early intervention, with a further reshaping of services to meet this end.

In 2003, the NHS in Wales underwent further reform when Health Authorities were scrapped and replaced by 22 Local Health Boards, however the overall commitment to a localised approach to the organisation of services remained. Some, however, pointed out that this commitment actually resulted in fragmentation and difficulty in making Wales-wide decisions (Smith and Babbington, 2006).

Designed for Life (WAG, 2005b) announced the decision to introduce a new planning system for health and social care in Wales. This was to be user centred, with both service users and service providers to be involved in the process. As in the rest of the UK, not only an ageing population, but increased levels of chronic illness, were acknowledged as an additional problem to future health service provision, and so supported self-care in the community was to become an important component. Access to services was also to be improved, and since 2001 several practical measures had been put in place with relation to this, with free dental and eye examinations and, perhaps most importantly, prescription charges first frozen then to be phased out entirely by 2007. Overall, the aim remained constant, however, in terms of a focus to be kept on achievement of sustainable health and wellbeing, and reduction in levels of inequalities.

Despite the Welsh Assembly's chosen policy path, however, in 2005 a further report by Peter Townsend, *Inequalities in Health: The Welsh Dimension 2002–2005* (WAG, 2005c), indicated that levels of inequalities in Wales remained high, and in some cases had become worse. The dual strategy proposed in 2001, along with partnership and joined-up policy making were all included as recommendations to continue with, with local action by Health Boards highlighted as a key action in the implementation of these.

Therefore, despite an apparent lack of progress in dealing with inequalities by dealing with the underlying determinants, Welsh policy resolutely stuck to the path chosen immediately following devolution. More recent policies, such as *One Wales* (Plaid Cymru, 2007), indicated that this resolution was set to continue, though services were set to be restructured yet again. The latest service reforms took place in 2009, when the 22 Local Health Boards were replaced by seven integrated Local Health Boards. Public Health Wales was established as an NHS Trust on 1 October 2009.

In 2010 policies such as *Setting the Direction* (WAG, 2010e) and *Doing Well, Doing Better* (WAG, 2010b) were still espousing the principles of localism, partnership and reduction of health inequalities through Health Promotion, Protection and Improvement. It would appear that these will remain the staples of Welsh policy for some time to come.

Recent change in central government may well prove problematic, however, for future Welsh health policy. The devolution agreement for Wales means that the Welsh Assembly cannot make legislative change without ratification from Westminster. While a Labour government was in power within the Welsh Assembly and Westminster this might have been easier to achieve than the current situation with a Plaid Cymru and Labour alliance in the Assembly and now a Conservative government in Westminster. The gap in political ideologies may prove a difficult barrier for the Welsh Assembly to overcome.

ACTIVITY 3.3

Welsh health policy has focused largely on local solutions for local problems.

- What are the potential advantages/disadvantages to such a focus?
- How might such a focus influence partnership working?

Additionally, Welsh policy has concentrated more on health than healthcare.

- What justification could you suggest for this?
- What might be potential barriers to continuing this approach in the future?

English health policy

There have been numerous changes within English health policy since 1998, and structures have changed frequently. Traditionally England was the dominant 'force' within the UK, and whatever happened in London set the UK agenda. However, since devolution, there have been growing divergences from England to the other three UK countries. This can mainly be attributed to their stance of 'markets' (Greer, 2004a) and the political views that have not been shared by the devolved governments.

One of the most significant English policies published in this time was the Acheson Report, *Independent Inquiry into Inequalities in Health* (1998) as mentioned previously. It identified some of the key inequalities and provided 39 recommendations to influence future policy. This informed the publication of *Saving Lives: Our Healthier Nation* (DoH, 1999b). This in particular set targets to reduce death rates from cancer, heart disease, stroke, accidents and mental health by the year 2010. It also informed government strategy, as outlined in *Tackling Health Inequalities: A Programme for Action* (DoH, 2003).

The NHS Plan (NHS, 2000) and *Delivering the NHS Plan – Next Steps on Investment; Next Steps in Reform* (DoH, 2002) outlined the principles of shorter waiting times, recruitment of more health professionals, creating more beds and establishing a better NHS system. It accepted that the setting up of the Primary Care Trusts in the late 1990s was the right approach, but that stronger incentives were required to ensure the extra cash produces improved performance. New Strategic Health Authorities were to be implemented to manage the day-to-day business of the NHS and oversee local health services. The term 'market' was avoided, however the plan was full of market-type terminology (Jervis and Plowden, 2003). This paper accepted the Wanless Report's (Wanless, 2002) proposals to involve local authorities to reduce hospital bed blocking by making them financially responsible. There was a major commitment to involvement with the private sector in this paper. This was followed by the *NHS Improvement Plan* (DoH, 2004c), which set out the priorities for the NHS between 2004 and 2008. It supported the ongoing commitment to a ten-year process of reform first set out in *The NHS Plan* (DoH, 2000).

Wanless, in 2004, published a second report, *Securing Good Health for the Whole Population*, which proposed a strategy for reducing preventable illness and improving healthcare. This report fed into *Choosing Health* (DoH, 2004b), presenting a new approach to public health, and focused on empowering and educational approaches to individuals' public health issues with the support of national and local organisations. For example, it proposed the start of the smoking ban in public places, along with increased support for smokers to quit. This was not fully implemented in England until July 2007, but was implemented in Scotland the previous year.

Due to financial pressure within the English NHS around 2006, redesign of services was required. *Our Health, Our Care, Our Say* (DoH, 2006b) was one of a number of policies to provide a framework to guide this recent shift in focus. In particular it focused on the management of long-term conditions, with the principles of keeping people well and avoiding the need for clinical care. This would be achieved in the context of system reform with incentives to move care from acute to community settings. Within these recent NHS reform policies, *Practice Based Commissioning* (DoH, 2005c) was regarded as a key concept allowing primary care teams incentives to look after their population effectively. This could be seen to be another English marketing model in preference to Scotland's partnership working approach. From another perspective, one could argue it is a positive move to take a population approach to address long-term conditions.

In 2008, *High Quality Care For All: NHS Next Stage Review Final Report* (DoH, 2008c) published a strategy for the NHS over the subsequent ten years. Its main principles were a focus on clinical care, quality and patient safety, with a continuation of the previous agendas. With the run-up to a general election, despite different policy initiatives, neither of the major parties questioned the market and strategic direction of health policy (BMA, 2010).

Three months prior to the general election, *Fair Society, Healthy Lives*, the Marmot Review (Marmot, 2010), an independent review into health inequalities in England which Professor Sir Michael Marmot was asked to chair by the Secretary of State for Health, was published. Many of its recommendations have been seen in previous reports on inequalities but what it does differently is to place the responsibility on all parts of society and, like Acheson, suggest that inequalities is a wider issue than that of the NHS. This strategic review of health inequalities concluded that a social gradient in health persists and that interventions should focus on reducing it across all the social determinants of health. It also proposed that progress should in future be monitored nationally against three main targets, including one on health outcomes as measured by life expectancy, healthy life expectancy and wellbeing. It will be interesting to see how this influences future national and local policy.

The general election in 2010 resulted in a coalition government between the Conservatives and the Liberal Democrats, and another new health policy was quickly developed. *Equity and Excellence: Liberating the NHS* (DoH, 2010a) builds on the core values and principles of the NHS – a comprehensive service, available to all, free at the point of use, based on need, not ability to pay. The White Paper focuses on five key areas:

1. the GP commissioning revolution;

2. quality and outcomes;

3. public health and prevention;

4. efficiency savings;

5. value and innovation.

While there are relatively few changes from a patient perspective, the proposals to introduce GP consortia to carry out the bulk of NHS commissioning, and to reduce bureaucracy, constitutes a radical and bold step. Primary Care Trusts and Strategic Health Authorities are to be abolished. This has the potential to bring primary care closer to patients, with a stronger focus on prevention. There is the concept that public health and prevention are at the centre of the NHS and a new Public Health Service is proposed. This move is much needed to safeguard the future health of the country, and embraces some of what was included within *Fair Society, Healthy Lives* (Marmot, 2010).

It is clear that the status quo is not an option, however whether the English model will achieve what it set out to do is debatable. The recent change in government has resulted in a change of thinking, with a shift from state intervention to individual responsibility. This may in fact reinforce the 'market' philosophy. As both Labour and the Conservatives readjust their political stances after the 2010 election, it seems that both may be moving away from the centre and back towards a more 'traditional' standpoint. The unknown factor is how much influence the Liberals will have in affecting this drift back to a more right-wing perspective. *Healthy Lives, Healthy People* (DoH, 2010c) adds to this debate. However, no matter what, it would appear that the divergence from the remaining countries of the UK is set to continue.

ACTIVITY 3.4

Access a copy of *Fair Society, Healthy Lives* (2010) (the Marmot Review).

- Consider the range of policy objectives and recommendations in Chapter 4. Does the evidence suggest that these would be effective in reducing the social gradient if fully implemented?
- Given the change in government in Westminster following the publication of the Marmot Review, how might the accompanying change in the political agenda have an effect on the implementation of the Review's recommendations?

Northern Ireland health policy

Northern Ireland is much more complex than the rest of the UK due to its geographical and political circumstances. It does not share a border with any of the other UK countries but with the Republic of Ireland, with which it has experienced political unrest for many years. Devolution for Northern Ireland was seen by many to be more about the start of the peace process rather than to allow self-government (Greer, 2004a; BMA, 2010). The Belfast Agreement (Northern Ireland Office, 1998), otherwise known as the Good Friday Agreement, permitted devolution, however more significantly its aim was not to solve conflict, but to establish democratic procedures to address the conflict. The Democratic Unionist Party was the only large party that opposed the Agreement. Its content acknowledged Northern Ireland as being part of the UK, but also that the population needed to work towards a united Ireland. Therefore it had three strands that led to the establishment of:

1. a North–South Ministerial Council to bring together those with executive responsibilities in Northern Ireland and the Irish governments to develop consultation, co-operation and action on six cross-border issues, one being health – focusing on accident and emergency planning, co-operation on high-technology equipment, cancer research and health promotion;

2. a British–Irish Council to exchange information, discuss, consult and use best endeavours to reach agreement on co-operation on matters of mutual interest within the competence of the relevant administrations; membership comprises representatives of the British and Irish governments, devolved institutions in Northern Ireland, Scotland and Wales, together with representatives of the Isle of Man and the Channel Islands;

3. a British–Irish Intergovernmental Conference comprising senior representatives from both governments to promote bilateral co-operation at all levels on matters of mutual interest.

Although the Belfast Agreement was a historic compromise in 1998, its implementation has been challenging and the different political parties interpreted it in different ways. Northern Ireland's politicians were unprepared to work in a democracy. This resulted in continued political unrest and, from 2002 to 2007, Northern Ireland's powers were suspended and the British government stepped in. During this period, the focus from the British government was on peace rather than developing health policy to address the needs of Northern Ireland's population. Consequently change has been slower in Ireland than in other UK countries.

Northern Ireland was said to be repackaging English health policy (Jervis, 2008) and the internal market continued much longer following devolution than in Scotland or Wales. Greer (2004a) describes this model for the NHS as permissive *managerialism*, whereby the focus is on maintaining services in challenging conditions and produces little policy. However, one significant difference in Northern Ireland since the start of devolution is that the health service is integrated with the social care structures under the Department of Health, Social Services and Public Safety.

The main policy initiative during the time when Northern Ireland's powers were suspended was the Review of Public Administration. This examined all public services, including health, and followed on from the Wanless Review in England (2003). Appleby was commissioned to the review in Northern Ireland. *The Appleby Report: An Independent Review of Health and Social Care Services in Northern Ireland* (Appleby, 2005) focused on three main areas: funding, use of resources and performance management. It identified that many of the countries' problems were related to the use of resources rather than what was available. For example, he identified that there was little improvement in waiting times despite the additional resources. Overall he made 25 recommendations and the main focus of the report was that efficient use of resources would improve health outcomes. The differences from England were recognised and in particular it was stated that *the competitive economic environment is unlikely to be appropriate in Northern Ireland*. However, despite rejecting GP fund holding, Appleby argues that explicit performance management systems would promote positive change in health and social care (Jervis, 2008). As a result of this report there was trust reconfiguration in 2007, and work started on a new commissioning system and the establishment of seven local commissioning groups.

At this time the devolved government was restored to the Northern Ireland Assembly on Tuesday 8 May 2007 following the election of a four-party Executive. This decision was a result of many English policies, such as the proposal of water charges being unacceptable to Northern Ireland, and it was the way to avoid policies being enforced by direct rule from Westminster. Since then Appleby's recommendations have been refined and implementation begun (BMA, 2010).

In 2002, *Investing for Health Strategy* (Department of Health, Social Services & Public Safety Northern Ireland (DHSSPS NI) was published by the previously devolved government. This policy was Northern Ireland's equivalent to other UK policy to reduce health inequalities, based on partnership working similar to that of Scotland and Wales. It focused on two overarching goals:

1. to improve the health of the people by increasing the length of their lives, and increasing the amount of years they spend free from disease, illness and disability;

2. to reduce inequalities in health between geographic areas, socioeconomic and minority groups.

The new devolved government still has this strategy underpinning its health improvement plans (Northern Investing for Health Partnership, 2008). Due to the nature of the original goals, the achievement of them will not be seen in early years. However, many of the actions working towards the end goals have been implemented. It has been recognised that this public health strategy focusing on addressing health improvements and health inequalities is a positive outcome during a period of uncertainty.

ACTIVITY 3.5

- How has the period of political unrest in Northern Ireland contributed to the development of health policy since devolution?
- Consider the other three countries within the UK. Do trends seem to suggest that health policy in Northern Ireland is moving into line with any of them, or is it following a distinct course of its own?

Comment

As a result of Northern Ireland's Assembly only being in place for a short time in comparison to that of Scotland and Wales there has been significantly less health policy produced and little has changed since 1998. However, since the Northern Ireland Executive was reformed, work from the Department of Health and Social Services and Public Safety has moved forwards, mirroring some of the strategies from Scotland and Wales. For example, on 1 April 2010, the charge for prescriptions was abolished in Northern Ireland. However, on some issues there have been challenges. Although Northern Ireland is committed to the concept of 'free personal care', unfortunately at this point in time it cannot afford to commit to it. It is expected that Northern Ireland will move forward with a strong public health agenda focusing on care in the community.

Chapter 3 summary

In this chapter the effects of diverging health policy across the UK were examined. It could be concluded that the broad aims for services across the four countries are similar. All recognise the shifting balance of care from the acute sector to the community, with an increasing focus on the management of long-term conditions to avoid hospital admission. However, the various political stances provide differing opinions on how to develop health services considering the demographics of the four countries. As Jervis concluded in 2008, different values do exist, which include:

- collaboration and collectivism in Scotland;

- similar communication and collectivism in Wales;

- democratic participation, neutrality in Northern Ireland;

- markets and technical solutions in England.

With the recent change in UK government it is expected that this divergence will escalate.

GOING FURTHER

Alcock, P (2008) *Social Policy in Britain* (3rd edn). Basingstoke: Palgrave Macmillan, Chapter 15. This is one of the key texts on social policy, covering the basics on policy and how policies are made.

Baggott, R (2010) *Public Health Policy and Politics* (2nd edn). Oxford: Wiley Blackwell. This new edition discusses the contemporary debate surrounding public health, exploring the many facets of health improvement and promotion within their historical, socioeconomic and political contexts.

Cowley, S (ed.) (2008) *Community Public Health in Policy and Practice* (2nd edn). Edinburgh: Bailliere Tindall. The positive emphasis on developing and describing all services in relation to their purpose and client/user group is reflected in this second edition, emphasising a non-integrative mixture of disciplines and service focus rather than individual professions.

Key UK health policies and reports

The following provide an overview of the current and proposed organisation of healthcare and the policies that seek to ensure its continuance and improvement in all parts of the UK.

Scotland
Scottish Legislation since devolution: www.legislation.gov.uk/browse/Scotland.

Wales
Health Social Care and Well-being Strategy Guidance 2010: wales.gov. uk/consultations/healthsocialcare/hscandwbstrategyandcypplan/?lang=en.

England
Health and Social Care Bill 2010–2011: http://services.parliament.uk/ bills/2010-11/healthandsocialcare.html.

Northern Ireland
Health Improvement Plan (2008): www.northernifhpartners.co.uk/health_ improvement_plan.aspx?dataid=416412.

chapter 4

Communicating and Implementing Policy and Strategy to Improve Health and Wellbeing
Marcus Longley

Meeting the Public Health Competences

Core area 3: Policy and strategy development and implementation to improve population health and wellbeing

This chapter will help you to evidence the following competences for public health (Public Health Skills and Careers Framework):

- Level 5(a): Knowledge of the policies and strategies that affect the overall area in which one works;
- Level 5(b): Awareness of the complexity of the policy context and how policy is made;
- Level 7(f): Understanding of how to communicate and implement policy and strategy to improve the population's health and wellbeing;
- Level 7(1): Interpret and communicate local, regional and national policies and strategies within own area of work;
- Level 8(1): Interpret and apply local, regional and national policies and strategies.

This chapter will also assist you in demonstrating the following National Occupational Standard(s) for public health:

- PHP39: Present information and arguments to others on how policies affect health and wellbeing.

This chapter should also be useful in demonstrating Standard 10 of the Public Health Practitioner Standards:

Standard 10: Support the implementation of policies and strategies to improve health and wellbeing outcomes – demonstrating:

a. knowledge of the main public health policies and strategies relevant to own area of work and the organisations that are responsible for them;
b. how different policies, strategies and priorities affect own specific work and how to influence their development or implementation in own area of work;
c. critical reflection and constructive suggestions for how policies, strategies and priorities could be improved in terms of improving health and wellbeing and reducing health inequalities in own area of work.

Overview

This chapter looks at the different explanations for the difficulties of policy communication and implementation, both generally and in the context of public health and wellbeing, and at how 'implementation' and 'policy' are intimately interrelated. It explores different approaches to tackling these challenges, and looks at how devolution within the UK might change the picture. It considers the roles played by ideology, citizen engagement and the professions in making implementation more effective.

Introduction

'There's many a slip 'twixt cup and lip' could serve as a summary (albeit rather trite!) of this chapter: public health strategy often seems to disappoint when it comes to implementation. Why, and what can be done about it? What are the challenges of communicating and implementing such policy?

Evidence of implementation failure

This is partly a cup half full/cup half empty conundrum: how successful does the implementation of a policy have to be for it to be pronounced a success? It is also a cause/effect conundrum: how do we know whether success (or failure) is due to the policy, or its implementation?

The answer to the first is a matter of personal judgement. The answer to the second, as the next section will argue, is that policy versus implementation is a false dichotomy – they are intimately connected.

Both conundrums become clearer if we consider an example of the problem: reducing health inequalities. This is a complex and contested area, but consider the following facts (Strategic Review of Health Inequalities in England post-2010, 2010). Between 1971 and 2005, the gap in life expectancy by social class for both men and women has persisted, with some widening taking place in the 1980s and 1990s, despite determined attempts over prolonged periods to reduce them. More recently, a national health inequalities Public Service Agreement (PSA) target was set in 2001. Updated in 2004, it was supported by two more detailed objectives around infant mortality and life expectancy. The infant mortality target was, starting with children under one year, to reduce by at least 10 per cent the gap in mortality between the routine and manual occupation group and the population as a whole by 2010. The life expectancy target was, by 2010 (Marmot Review, 2010), to reduce by at least 10 per cent the gap between the fifth of areas with the worst health and deprivation indicators (the 'spearhead' group) and the population as a whole.

The next section considers some of the explanations for implementation failure, and the difficulty of separating 'policy' from its 'implementation'.

ACTIVITY 4.1

The data for the two targets show that the gaps in infant mortality and male and female life expectancy remain. The infant mortality gap reached a peak of 19 per cent in 2002–04 and narrowed slightly in each of the subsequent periods to 16 per cent in 2006–08. Is this a success or failure?

Comment

Based on these data, it looks rather like the latter. However, during both the periods discussed here, overall life expectancy for all social classes in England increased – it's just that the gap between them did not narrow.

If you take the cup-half-empty view, is this a failure of policy or of implementation? Again, different interpretations are possible. In an independent review of policy in different countries, one expert concluded that Britain was ahead of other countries in implementing policies to reduce health inequalities (Mackenbach, 2006). Some would argue that the policies were misconceived, in that they were targeting the wrong issues; others that greater and smarter effort was required to implement them better.

Different explanations for disappointment

In order to understand some of the complexity and challenge of communicating and implementing health and wellbeing strategy it is helpful to understand why it is that public policy and strategy *generally* seems to falter at the implementation stage. This section looks at the various approaches that scholars have taken to this problem.

It is useful to start by understanding the relationship between policy – as the formal expression of a government's intent – and three other factors: demand, supply and 'events'. First, *demand* for services – in our case, health and those elements of public provision that bear directly upon it – is to some extent an independent variable. In other words, it will vary independently of the others, as epidemiological, demographic and other factors change, and as people's expectations alter. Similarly, the *supply* of healthcare and other services relevant to wellbeing, including new technologies for diagnosis and treatment, and new understandings of the causes of disease, will alter in response to its own sets of dynamics. But both supply and demand also influence each other. For example, a treatment for a previously incurable disease stimulates a demand for that treatment; and demand for better diagnosis provides an incentive for more research and development, and eventually a new category of supply.

Policy seeks simultaneously to achieve a sustainable balance between supply and demand, and also to achieve its own objectives. Thus a government may wish to ensure that new technologies are introduced to meet public demand, while also pursuing a reduction in health inequalities.

Finally, there is the unpredictable. Prime Minister Harold Macmillan apparently once responded to a journalist's question about what kept him awake at night by replying: 'Events, dear boy, events' (Figure 4.1). This can affect supply, demand and policy, but particularly the latter.

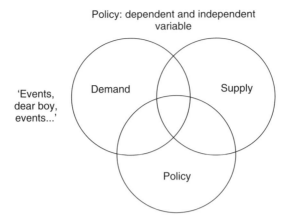

Figure 4.1 Policy: dependent and independent variable

The 'top down' approach

'Why is implementation so difficult?' was the title of a seminal article by Lewis A. Gunn as long ago as 1978. The answer starts to become clear when you consider how demanding are his ten pre-conditions for success in policy implementation (Gunn, 1978).

1. There are no crippling external circumstances.

2. Adequate time and resources are available.

3. The necessary resources are available as needed during implementation.

4. The policy is based on a valid theory of cause and effect.

5. Cause and effect are closely linked.

6. A single agency can control the whole programme, with minimal dependency on others.

7. Everyone involved agrees on the objectives.

8. It is possible to specify in advance who needs to do what, and when.

9. All those involve communicate and co-ordinate well throughout.

10. Those in authority can obtain obedience throughout.

This is, in a sense, the 'perfect type': a set of parameters that, although probably never realised in practice, at least highlights the important issues that need to be addressed if the intentions of the policy makers are to be realised. But the problem remains: if they can never be achieved, does that mean the implementation will always be characterised by various degrees of failure?

Gunn's exposition is an example of the 'top down' approach to policy implementation: getting everything in place so that those at the top can ensure that those at the bottom (and all those in between) do the right thing. During the 1980s, this approach to implementation began increasingly to be questioned. First, there was a general re-evaluation of the role of government, and how it should go about its job. Particularly in the UK and USA, economic austerity and an ideological shift in politics led to a new orthodoxy, which saw government not as a system of command and control but rather as a way of setting up a self-sustaining set of incentives and mechanisms that could be relied upon to deliver the goods. Typically, they adopted characteristics of the market, with the NHS, for example, seeing the emergence of quasi-markets, with GPs and others commissioning elements of care from other parts of the NHS. In this climate, Gunn's perfect model appears both unrealistic and undesirable. Thus, Osborne and Gaebler, for example, writing in the USA in the early 1990s (Osborne and Gaebler, 1992), were able to have great influence over the Clinton administration by arguing that government should be 'reinvented' based on a number of principles, including those listed below.

- Governments should steer more than they row.

- Policy making should be about empowering communities, rather than simply delivering services.

- Governments should encourage competition in the delivery of service rather than monopoly.

- Funding should be focused on outputs rather than inputs.

- The needs of the customer should be the priority, not those of the bureaucrats.

- Invest in prevention, rather than cures.

These principles would clearly still resonate with governments in the UK and USA today.

The 'bottom up' approach

What they also serve to do is highlight the fact that 'policy making' is not simply the act of the people at the top. 'Policy' is not just what it says in the official policy document; rather it is the result of the combination of the policy document and how it is implemented in practice: *Policy is being made as it is being administered and administered as it is being made* (Anderson, 1975, p98).

And therein lies the frustration of the politician who, like a demented railway signalman confidently pulling on his or her policy levers in the Ministry, finds at best that they are only weakly connected to the signals, and at worst, end in a broken wire!

The top-down approach of Gunn and others was challenged by a variety of analysts who instead focused on a 'bottom up' approach to policy making, very much building on Anderson's insight that policy is in part made by those who administer it. Perhaps the most famous formulation of this approach is in the concept of the *street-level bureaucrat*, coined by Michael Lipsky (1971). He described how doctors, teachers, social workers, welfare clerks and others at the 'front line' of public services shape what policy becomes in a process of negotiation and consensus building, which reconciles their own organisational and professional cultures with the political context in which they work. In reality, what a doctor or social worker does in the privacy of their interaction with a patient or client can only ever be shaped in part by what government tells them to do; the rest will come from factors such as their own education, culture, professional mores and personality, and from what the client demands.

Understanding how to achieve policy goals, therefore, requires a process of *backward mapping* (Elmore, 1979), taking full account of the human factors that will shape implementation. Thus the question should not be how best to pass the message clearly down the chain of command and address the other concerns of Gunn and the 'top down' advocates; rather it should be how to encourage and enable the street-level bureaucrat to behave in ways conducive to the overall policy aims.

Further complications

While the 'top down' approach now seems rather naive, one might also worry that an exclusive focus on the 'bottom up' is also a little limited. Other scholars have highlighted different factors in implementation that further complicate the picture.

One concerns the games people play. At all stages in the implementation process, and at all levels in the hierarchy, there are groups of people with particular perspectives and agendas, all trying their best to maximise their influence on the outcome in order to advance what they believe in. Implementation, therefore, becomes a game of *bargaining, persuasion, and manoeuvring under conditions of uncertainty* (Bardach, 1977, p56).

Another highlights the *inherent* complexity of policy implementation (Lewis and Flynn, 1979). A whole series of factors make the command-and-control model all but impossible, including:

- disagreement about policy objectives and their respective priorities;

- ambiguity and uncertainty about processes and outcomes;

- procedural complexity;

- insufficient power to address some aspects;

- challenge from service users/recipients.

Finally, many of these considerations need to be seen in the context of the 'culture' of the organisation. This is a notoriously slippery concept, but Charles Handy has helpfully defined four types of culture, which turn organisations into coherent tribes, with their own values, private languages, tales and heroes (Handy, 1985). He gives each its patron god as follows.

- Power culture: decisions are the outcome of power and influence. Patron god: Zeus, who rules by impulse and whim.

- Role culture: decisions come from rationality. Patron god: Apollo, god of reason.

- Task culture: the priority is to 'get things done'; efficient, responsive to consumers. Handy believes it has no patron god.

- Person culture: individuals dominate structure and organisation. Patron god: Dionysus.

Towards a solution

Managing the way to a solution

Each of these perspectives is helpful in highlighting different aspects of the 'implementation problem'. But what to do about it?

Public services in the UK and USA have, since the 1970s, started to explore whether the tools in the management toolkit might help. In the NHS, the determination to break with the ways of consensus and really get to grips with independent-minded street-level bureaucrats through general management came in the early 1980s, when Roy Griffiths delivered a 24-page blueprint for the future (NHS Management Inquiry, 1983), from which the NHS has not looked back (Harrison and McDonald, 2008).

This 'managerialism' has operated on a variety of levels. At its most specific, a variety of managerial techniques have been imported into the NHS, ranging from project management techniques such as PRINCE, to personnel management approaches such as individual performance review and job planning. At a system level, successive governments have sought to apply Osborne and Gaebler's advice to put the needs of the customer first, and to encourage a diversity of suppliers – although these aspects have been interpreted differently in the different countries of the UK (Greer, 2004b).

A lot of thought has also gone into the management of inter-agency relationships. The top-down school rightly identified the difficulties for implementation posed by having more than one agency involved, but this is often unavoidable in health and wellbeing. Work has focused on:

- the macro level – for example, ensuring clarity and consistency of policy across departments;

- the meso level – for example, providing specific mechanisms (such as joint funding) that brings agencies together for mutual benefit; and

- the micro – for example, co-locating staff from different agencies.

A synthesis

It should not be surprising, of course, that there is no one simple answer to the problem of implementation: why should one expect something so complex to have a single solution? As so often in the social sciences, progress depends upon better understanding and intelligent synthesis. In terms of understanding, Gareth Morgan offers a very helpful set of 'metaphors', each of which offers a different and complementary insight into implementation failure (Morgan, 1986) (Figure 4.2).

In terms of positive steps to improve implementation, one useful synthesis of the insights of the top-down and the bottom-up approaches was developed by Sabatier in the 1980s (Sabatier, 1986), and has stood the test of time. It posits six sufficient and necessary conditions for successful implementation:

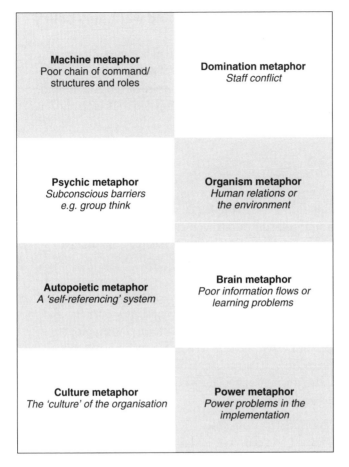

Figure 4.2 Implementation failure

Source: adapted from Morgan (1986)

1. clear and consistent objectives;

2. adequate causal theory;

3. legal structures that require joint working by agencies, and with recipients;

4. committed and skilful implementers;

5. support of interest groups, the legislature and executive;

6. stability in the external socio-political-economic environment.

ACTIVITY 4.2

Choose a policy implemented by your organisation and evaluate its success or failure using the six conditions identified by Sabatier.

Particular problems in implementing health and wellbeing policy

Each of the issues identified so far in this chapter bears upon policy and strategy for health and wellbeing just as much as they do on other areas of public policy. The same approaches to their resolution (or at least minimisation) will also be relevant. In addition, there are other issues which are more particular to health and wellbeing, and it is to these that we now turn.

Ideology

One of Sabatier's pre-conditions for successful implementation was a set of clear and consistent objectives. Health and wellbeing can struggle even to cross this hurdle. Three of the most obvious sets of objectives are ruled out by ideology, as outlined below.

1. No major redistribution of wealth: it now seems fairly clear that more equal societies tend to enjoy better health and wellbeing than less equal ones. But none of the major political parties in the UK with a chance of national power is proposing major wealth redistribution. Despite the fact that greater equality has the potential to benefit *everyone* in society – so the message is not necessarily as divisive as the rich vs poor polarisations of previous politics – nevertheless the scale of the change should not be underestimated.

2. Minimal role for fiscal measures: for many years, UK governments have been reluctant to use fiscal measures in a consistent and determined attempt to shift the determinants of ill health. In some areas – such as tobacco – taxation has been an effective part of the armoury, but governments have been reluctant to penalise or incentivise other aspects of life that might affect, for example, obesity, oral health or physical activity. In general, health is not regarded as a legitimate prime objective of tax policy, especially in times of fiscal austerity. This latter demonstrates the sixth of Sabatier's conditions: the need for stability in the external environment.

3. Little appetite for direct intervention in people's lives: there is a general aversion to what is derogatively branded the 'nanny state', and individual autonomy is regarded as more precious than effective health promotion. In fact, many argue that direct intervention simply does not work.

An interesting trilogy of publications emerged from the English Department of Health in early 2010, which summarises the consensus in the policy-making elite about what implementation can mean. These define the boundaries of what governments can and cannot do, on both ideological and practical grounds. While they do not officially constitute government policy, nevertheless they were commissioned and published by a government department, and are clearly consonant with the views of ministers. They also fit quite comfortably with the pronouncements of politicians of the other two major parties in England.

The first addresses what *should* be the role of the state, from an ideological perspective (Reeves, 2010). Given the potential repressiveness and clumsiness of the state trying to change people's behaviour, it suggests three key questions to be answered before the state seeks to influence health and wellbeing.

1. Legitimacy – is there really no alternative to the state becoming involved? State intervention is a last, not a first, resort.

2. Autonomy – does what is proposed support individual autonomy, or the reverse? If the latter, it probably should not be adopted.

3. Effectiveness – is there good reason to believe that it will work? Too many policies are implemented more in hope than realistic expectation.

In general, the *tone* of government intervention in health and wellbeing needs to emphasise informed choice and individual capacity.

The second (Mulgan, 2010) argues that implementation should emphasise the benefits of change for the individual and community, echoing the influential work by Thaler and Sunstein (2008), rather than the negative consequences of no change, and recognise that hard incentives may be needed. Thus it praises a scheme that offers financial rewards to pregnant women who gave up smoking. It also points out the importance of all the relevant arms of government acting together to achieve health objectives, and cites good examples of the work of the Food Standards Agency on food labelling and the efforts of HM Revenue & Customs to combat tobacco smuggling. However, it also points out the paucity of evidence on what actually works.

ACTIVITY 4.3

Look at some locally initiated schemes in your area of work or organisation, and explore if they have been a success or failure and why. Interpret any relevant research that supports your findings.

The final publication, by an eminent trio from local government, public health and the NHS (Bernstein *et al.*, 2010), argues that the overall goals of public health policy need to shift fundamentally from extending life to improving the quality of life and increasing disability-free years, and measuring success in these terms. They recommend various changes to the mechanisms of policy delivery, including:

- better cross-government working;
- local consistency in goals, and a unified inspection regime;
- a renewed vision for general practice, emphasising its public health role;
- more integration of the workforce for children's health and wellbeing.

The theme of greater integration – nationally and locally – echoes one of Mulgan's concerns.

The issue of health inequalities remains the ultimate challenge for all of these nostra. It remains stubbornly resistant to government policy, is quintessentially cross-agency and challenges many ideological sacred cows. Wilkinson and Pickett (2010), in their plea for a fundamental shift in thinking about the impact of inequality on health, point out that the problem really does lie with the 'how?' implementation:

> *Everyone will agree that a good society would have fewer of all the health and social problems ... The argument is therefore about solutions.*
>
> (Wilkinson and Pickett, 2010, p248)

Given politicians' refusal to use some of the measures set out here, their plea for a new politics is by no means an easy panacea:

> *Political will is dependent on the development of a vision of a better society which is both achievable and inspiring ... The task is now to develop a politics based on a recognition of the kind of society we need to create and committed to making use of the institutional and technological opportunities to realise it.*
>
> (Wilkinson and Pickett, 2010, p271)

Co-ordination of effort

There has been some progress against Sabatier's requirement for a legal injunction on agencies to work together for health. In each country of the UK, both legislative and policy imperatives have encouraged the NHS, local government and others to develop joint plans, share resources and consider the impact of their actions on each other. But there is still a long way to go here, especially while different funding and charging regimes, different governance arrangements and long histories of separation are all pushing in the opposite direction.

Engaging with citizens

Sabatier points out the importance of implementation engaging with recipients. This is especially the case with health and wellbeing, but here the term 'recipients' is far too passive. Central to the notion of improving people's health is the concept of *co-production* – professionals, agencies and others working in partnership with lay people to effect sustainable change jointly:

> *... delivering public services in an equal and reciprocal relationship between professionals, people using services, their families and their neighbours. Where activities are co-produced in this way, both services and neighbourhoods become far more effective agents of change.*
>
> (Boyle and Harris, 2009, p1)

The implementation challenges here are significant (Needham and Carr, 2009). Rather than offering an off-the-shelf model, it:

- challenges existing service models and delivery patterns;
- questions assumptions of users as the passive consumers rather than the active producers of care;
- supports collective rather than primarily one-to-one service relationships;
- demands renegotiation and restructuring of relationships between people who use services and professionals, which in turn requires the empowerment of both parties;
- recognises that working with people is an iterative and negotiated process, not a simple delivery chain from government to the front room; the concept can be combined with various forms of user involvement and service redesign, so long as there is a commitment to power sharing, an active and productive role for the user, and a recognition of the importance of collaborative relationships in delivering service outcomes.

These are all challenges within the 'provider' side. Another challenge comes directly from the putative recipient: scepticism about much that they hear from the professionals and politicians, and a challenge to the veracity of their health messages.

In part, this is one aspect of a much wider change in society, characterised variously as 'post-', 'late-' or 'reflexive-modernity' (see, for example, Beck, 1992; Beck *et al.*, 1994), in which people have very different perspectives on external authority. At a mundane level, this might translate into greater scepticism about simple 'do' and 'don't' health promotion messages, and a more complex personal calculus of risks and benefits.

More specifically, it is a product of a general challenging of professional dominance, in health and in other aspects of life. For many years – about a century and a half in the case of medicine – professional power has been accumulating, buttressed at various points by statutory protection. It has accumulated at three levels (Figure 4.3). Government, with doctors and others influencing policy, directly and indirectly; institutional (embodied, for example, in the post of Medical Director in Trusts); and at the one-to-one interaction with patients (for example, the doctor has to approve the prescription). It all rested on two planks: an acceptance that doctors (and other professionals) had a unique *competence*, a body of knowledge which meant that no outsider could regulate them; and that we could have *confidence* in the fact that doctors could be generally trusted to exercise their autonomy in the interests of their patients. But over the last decade or two this has been gradually eaten away from below, as scandals such as the Bristol babies' heart surgery disaster and others have suggested that both planks may be rotten. This has resonated with patients, governments and many professionals, and been amplified by the media, lawyers and politicians.

The causal theories in health and wellbeing are often contested. The medical model still exercises considerable hegemony, both in the expressed and implicit policy of the NHS, and also in the minds of citizens. Thus the vast majority of 'health'

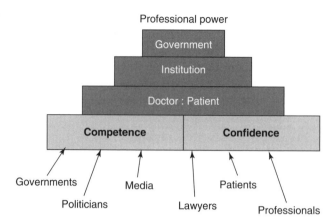

Figure 4.3 Dominance of the medical model

investment is channelled into the conventional approaches of healthcare, with very little left for the development of social infrastructure, or for the effective support of patient empowerment or co-production.

While patients – as we have seen above – increasingly express their doubts about the efficacy of such approaches (and vote with their own wallets by, for example, purchasing complementary therapies of various sorts), most popular pressure on the health service is directed at *more* conventional therapy – the latest drugs, technological interventions – rather than less. In such a climate it is difficult to generate enthusiasm for a different approach to health and (especially) wellbeing. In Sabatier's terms, there is little support for a different approach among interest groups or the legislature.

The future: devolution and diversity

The devolution of responsibility for health policy to the nations of the UK is a process not an event: we are seeing a gradual working-out of the consequences of the statutory settlement of 1999, and subsequent constitutional changes. Further changes will probably result from the recent shift in the political orientation of the Westminster government, from the impact of public-sector spending cuts, and from the ongoing process of 'learning by doing', as differences in policy and approach in turn lead to further changes. The four nations will share at least three key factors in common:

1. similar demography and epidemiology;

2. the ideological and structural dominance of the medical model in much of the public health discourse;

3. fiscal pressures.

But, in other respects, the gaps between the nations in the implementation of public health policy will continue to widen:

- ideology, with left-of-centre politics in Scotland and Wales, and right-of-centre in England, challenging the consensus described earlier;

- different legislation;

- local experimentation will in turn stimulate other new approaches;

- influence of enthusiastic and visionary public health professionals and alliances, which can be particularly influential in the smaller nations.

Chapter 4 summary

Communicating and implementing policy is challenging, for a variety of structural, ideological, cultural and historical reasons, and public health and wellbeing has these problems in spades. This chapter has considered the different explanations for the difficulties of policy implementation, both generally and in the context of public health and wellbeing, and how 'implementation' and 'policy' are intimately interrelated. Various different approaches to tackling these challenges have been tried over the years. For the future, key influences will include ideology, citizen engagement and the contribution of the health professions, and devolution is likely to crystallise four rather different contexts in which these elements play themselves out.

GOING FURTHER

A ladder of citizen participation. Online at: www.lithgow-schmidt.dk/sherry-arn-stein/ladder-of-citizen-participation.html. Originally published as Arnstein, SR (1969) A ladder of citizen participation, *Journal of the American Institute of Planners*, 35(4), July: 216–24. *This article demonstrates how power structures in society interact, showing who actually has power when important decisions are being made.*

Harrison, S and McDonald, R (2008) *The Politics of Healthcare in Britain*. London: Sage. *This book provides a clear and considered overview of the politics of healthcare in Britain, combining theory, historical detail and analysis of contemporary events.*

Hunter, DJ (2003) *Public Health Policy*. Cambridge: Polity Press. *An analysis of the links of policy to the history and weaknesses of the public health profession, with suggested solutions for management and public health, which shift the focus to health.*

Parsons, W (1996) *Public Policy: An Introduction to the Theory and Practice of Policy Analysis*. Cheltenham: Edward Elgar Publishing. *A comprehensive review of the vast and varied literature on public policy, presenting a wide range of arguments and theories.*

chapter 5

Developing a Strategy for Implementation of Policy

Yvette Cox

Meeting the Public Health Competences

Core area 3: Policy and strategy development and implementation to improve population health and wellbeing

This chapter will help you to evidence the following competences for public health (Public Health Skills and Careers Framework):

- Level 6(e): Knowledge of tools used in strategic decision-making and planning;
- Level 7(a): Understanding of various methods to assess the impact of policies on health and wellbeing;
- Level 7(c): Understanding of the variety of tools that can be used to aid strategic decision-making and planning;
- Level 8(b): Understanding of the strategic context of policy development;
- Level 5(3): Contribute to development of specific policies and strategies;
- Level 6(3): Appraise draft policies and strategies and recommend changes to improve their development.

This chapter will also assist you in demonstrating the following National Occupational Standard(s) for public health:

- PHP15: Implement strategies for putting policies to improve health and wellbeing into effect;
- PHP39: Present information and arguments to others on how how policies affect health and wellbeing.

This chapter should also be useful in demonstrating Standard 10 of the Public Health Practitioner Standards:

Standard 10: Support the implementation of policies and strategies to improve health and wellbeing outcomes – demonstrating:

a. knowledge of the main public health policies and strategies relevant to own area of work and the organisations that are responsible for them;
b. how different policies, strategies and priorities affect own specific work and how to influence their development or implementation in own area of work;
c. critical reflection and constructive suggestions for how policies, strategies and priorities could be improved in terms of improving health and wellbeing and reducing health inequalities in own area of work.

Overview

This chapter will provide practical guidance on how to develop local strategies aimed at achieving policies for improving health and wellbeing. The key stages of strategy development will be explored and the chapter will help you to develop your thinking about strategic management, and in particular strategies to improve the services you are involved in delivering.

Introduction

Health and social care in the UK is funded publicly via taxation and it is therefore the responsibility of the government to establish policies that guide the way in which it operates and the services that are provided (Capon, 2008). Policy making is described as *the process by which governments translate their political vision into programmes and actions to deliver 'outcomes' – desired changes in the real world* (Moran *et al.*, 2006, p153).

Hunter (2003) suggests that health policy has two elements: the first is *health care policy*, which focuses on the issues of financing and providing healthcare services; the second is *policy for health*, which concentrates on improving the health of the population. When defining a strategy for a department or publicly funded organisation, the strategist has to take into account the policies laid down by the government of the day (Rowe 2002). The term 'strategy' means:

> . . . the direction [and] scope of an organisation over the long term, which achieves advantage in a changing environment through its configuration of resources [and] competences with the aim of fulfilling stakeholder expectations.
>
> (Johnson *et al.*, 2006, p9)

The strategic management process

Strategic management is a process that establishes what services an organisation will provide and how these will be delivered. The strategy enables engagement with current challenges and prepares the organisation for the future (Johnson *et al.*, 2006). Strategic management transforms ideas (or policies) into reality, and determines the ultimate success or failure of an organisation. Figure 5.1 outlines the stages involved in the strategic management process.

Public health and wellbeing strategies need to ensure that available resources are used effectively in the delivery of the service (Cox and Rawlinson, 2008). The current emphasis tends to be on achieving governmental policies while at the same time improving efficiency in order to develop or retain services on a limited budget (Johnson *et al.*, 2006).

There are a lot of factors that need to be considered when developing a strategy. For example:

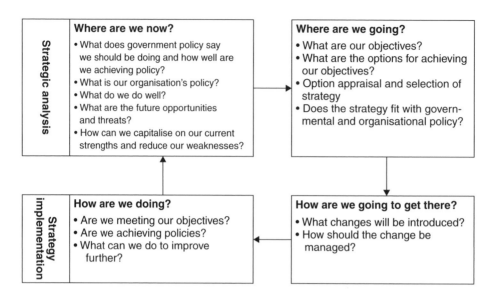

Figure 5.1 The strategic management process

- the organisation's objectives and local policies, and how these relate to policies set by government for public health and wellbeing;

- the scope of the services provided, e.g. what and where services will be provided, and which services will not be offered; these decisions define the boundaries for the organisation;

- the needs of the population served by the organisation, and how best to satisfy those needs;

- availability of resources to meet the changing needs of the population (Cox and Rawlinson, 2008); this may include identification of resources that can be redeployed;

- opportunities that exist to build on organisational competencies and gain competitive advantage over other service providers;

- the values and expectations of powerful stakeholders, as these will influence the type of strategy that would be supported or rejected.

The remainder of this chapter will focus on the first two stages of the strategic management process: strategic analysis of the present situation (Where are we now?), and identification of options leading to the selection of a strategy for achieving government policy and improving current service delivery (Where are we going?). Chapter 4 looks at how to communicate and implement strategy (How are we going to get there?).

ACTIVITY 5.1

As this chapter aims to help you to develop a strategy to improve services within your area of work, specifically to develop a strategy that is in line with governmental policy, it is recommended that you identify an aspect of your service to use as a case study while you read this chapter. Use the following as a guide.

- Briefly describe your organisation in terms of:
  - the nature of its business;
  - the services it delivers;
  - the key recipients of the service.
- Identify other organisations in your area that deliver similar services and with which you may be competing.
- What is the main objective of your organisation (you may find it helpful to refer to your organisation's mission or vision statement)?
- What is the main objective of your part of the service?
- Do you think the services you are involved in delivering are meeting the needs of the consumers and could be called successful?
- What evidence do you have to support your view (e.g. feedback, achieving targets, delivering services within budget)?
- Identify **one** part of the service that is not being delivered effectively on which to focus. What are the key policies that have to be taken into consideration when delivering this part of the service?

Comment

If you could answer all of the questions above from your existing knowledge, then you have selected an appropriate service to focus your thinking on. If you were unable to answer some of the questions, identify how easy it is to access the information and make a judgement on its suitability as an area to use as a case study.

Analysing the current situation: Where are we now?

All too often, busy managers make decisions about changes to be introduced in order to achieve policy drivers or improve services, without first analysing the current situation. A thorough analysis will enable the manager to identify strengths in the way services are delivered now that can be built upon and weaknesses that need to be addressed. In addition, the analysis will ensure that all relevant factors that need to be taken into account (e.g. national or local policies, the needs of service users) are considered. Hence, a good analysis should enable the manager to set aside preconceived ideas and develop sound strategies for the future. Jenkins and Ambrosini (2002) recommend that, when analysing the current situation, three core levels of the strategic environment should be scrutinised. These are outlined in Table 5.1.

Table 5.1 Three core levels of strategic analysis

Level of strategic analysis	Examples
External environmental analysis	Governmental policies Regulatory influences Competing organisations
Organisational analysis	Organisational policies Current processes Use made of physical resources Current structure and culture Financial issues Stakeholder and client satisfaction
Individual analysis	Capability of staff Training needs Culture/willingness to change

There are a number of models/tools described within the strategic management literature that can assist with analysing the current situation, and it is recommended that several are used as each provides a different perspective and so enables the user to gain a more thorough view of the current situation. The models/tools that will be described in this chapter include:

- PESTLE;

- SWOT;

- combined PESTLE/SWOT;

- adaptation of Porter's (1980) five forces framework;

- adapted public-sector BCG matrix.

Prior to starting to analyse the current situation, it is vital that the scope of the analysis is clearly defined – for instance, an analysis of how a whole organisation or department functions will give a very different perspective to a more specific analysis of just one aspect of the service being delivered (Sheffield Hallam University, 2010).

PESTLE analysis

PESTLE (political, economic, social, technological, legal and environmental) analysis identifies external environmental factors that are having an impact upon the service and the way in which it is being delivered. PESTLE analysis may also be referred to as PEST (political, economic, social, technological); STEEP (social, technological, environmental, economic, political); or STEP (social, technological, economic, political), depending on the elements that are being reviewed using this tool.

Within publicly funded organisations, this analysis is important because, among other things, the user is encouraged to consider how well the service is achieving current policy, and how economic factors impact upon delivery of cost-effective services. While the tool is useful, it can lead to a long list of all the influencing factors. In order to maximise its usefulness, the focus should be on the current *key* factors that are likely to have an impact on the service. In addition, the combined effect of any of the factors on the service should be examined, as these will have more of an impact than would individual factors (Johnson *et al.*, 2006).

Table 5.2 provides an illustration of some of the factors to consider when undertaking a PESTLE analysis (it is not an exhaustive list). PESTLE is widely acknowledged as a useful tool for analysing the external environment, however in Table 5.2 the PESTLE has been adapted and combined with the first two levels of strategic analysis proposed by Jenkins and Ambrosini (2002) (external environmental and organisational analysis). This model acknowledges the fact that political, economic, social, technological, legal and environmental factors impact on services in different ways if they are part of the external environment as opposed to the internal environment. For instance, the governmental policies indicate *what* the organisation should be doing, but organisational policy will influence *what* and *how* services are delivered.

Table 5.2 Example questions to ask when undertaking a PESTLE analysis

	External environmental analysis	*Organisational/individual analysis*
Political	What are the **key** policies saying we should be doing in relation to the service (worldwide/European/national/Department of Health policies? Is governmental policy stable or subject to change? How does the current political agenda impact on this service?	What are the **key** organisational policies saying we should be doing in relation to the service? How does the current organisation strategy impact upon this service? Does this service fit with the organisation's mission statement?
Economic	How are national funding policies impacting on this service? Has funding been specifically earmarked for this service? How are interest rates/inflation/petrol prices etc. impacting upon the service? Do factors such as unemployment have an impact on this service? Is there a correlation between level of income and the needs of the local population?	How is local funding impacting on this service? Is there any other local source of funding for this service? Are the local costs of energy, transport, communication and raw materials impacting on this service?
Social	What are the expectations of society that impact on how services	Are we able to satisfy the needs of the local population via this service?

are delivered currently?
What are the needs of our local population in relation to this service?
Is there a high local demand for this service?
Are the consumers of our service demanding changes to the way in which it is being delivered, e.g. access to GPs in the evenings/at weekends?
Are the public well educated/informed regarding health matters?

How do the social needs of staff impact upon this service (lone working/European working hour directive/equal opportunities legislation etc.)?
Is there a good work/leisure balance for all our staff?

Technological

Is there government or EU investment in technology to support this service, e.g. IT?
Is there any national research into aspects of this service?
Is there new technology being developed that would improve service delivery?

Is there local investment in technology to support this service, e.g. IT?
Is there any local research into aspects of this service?
What is the local policy in relation to introducing new technology to enhance services?
Is our current technology adequate or becoming obsolete?
Are all staff able to use the available technology?

Legal

Is our service adhering to legislation such as health and safety/employment law in delivery of the service?
How does professional regulation impact upon this service?

Are the managers of the service enabling staff to adhere to their professional codes of conduct?
Is there a possibility of litigation because the service is not meeting current needs?

Environmental

Who are our competitors and how good are they at delivering their services?
Are there any environmental laws that we need to address, e.g. disposal of clinical waste?
Are there any major health issues likely to impact on the service, e.g. pandemic flu?

What are we doing that differentiates our services from those of our competitors?
What is our current energy consumption and can it be reduced?
Are the estates and facilities fit for purpose?

ACTIVITY 5.2

Try to undertake a PESTLE analysis for the part of the service you are focusing on.

First of all, undertake the PESTLE analysis based on the knowledge you currently have about the service. Then review each of the PESTLE headings and identify where you may seek further information to assist you to analyse in more depth, e.g. policies, other staff, service users, contacting other organisations.

Comment

When analysing your service it is better to seek a number of different sources of information rather than rely on one source. Try to find a number of sources that are all saying the same thing, as this triangulation of information will lend more credence to your analysis.

SWOT analysis

PESTLE is a useful tool to assist with understanding the wider issues impacting on the service and also for predicting changes that may have an impact in the future. However, this tool does not enable thorough analysis of the strengths, weaknesses, opportunities and threats (SWOT) of the service.

SWOT focuses on the three levels of strategic analysis (external, organisational or individual). This enables a picture to be developed of:

- how well the service is being provided in relation to other providers;

- how internal processes help or hinder delivery of the service;

- the threats associated with poor delivery of service in terms of the impact on competing organisations, the organisation and individual staff.

For instance, there may be opportunities to improve the way services are delivered or to expand or take over services from a competing organisation. Figure 5.2 provides an illustration of the types of questions that may be asked when undertaking a SWOT analysis.

Strengths	Weaknesses
How good are our internal processes for delivery of the service? How good are we at keeping staff informed? Are we making the best use of our resources, e.g. staff / buildings / IT / equipment? How satisfied are the consumers of our service? How well are financial targets being met?	What are the weaknesses in relation to: • current processes, e.g. bottlenecks • provision of information • utilisation of current resources • consumer satisfaction, e.g. unmet needs • overspending / budget cuts, etc.?
Opportunities	**Threats**
What are the opportunities for: • improving processes • improving information to staff • improving utilisation of resources • improving consumer satisfaction • improving cost effectiveness?	What threats may impact on our services: • recruitment issues • competition from other service providers • funding cuts • change of government?

Figure 5.2 SWOT analysis

ACTIVITY 5.3

Undertake a SWOT analysis for your service based on your current understanding of the service. Identify other sources of information and test your understanding of the current situation with other staff.

What are the *key* factors currently impacting on your service?

Comment

There is a danger that the SWOT analysis may be too general or superficial, and it can generate long lists that make it difficult to identify the important factors. It is important to focus the analysis on the particular service or issue and to identify the *key* factors that have an impact.

SWOT/PESTLE analysis

In practice, a SWOT analysis is often undertaken without regard to the PESTLE. However, combining the PESTLE with the SWOT provides a different perspective as it makes the user examine the strengths, weaknesses, opportunities and threats in relation to the *key* PESTLE elements. In addition, it should help to identify the extent to which the service is capable of meeting the challenges posed. For example, the PESTLE analysis should have identified relevant policies, and the combined SWOT/PESTLE enables the user to consider how well these policies are being achieved or what the weaknesses are in relation to meeting the political agenda.

The tool also assists with the identification of options that will enable the service to better achieve the political agenda and overcome weaknesses. In addition, the current threats to the service can be identified – these can be used at a later date to strengthen the argument for the need to change the way services are delivered. Table 5.3 provides an example SWOT/PESTLE; again the questions are not exhaustive and are designed to get you thinking along the right lines.

Table 5.3 Combined SWOT/PESTLE

	Strengths	*Weaknesses*	*Opportunities*	*Threats*
Political	How well are we achieving the political agenda/what do we do well in relation to current policy?	What aspects of the political agenda are we not achieving well?	How can we improve services so they achieve the political agenda?	What are the current threats associated with the political agenda?
Economic	How good are we at providing value for money? What are the strengths in relation to current funding/budgeting?	Where are resources being wasted/under-utilised?	How can we reduce costs/increase productivity? Are there any sources of funding we are not tapping into?	What are the consequences if we do not make better use of our current resources?
Social	How well are we satisfying the needs of our stakeholders? Are we providing the right services to meet the needs of our users?	Which aspects of the service are not meeting the needs of our stakeholders?	How can we improve our services to meet the needs of our stakeholders?	What are the consequences if we do not change the way we currently deliver our service?
Technological	How are we making the best use of available technology in providing our service?	Is there any technology that is not being used to the maximum in support of our service?	What technological advances could we use to enhance our service?	What are the likely consequences if we do not embrace and utilise technology to the full?

Legal	How good are we at adhering to legislation and professional standards?	What aspects of legislation/ professional standards are we not achieving well?	What do we need to improve in order to ensure we adhere to legislation/ professional standards?	What are the likely consequences if we do not change?
Environmental	How good are we in comparison to our competitors?	What do our competitors do better than us?	How can we ensure our services are better than those of our competitors?	What are the consequences if we do not ensure we are as good as or better than our competitors?

So far, this chapter has presented three tools to help you analyse the factors that influence/need to be taken account of when developing a strategy. The focus on PES-TLE is deliberate because this tool makes the user consider the political agenda that is central to managing in health and social care within the UK. However, there are other issues that must also be taken into consideration, such as the factors within the environment that impact on how good you are at delivering services in comparison with other providers.

ACTIVITY 5.4

Examine the strengths, weaknesses, opportunities and threats associated with each of the key elements identified via the PESTLE undertaken in Activity 5.2. Check your understanding of the current situation with other members of staff.

Comment

When using the tool, try to avoid looking for opposites, e.g. an opportunity may be identified and then the threat is seen as that opportunity not being taken up. This is not a threat, as threats are things that exist in the present. Instead it is a risk – something that may or may not occur in the future (Northumbria University, 2009). It is important to focus the analysis on the *current* situation.

Five forces framework

Porter (1980) developed the 'five forces framework' to enable managers to assess the factors influencing competition and the potential success of different organisa-tions. The notion of competition within public sector organisations was unfamiliar

Table 5.4 Adaptation of Porter's (1980) five forces framework

Porter's (1980) five forces	*Public service adaptation (Cox and Fenech, 2010)*
Threat of new entrants:	Other providers offering or planning to offer the services that your organisation has traditionally provided
Bargaining power of buyers:	**Purchaser choice (demand)** This includes factors that influence whether clients will be referred to your services, e.g. • reputation • waiting times for treatment • quality of care • added value • preference for venue
Bargaining power of suppliers:	**The costs involved in supply of services, e.g.:** • costs of equipment • recruitment and retention • resources matching demand • political priorities • budget restraints
Threat of substitute products:	Services being offered that can achieve the same outcome via different means
Competitive rivalry:	Cost-effective high-quality services

until governmental policies in 1989–97 and post-2002 were aimed at making providers more responsive by developing competition within the NHS via the internal or 'quasi' market. The overall intention was to improve cost effectiveness, quality, efficiency and innovation (Brereton and Vasoodaven, 2010). The concept of providing high-quality and cost-effective services is seen as increasingly important (DoH, 2008c), and providers of these services are more likely to receive referrals and hence take business away from other providers.

Cox and Fenech (2010) have adapted Porter's (1980) five forces to enable an analysis of the factors that influence health and social services' ability to provide cost-effective high-quality services. The framework also enables managers to:

- consider why clients may be referred to their service as opposed to another service;

- assess other providers of services who may be able to take referrals away, or provide substitute services.

Each of the forces will now be explored in more depth.

Threat of other providers offering the same services

Other neighbouring health and social care providers or the private sector may be competing by providing (or planning to provide) the same services as your organisation. An example of a competitive service development is a GP practice that offers a 'commuter service' from 7–10 p.m. one night a week to improve access for those people that work away from home. This may be an attractive option for some patients, who then choose to move to that GP practice.

There are some aspects, as noted below, that make it more difficult for others to establish services and take business away from the traditional supplier.

- Set-up costs may be prohibitive, especially if there is a need to purchase lots of expensive equipment.

- Capital investment may be required, commercial organisations may finance the capital costs from profits from other parts of the organisation, but this option may not be available to NHS organisations or local government.

- There may be penalties if purchasers want to switch to a different provider (switching costs), so purchasers may prefer to remain with the existing service provider until the end of the current contract.

- Established and successful working relationships between purchasers and providers make it more difficult for another service provider to get referrals.

- The experience and expertise of existing suppliers can result in better outcomes and more cost-effective provision of the service. This makes it harder for inexperienced newcomers to compete.

Threat of alternative (substitute) services

Alternative services reduce demand (or referrals) to existing services and can even lead to that service becoming obsolete if the alternative service provides a higher benefit or better value for money (Thompson, 2001).

Examples of substitutions may be:

- offering exactly the same service, but in a different way or at a lower cost, e.g. mobile breast screening versus outpatient breast screening clinic;

- replacing an existing service with another service, e.g. providing homeopathic medicine/alternative therapies instead of conventional medicine/therapy;

- developing new ways of delivering a service that make existing practices redundant, e.g. computerised records reducing the need for records departments.

Costs involved in supplying services

Purchasers demand value for money, and decisions regarding where to purchase services will include considerations of the cost. There are a number of factors that can directly impact on how costly it is to provide a service.

- The costs of purchasing materials and supplies will directly affect the cost of providing a service. If there are a number of suppliers of the same product they will be more likely to compete against one another by reducing prices in order to gain business. However, if a supplier produces a unique product that is essential to the service, then it can charge more for it, hence driving up the cost of provision.

- Concentration of buyers: health and social care providers may club together in order to benefit from bulk purchasing of supplies and therefore drive down the costs of their provision.

- Costs of switching suppliers: contractual arrangements may make it difficult for providers to purchase goods more cheaply elsewhere without incurring penalties from their normal supplier.

- Ability to recruit and retain staff: suitably qualified and experienced staff are more likely to provide high-quality services. If a particular expertise is in short supply it may be necessary to offer incentives in order to recruit and retain the appropriate staff.

- Budgetary restraints and cost-saving measures are aimed at reducing the costs involved in the delivery of services and may result in innovative ways of providing the service more cost effectively.

- Demand exceeding capacity to provide the service: in health and social care, demand is affected by things that are not in the direct control of either the purchaser or provider, e.g. emergency admissions resulting in a lack of space for booked admissions. In order to meet contractual obligations and avoid penalties it may be necessary to create more capacity, e.g. open closed ward areas, with the associated cost implications. Only through monitoring trends can managers make plans to accommodate demand for services.

- High fixed costs: if the fixed costs (e.g. for buildings) are high it makes it more difficult for service providers to reduce the costs associated with delivering the service.

- Political priorities can sometimes result in providers having to supply services without funding to support the provision. In order to achieve this, costs have to be spread across other services.

Purchaser choice (demand)

Purchasers have an influence on the quality and cost of the services they buy, e.g. through establishing criteria for the quality of service they demand. A number of other factors will also influence purchaser decisions. For example:

- the quality and price of the service in comparison with similar services being offered elsewhere;

- the reputation of the service provider – factors such as waiting times, complaints and preferences for venue influence the choice made by purchasers/referrers and clients;

- concentration of purchasers – purchasers may join together to purchase services, and in doing so negotiate a lower price for those services.

Provision of high-quality cost-effective services

Through analysis of the above factors, the issues impacting on the ability of the organisation to provide cost-effective high-quality services can be identified. Differentiation of services becomes important when there is direct competition or a threat of substitute services. Where there is minimal or no differentiation between services there is little to prevent purchasers from switching to another service provider, with the resultant loss of income.

ACTIVITY 5.5

Using the adapted five forces model, analyse the factors that impact upon your service's ability to promote health and wellbeing, for example smoking cessation.

Comment

The following four principles must be considered when using the five forces framework.

1. The five forces framework should be applied at the level of division/service or business units (as opposed to across the whole organisation) because each area will be delivering different services and the impact of the forces will differ (e.g. a regional neurological service has different challenges to a local orthopaedic service).
2. It is important to understand the connections between the different forces and the key drivers within the environment (e.g. political changes can have a major impact on all the forces within the framework).
3. The five forces are interconnected and a change in one may result in changes in another (e.g. an inability to recruit suitably qualified staff may lead to referrals being made to another provider).
4. In order to achieve value for money, the focus should be on disrupting the forces rather than merely accepting them.

When undertaking strategic analysis, information identified using one model may be applied and further analysed within another model (e.g. the PESTLE may have identified that there is a lack of health and social care facilities for the elderly in the local area, which results in delays in discharging elderly patients from acute services). This in turn affects the costs of providing the acute services and the ability to meet demand due to overcapacity.

The final model to be introduced is the Boston Consulting Group (BCG) matrix. This model enables the user to analyse the services provided and identify appropriate strategies for managing the different services.

Public-sector adaptation of the Boston Consulting Group (BCG) matrix

The BCG matrix was originally developed to enable profit-making companies to examine the balance of their portfolio of products or business units in terms of market share and market growth. Analysis of the different business units/products enables identification of those aspects of the business that are making a profit, those that require more investment in order to increase market share and profitability, and finally those aspects that are not viable. A balanced portfolio within a profit-making company would enable the company to reinvest profits from some parts of the business in order to support the development of new products. It is important to achieve a balanced portfolio in order to ensure the viability of the business and continued profitability.

Montanari and Bracker (1986), cited in Johnson *et al.* (2006), adapted a public-sector BCG matrix that enables the user to analyse public-sector services in terms of their ability to provide value for money with available resources. This is affected by:

- the need or attractiveness of the service (degree of political/public support and funding);

- the ability to serve effectively (the 'fit' of that service with the organisation's aims).

The aim is to achieve a balance of services within each sector of the portfolio – it is more expensive to deliver new or different services because of the set-up costs involved and the staff's lack of experience. Over time, as experience grows, the service can be delivered more cost effectively (Golden Fleece – see Figure 5.3), and as the cost of providing that service goes down, funds can be redirected to support other services that are either new (Public Sector Star) or lack sufficient funding support (Political Hot Box). Sometimes, difficult decisions have to be made regarding discontinuing services when there is insufficient support or resources for those services (Back Drawer Issues).

The adapted public-sector BCG matrix enables analysis of the options for services, depending on where they sit within the matrix, as outlined below.

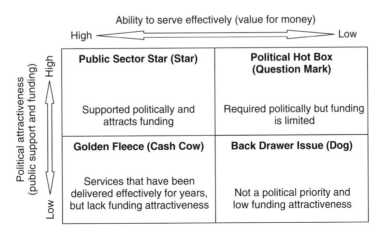

Figure 5.3 Public-sector portfolio (adaptation of the BCG matrix)

Public Sector Stars

These are seen as being able to serve effectively, and have political support and funding. The principal aim with the services that fall into this category is to increase the efficiency and cost effectiveness of their delivery. By doing so some of the funding associated with these services may be diverted towards the services that fit within the Political Hot Box category.

Political Hot Box

This is where many services in health and social care are situated because there is a political need for the service, but limited resources for delivery. The options available for these services are to:

- improve efficiency in delivering the service (e.g. by applying lean thinking principles) and hence reduce costs/wastage;

- increase funding attractiveness by lobbying for public support;

- divert resources from services that are able to deliver efficiently and under budget, e.g. Public Sector Stars or Golden Fleece services, with the aim of developing the service so it becomes more effective and less costly.

Golden Fleeces

These are those services that have been delivered for some time, and so benefit from experienced staff being able to deliver cost-effective services. These services are necessary, but do not enjoy political or public support and funding. The aim with these services is to constantly seek to deliver them in the most cost-effective way possible.

Back Drawer Issues

These are those services that are difficult to deliver effectively and are not politically or publicly supported, so funding is limited (or in some cases non-existent). It may be necessary to consider discontinuing provision; alternatively, consideration could be given as to whether to invest in developing the service so it becomes a Golden Fleece.

The analysis of the current situation will have revealed the key factors impacting upon the service and any constraints that exist. A thorough analysis is important in order to support sound decision making, and ensure a robust strategy is implemented. The analysis should also provide some ideas for improving the current situation, and these options need to be considered further.

ACTIVITY 5.6

Using the adapted public-sector BCG matrix, try to position your services within the matrix. Consider how you may improve ability to serve effectively or increase the public support and funding attractiveness of the service.

Comment

There always will be services that provide good value for money, while other services are more costly to deliver because of the stage at which they are within their life cycle. It can be argued that most public-sector organisations have an imbalanced portfolio of services because many services are politically attractive but lack funding support.

Option appraisal

The analysis may have led to a number of options being identified and a thorough analysis of the different options is important in order to ensure the most appropriate strategy is pursued. Before the strategic options can be appraised the criteria for evaluating the options must be clear. Setting objectives (or goals) is useful at this stage because it helps to focus on what the new strategy aims to achieve, and provides a means by which to evaluate success at a later date. In addition, any constraints that exist need to be clarified because whatever strategy is selected must be able to work within these constraints.

SMART (specific, measurable, achievable, relevant, time-bounded) objectives can be used to evaluate the strategic options. However, Johnson *et al.* (2006) argue that there may be some objectives that are difficult to quantify but are still important, and these should be included. Other criteria for evaluating the options may be considered, such as suitability, acceptability and feasibility (SAF). Listed below are some example questions to consider.

Suitability

Do the proposed options:

- enable achievement of governmental policies (political drivers);
- build upon strengths, overcome weaknesses/threats and capitalise on opportunities identified within the SWOT?

Acceptability

Are the proposed options in line with:

- the organisational strategy and mission;

- stakeholder expectations;
- the culture?

Feasibility

Is the proposed strategy likely to work in practice?

- Do the options fit within current financial constraints?
- Are the necessary resources available (e.g. staff/venue)?
- Do staff have the necessary skills? If not can they be trained/recruited?

ACTIVITY 5.7

- Identify at least three different options for improving the current situation (one of these options may be to do nothing).
- Identify the objectives or goals that you want to achieve through your strategic change.
- Analyse each of the options against your objectives/goals or the SAF criteria, and rank the options in order of preference.
- Examine whether it is feasible to combine options or elements of the options in order to create a better strategy.

Comment

It is important to suspend any preconceived ideas as to what needs to be done in order to improve your services because this can prevent you from exploring alternative options and being more creative in considering the available options.

Chapter 5 summary

Policies provide direction for public-sector organisations, but knowing what strategies to implement in order to achieve policy is often difficult. This chapter has provided a practical introduction to the first two stages in the strategic management process: analysis of the current situation and identifying suitable strategies to pursue in order to improve services in the future. A number of different tools were introduced to assist the user to undertake an in-depth analysis of the current situation within the workplace. The analysis is seen as important in order to ensure sound decision making, and the importance of suspending preconceived ideas throughout the process has been stressed. The selection of an appropriate strategy is dependent on reviewing each option against criteria or objectives; these criteria can be revisited following implementation of the strategic change to review the success of the changes made.

GOING FURTHER

Brereton, L and Vasoodaven, V (2010) *The Impact of the NHS Market.* London: CIVI-TAS; Institute for the Study of Civil Society. *This briefing presents the results of a large-scale literature search on the effectiveness of NHS 'market policies' in England, which have, since the 1990s, aimed to promote competition among providers in the hope of replicating the benefits of market efficiencies.*

Cox, Y and Rawlinson, M (2008) Strategic leadership for health and wellbeing, in Coles, L and Porter, E (2008) *Public Health Skills: A Practical Guide for Nurses and Public Health Practitioners.* Oxford: Blackwell Wiley.

Gillespie, A (2007) *Foundations of Economics, Additional Chapter on Business Strategy.* Oxford: Oxford University Press. Online at: www.oup.com/uk/orc/bin/9780199296378/01student/additional/ (accessed June 2010). *Looks at how the analysis of economic issues fits in with the study of business, and SWOT analysis.*

Johnson, G, Scholes, K and Whittington, R (2006) *Exploring Corporate Strategy.* Harlow: Prentice Hall. *Understanding and exploring the issues of strategic management.*

chapter 6

Tackling Health and Social Inequalities
Steve Tee

Meeting the Public Health Competences

Core area 3: Policy and strategy development and implementation to improve population health and wellbeing

This chapter will help you to evidence the following competences for public health (Public Health Skills and Careers Framework):

- Level 6(2): Implement relevant aspects of policies and strategies in own area of work;
- Level 6(3): Appraise draft policies and strategies and recommend changes to improve their development;
- Level 6(4): Contribute to assessing the potential or actual impact of policies and strategies on health and wellbeing in own area of work;
- Level 7(1): Interpret and communicate local, regional and national policies and strategies within own area of work;
- Level 7(4): Contribute to the development of policies and strategies within own area of work;
- Level 7(5): Assess the actual or potential impact of policies and strategies on health and wellbeing;
- Level 7(6): Provide specialist input to policies and strategies that are under development;
- Level 7(7): Alert the relevant people to issues and gaps in policies and strategies that are affecting health and wellbeing;
- Level 8(1): Interpret and apply local, regional and national policies and strategies;
- Level 8(2): Influence the development of policies and strategies at other levels and/or within own area of work;
- Level 8(3): Develop and implement policies and strategies in own area of work;
- Level 8(4): Identify opportunities for policy development that will improve health and wellbeing and reduce inequalites.

This chapter will also assist you in demonstrating the following National Occupational Standard(s) for public health:

- PHP30: Work in partnership with others to plan how to put strategies for improving health and wellbeing into effect;
- PHP31: Work in partnership with others to implement strategies for improving health and wellbeing;

- PHP33: Work in partnership with others to make a preliminary assessment of the impact of policies and strategies on health and wellbeing;
- PHP35: Advise how health improvement can be promoted in policy;
- PHP39: Present information and arguments to others on how policies affect health and wellbeing;
- PHP40: Evaluate and recommend changes to policies to improve health and well-being;
- DA AB 3: Contribute to the development of organisational policy and practice.

This chapter should also be useful in demonstrating Standard 10 of the Public Health Practitioner Standards:

Standard 10: Support the implementation of policies and strategies to improve health and wellbeing outcomes – demonstrating:

a. knowledge of the main public health policies and strategies relevant to own area of work and the organisations that are responsible for them;
b. how different policies, strategies and priorities affect own specific work and how to influence their development or implementation in own area of work;
c. critical reflection and constructive suggestions for how policies, strategies and priorities could be improved in terms of improving health and wellbeing and reducing health inequalities in own area of work.

Overview

This chapter considers how the development and implementation of policy can help to tackle health and social care inequalities. It will demonstrate how national policy aimed at reducing health inequalities can be translated into local action targeted at those populations most in need of services, with the objective of improving health, wellbeing and social functioning. This chapter considers how an effective national campaign can be implemented through local, regional and national partnerships involving organisations across the statutory, voluntary and private sectors.

Introduction

Health and social inequalities within populations arise as a consequence of many factors. Issues such as where an individual is born, where they grow up, where they work and where they age can all have implications for their long-term health and wellbeing. In the UK the health of the population has improved steadily over the last century, demonstrated in indicators such as a falling infant mortality rate in response to improved living conditions and availability of healthcare, illustrating successful public health campaigns. However, despite these successes, there remain significant differences in health and life expectancy due to the unequal distribution of money, power and resources at local and national levels.

To achieve an effective public health policy, services and resources should seek to address inequalities through developing a range of policies that can provide greater equity of provision.

Health and social care inequality

It is clear that the promotion of public health has been an important priority for successive UK governments, with the aim of addressing the rising demand for health-care and to encourage people to take preventative action towards avoidable illness. However, enabling equal access to services that will facilitate healthy choices and reduce the burden of ill health across large populations remains very problematic. This is because inequity arises as a result of a person's circumstances. As the Marmot Review (2010) points out in *Fair Society, Healthy Lives*, inequalities in health arise as a consequence of inequalities in society. In other words, where individuals are born, where they grow up, where they work and where they age will determine their health and life expectancy. As the Marmot Review (2010) further indicates, the degree of health inequality is an indication of how fair, or otherwise, society has become.

Health and social care inequality is also a European and worldwide concern, with EU-funded projects such as Determine (European Union, 2010) and the World Health Organization's (WHO, 2005a) Commission on Social Determinants of Health targeting action. The Determine project brings together over 50 health bodies within 26 European countries and is focused on taking action on the socioeconomic deter-minants of health. In addition, it aims to influence national governments towards ensuring there is a health perspective in all policies, with the central purpose of reducing health inequalities. In the UK, it has long been evident that there is uneven distribution of resources addressing health issues, which are borne out by detailed analysis of postcode data (Ordnance Survey, 2010). Such analysis clearly highlights health inequalities, but through partnerships with organisations like Ordnance Survey, healthcare organisations can begin to target limited resources and interven-tions where there is a clustering effect of health need.

Public health campaigns are most likely to be successful where they can dem-onstrate a cost benefit, as economic arguments tend to be the most influential in persuading governments to take action. It was essentially economic arguments that were used to persuade the UK government to invest in one particular area of public health concern, namely mental health. Health inequalities were highlighted in the 2006 *Depression Report* (Layard, 2006). This estimated that 16.5 per cent of people between the ages of 16 and 75 were suffering from mental illness, and argued that the biggest single cause of misery in UK society is not poverty but mental illness. It argued that, if advice, support and treatment of mental health problems were more widely and consistently available, then this would enable individuals to overcome their mental health problems and return to work, thus improving the individual's sense of wellbeing and reducing the financial burden on the state. It justified this increased investment as follows:

> . . . from the Treasury's narrow financial point of view, this is a good investment. From society's point of view it is an even better one, because the benefits to society include the extra output produced when someone works (which is more than the value of incapacity benefits and lost taxes), as well as the savings to the NHS, and, most important of all, the reduction in distress.
>
> (Layard, 2006, p8)

In conclusion, it argued that there was a very strong case for making services more available as it would ultimately be cost neutral for the government and would reduce individual suffering, making life more bearable. It further suggested that, if public health policy is concerned with fairness and equality, then greater priority should be given to those most disadvantaged by mental illness. This mental health case study will be further examined throughout this chapter, the remainder of which will use a case study approach to explore and develop these ideas/themes.

Policy context to health and social inequalities

In the *Strategic Review of Health Inequalities in England post-2010* (Marmot Review, 2010), the point is made that the reduction of health and social inequalities is a matter of fairness and social justice. It is argued that health inequality is not just down to individual genetics or unhealthy behaviour but due as much to social and economic inequalities, which create a 'social gradient' in health.

The WHO (2005a) identified a range of interactive factors that shape health and wellbeing, which include:

- a person's material circumstances – their home, income and possessions;

- the social environment in which they live and where children grow up;

- psychosocial factors, including a person's sense of purpose and wellbeing;

- behaviours including those that lead to decisions about health;

- biological factors, including genetics and family history.

These factors, as the Marmot Review (2010) points out, are then further influenced by a person's position in society shaped by education, income, gender, ethnicity and race. An example of how these differences manifest themselves is reflected in indicators of health for particular social groups. For instance, if we consider data on an age-standardised basis, it is found that the reporting of poor health tends to be highest among the long-term unemployed and the 'never worked' group (19 per cent for men and 20 per cent for women), whereas in contrast it is lowest among those in the professional and managerial occupations (4 per cent and 5 per cent, respectively) (Marmot Review, 2010).

Such data clearly illustrate how early opportunities and advantage can have a favourable effect on health and wellbeing, and that by reducing health inequalities there are significant economic, as well as social, benefits to be gained. For example, according to the Marmot Review (2010), in the UK health inequality in illness costs the UK £31–£33 billion in productivity losses, and welfare payments in the region of £20–£30 billion. Reducing health inequalities will therefore have a beneficial effect on productivity and the wealth of the individual as well as the nation.

ACTIVITY 6.1

Think of your own circumstances. What have been the key factors that have shaped your life opportunities? Have these factors been predetermined by circumstance or have they arisen out of personal choice? What would you consider important if you were to begin to shape a policy that might address a health inequality?

Promoting change across all policy

The Marmot Review's (2010) ambition is to create conditions that will allow individuals to take greater control of their lives that in turn will influence their own health and that of their family. To this end, it sets out a conceptual framework (Figure 6.1) that identifies six policy objectives that seek to achieve health equity in all policies, and effective evidence-based interventions and delivery systems.

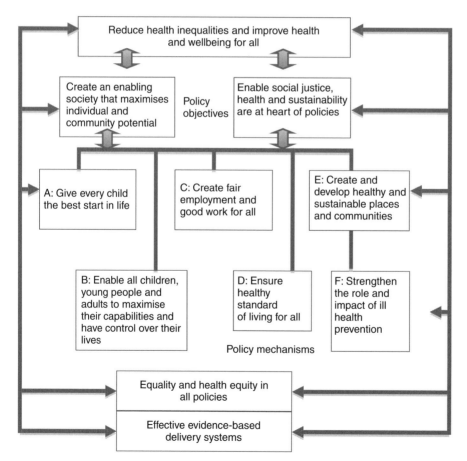

Figure 6.1 The conceptual framework from the Marmot Review (2010)

If we examine the policy objectives more closely we can see that no objective can be addressed by one single agency alone. Objective C identifies the reduction of long-term unemployment across the social gradient, and recommends that job quality can be improved through the implementation of guidance on stress management and the effective promotion of wellbeing and mental health. Objective E refers to the creation of healthy and sustainable communities through the reduction of social isolation and better co-ordinated planning between housing, health, environmental and transport systems. Objective F is focused on the prevention and early detection of conditions strongly related to health inequalities.

As the Marmot Review (2010) points out, although prevention has largely been seen as the domain of the NHS, effective policy implementation is dependent on a whole range of agencies working well together, including those from health, social care, the private and voluntary sectors, informal carers and higher education. The recent *Improving Access to Psychological Therapies* (IAPT) initiative (DoH, 2008d) is a case in point and will be used to illustrate how policy aimed at reducing health inequalities can be implemented. Although not strictly speaking a direct public health initiative, it is characterised by many of the key elements of a public health campaign, being focused on reducing health inequalities, reducing long-term unemployment, and promoting health and wellbeing, and entirely dependent on many agencies working together effectively.

The case study: mental health

The direction of mental health policy over the past two decades has led to the wider development of a range of community-based mental health services in the wake of the closure programme of the asylum system, which began in the early 1960s. The Labour government of 1997 increased funding to mental health services and quickly introduced the National Service Framework (NSF) for Mental Health (DoH, 1999a) that sought to address the mental health needs of working-age adults up to the age of 65. The NSF, for the first time, set national standards, service models and an underpinning implementation programme. In addition, the NSF established milestones, in order to assure progress, and related performance indicators to measure change.

However, despite these efforts, the London School of Economics' influential *Depression Report*, authored by Lord Layard (2006), indicated that mental illness was still accounting for more than 33 per cent of the burden of illness in the UK, with 40 per cent of disability being due to mental illness. This also equates to the numbers claiming incapacity benefit and those who regularly consult their GP. It is therefore very clear that the improvement of the UK population's mental health remains a very considerable public health challenge.

Mental health is key to individual and family health, and has wider economic implications. For example, it is evident that disorders such as depression and anxiety prevent some people from maintaining their employment. It is estimated by Layard (2006) that the loss of output due to depression and chronic anxiety is in the region of £12 billion a year, equating to 1 per cent of the UK's total national income.

At an international level, the WHO's MIND project (2010) highlighted the importance of promoting mental health in order for the population to realise the major improvements in their lives. In addition, the WHO, in partnership with World Family Doctors Caring for People (WONCA) (2008), stress the importance of people being able to access services, work and move out of poverty, and have particularly promoted the integration of mental health prevention into primary care. They state that, worldwide:

> *Mental disorders affect hundreds of millions of people and, if left untreated, create an enormous toll of suffering, disability and economic loss.*
>
> *Despite the potential to successfully treat mental disorders, only a small minority of those in need receive even the most basic treatment.*
>
> *Integrating mental health services into primary care is the most viable way of closing the treatment gap and ensuring that people get the mental health care they need.*
>
> (WONCA, 2008, p2)

The WHO and MIND (2010) further argue that, to achieve these important goals, there is a responsibility at national level to ensure there are human-rights-orientated mental health policies and legislation that enable individuals to receive treatment alongside prevention and promotion programmes targeted at those that need them.

The economic argument

In the UK, Layard (2006) argued that if funding for psychological therapies were increased and there was more even distribution, with access across the country through primary care, this would have a beneficial impact on the economy by increasing the number of people who were fit to work and reducing incapacity benefit claims. In other words, providing services that can detect, prevent and intervene early will reduce the likelihood of more intensive and expensive services further down the road. Layard (2006) reinforced this argument by highlighting the inequity of services, the long waiting times and inconsistency of provision.

Layard clearly made a good case for increased investment from central government as, in 2007, the UK government announced its plans to invest £130 million in primary mental healthcare cognitive behavioural therapy training aimed at Improving Access to Psychological Therapies (IAPT). This was targeted at individuals suffering from anxiety and depression, and was to be achieved through the development of services and the provision of new mental health practitioners who would deliver low- and high-intensity cognitive behavioural therapy (CBT) treatments, as well as advise on preventative measures and health promotion.

The Mental Health Foundation (2010) – an organisation that aims to ensure that mental health services meet the needs of populations, particularly in primary care – is keen to ensure that GPs and other staff have the knowledge and skills to be able to help people as early as possible who are experiencing mental health difficulties. It has welcomed the IAPT initiative given that mental health has not been the priority it should have been within primary care.

ACTIVITY 6.2

Within the evidence presented above by Lord Layard, he used economic, clinical and moral arguments to persuade government to invest in primary mental health services. Do you agree with his argument? Are there other perspectives to be considered here?

Analysing the broader picture

In the context of the broader policy drive towards ensuring healthy standards of living for all, strengthening the role and impact of ill health prevention and enabling greater control over people's lives, it is evident that the IAPT initiative was entirely consistent with these health equality aspirations. However, issuing and understanding a national policy initiative is one thing, translating this into a coherent local service that is valued, accessed and effective requires considerable skill and expertise, particularly in the areas of inter-agency working and achieving a shared vision.

As a public health practitioner who becomes aware of key national drivers it is necessary for you to begin to analyse the broader picture in order to more fully appreciate where it sits in terms of a wider policy framework. As discussed in earlier chapters, understanding the environment in which you are working when introducing a new policy will enable you to anticipate challenges and articulate a vision that is persuasive and realistic, thus increasing the likelihood of success.

The PESTLE analysis tool is the most helpful tool for this purpose. PESTLE will help you analyse and deconstruct the 'bigger picture' and is an orientation tool that will enable you to find out where policy sits in the context of what is happening in the national, regional and local environment. This is important as policies should always be seen as part of a broader overlapping patchwork rather than in isolation, particularly as other policies and initiatives will inevitably impact on what you and others are trying to achieve, and could affect the outcome.

As discussed in Chapter 5, PESTLE is an acronym that identifies political, environmental, social, technological, legal and environmental factors. The PESTLE model will assist you in analysing the context in which you are working.

The PESTLE as applied to the mental health case study

It is not possible to address all of these aspects in detail here, but the summary below provides the headline issues.

Political

The drive to address health inequalities has been gaining momentum at world (WHO, 2005a), European (European Union, 2010) and national levels (Marmot

Review, 2010), with emphasis on influencing national governments and local agencies to work in partnership (Smith *et al.*, 2009). There has also been a drive towards strengthening provision in primary care with intervention being closer to home (WONCA 2008; Health Committee, 2009).

In the context of mental health policy, there had been a strong political drive from the then Labour government towards implementing a new national approach to mental health. However, although in the UK there had been government investment, it was not clear whether any new government would still prioritise this initiative. If investment were to continue there would need to be considerable reshaping of service provision to accommodate the new approach, with greater focus on community/primary care commissioning, employment and inter-agency partnerships.

Economic

This new approach to achieving greater equality of mental healthcare provision coincided with one of the most challenging economic environments of modern times. The key factors specific to the case study were as follows:

- only three years' funding initially available for service development and training;
- deep recession putting significant pressure on public-sector finance that may result in a change of priority;
- public-sector cuts to staff and services;
- service improvements within primary service providers, causing change and uncertainty;
- new contractual arrangements involving voluntary and private providers;
- competitive environment involving tendering for service delivery.

Social

The IAPT initiative was going to involve reshaping and transforming existing primary care mental health provision. This would mean displacing existing roles and developing a whole cadre of new practitioners who had not been available locally before. Existing practitioners may also be suspicious of or sceptical about the value of the new service:

- services currently underrepresented by wider ethnic groups;
- existing staff will be displaced by new service;
- doubt among some GPs as to the value/effectiveness of potential services;
- training requirements of new practitioners.

Technological

As with many new healthcare initiatives, there was going to be a heavy reliance on technology for the delivery of treatments, training of practitioners and collection of data on effectiveness, including:

- approaches to the delivery of healthcare through Telehealth;
- support required for delivery of electronic psychological therapies such as cognitive behaviour therapy;
- data collection and storage;
- national curriculum available online to support the development of practitioners.

Legal

The psychological interventions required to bring about improvements in mental health require practitioners who are appropriately prepared using training that has been approved by a professionally regulated body. Existing staff working in primary care may have to upskill. Issues to be considered are:

- increasing regulation of practice;
- staff being displaced with potential TUPE arrangements;
- accreditation process for training programme.

Environmental

The primary care environment in which the service is to be provided will not have delivered such services before and so will need to be prepared in terms of both the training and service delivery. This will include:

- audit of local practice environment;
- training of staff who will be supervising trainees;
- local people being made aware of availability of the new service.

ACTIVITY 6.3

PESTLE analysis is a tool for analysing the external environment in which mental health policy and provision resides. Using the categories within PESTLE examine an area in which you currently practise. Are there any categories missing from the tool that you believe are important?

A SWOT analysis of the local context

The PESTLE revealed some important considerations in developing local policy. However, a more detailed SWOT analysis helped to clearly identify and prioritise the actions required.

The local SWOT analysis (Table 6.1) reveals a number of important strengths of the initiative in terms of the profile, resourcing and momentum for change. However, as can be seen, this needs to be balanced against recognition of some significant weaknesses that were not unique to but often characterise major change.

Table 6.1 Local SWOT analysis

Strengths	*Weaknesses*
Availability of local expertise in delivering programmes of mental health intervention	Lack of awareness among key stakeholders as this was a new service and was replacing existing services
Funding for a new initiative was available from the Department of Health	There was a perception that current practice was entrenched and not evidence based
A robust evidence base to support approach	
A national campaign that ensured the profile and purpose of the initiative was being widely communicated	There were generally poor systems of data collection to determine local need and outcomes of intervention
There was a momentum to the change and a desire among services to be part of something new and exciting	There was limited experience of using this specific approach among local service providers
Opportunities	*Threats*
The provision of high-quality training	Poor economic environment could threaten longer-term funding
The potential for future funding from the Department of Health	Suspicion and doubt as to the benefit and effectiveness of the approach
Inter-agency engagement and collaboration, which could build new partnerships for the future	Little history of inter-agency partnership in this specific area of work
Increased service provision targeting the most vulnerable and hard-to-reach groups	Future tendering process may put some services at risk
Raises the profile of mental health services	
Improved data sets that can more effectively target intervention where it is needed	The rapid speed of implementation, resulting in poor preparation of service providers and perceptions of 'failure'

Introduction of a new initiative will often mean existing services doing something different, staff being 'displaced' or requiring upskilling, and new systems of data collection, monitoring and reporting being implemented. It was important to acknowledge these weaknesses from the outset to ensure they could be managed or turned into strengths.

A new initiative such as IAPT clearly brings many opportunities for developing evidence-based services delivered through, previously absent, inter-agency partnerships that can target help to those that most need it. However, there were also significant threats from ongoing funding, and suspicion about the effectiveness of the proposed development, which can lead to sabotage, and the speed at which the changes needed to be in place.

The next important piece of work was to compose an action plan from the SWOT that would ensure that these weaknesses and threats were being addressed. Table 6.2 details the key actions that were needed. In essence there were three

Table 6.2 Action plan

1 Raise profile of new service, its aims and benefits, through a local communication strategy

- Undertake influencing activities in order to influence funding decisions and ensure long-term viability of this initiative at local level

- Implement locality-based communication strategy including inter-agency roadshows, newsletters, frequently asked questions, in order to demonstrate benefit for local populations

- Establish networks across agencies to support programme roll-out, to include representation from primary care, voluntary and independent sector, higher education and commissioners

- Target key staff in order to provide information and education about the new initiative in order to allay concerns

2 Provide training for the delivery of evidence-based interventions according the national guidelines and best practice

- Develop and accredit training programmes in partnership with key stakeholders to ensure co-operation and ownership of staff development process

- Audit and prepare local service providers for delivery of practice-based element of training

3 Develop data collection systems in partnership with service provider organisations that ensure effective monitoring and evaluation

- Benchmark progress against other national providers

- Establish process for communicating progress, highlighting successes and disseminating good practice, through local and national conferences and stakeholder events key elements to the action plan: the 'selling' of the project to stakeholders in order to convince them of the wider benefits and value of the service; the preparation of the training programme for the new practitioners; and, finally, the monitoring and evaluation of the service to ensure that it is effective and realises the anticipated benefits.

These actions particularly illustrate the importance of what is described as *strategic agility in a complex world* (Elementa Leadership, 2010, p1). This is characterised by intelligence, nimbleness and collaboration with others. The skills that can be identified to achieve this are communicator and relationship builder with the ability to adapt to circumstances at pace. Importantly, the individual can work well with ambiguity and uncertainty, and recognises the interdependence with others in order to successfully achieve strategic goals.

ACTIVITY 6.4 WORKING WITH OTHERS

Introducing a policy initiative invariably requires significant inter-agency working. You have decided on an event that will bring agencies together in small groups to identify approaches to the policy implementation. What techniques might you employ to enable the agencies to work together? How would you record and communicate outcomes?

Developing the communication strategy

Before embarking on a communication strategy it is important to identify to whom you will be communicating, how you will be communicating and what you will be communicating. Once again, there are some helpful tools that can support your work in this area. An example of each has been drawn from three UK countries.

1. Community profile (Belfast Healthy Cities, 2004);
2. Public Health Practitioner's Public Engagement Toolkit (Wales Centre for Heath, 2009);
3. Rapid Appraisal Tool for Health Impact Assessment (Ison, 2002).

Community profile

Key to successful policy implementation is effective partnership working and a communication strategy. The first step is to analyse the community in which the policy is to be delivered to help identify who the potential partners will need to be in implementing the policy and how stakeholders will be engaged. Table 6.3 outlines the range of stakeholders who worked together to establish the needs of the local community.

Table 6.3 Stakeholders involved in developing the community profile

- Statutory service providers – PCT Provider Trusts, NHS Foundation Trusts
- Primary care practitioners – counsellors, mental health practitioners
- Voluntary care service providers – mental health charities, link organisations
- Independent service providers – mental health trusts and private providers
- Service users – independent consultants, representatives from PALs
- Service commissioners – Strategic Health Authority, PCTs
- Higher education providers – universities involved in delivering the training

Community profiling is a useful method to assist in the process of identifying the specific needs of an area, and can provide baseline information to help with target setting. It was essential to establish a focus for the profile before deciding what information should be collected, otherwise the project could end up collecting irrelevant information. From the outset it was important that a partnership approach was taken in the development of the profile, to ensure ownership. Such an approach is essentially for achieving the competencies around partnership to plan how to put strategies for improving health and wellbeing into effect.

The full profile would take up many pages, however it consisted of clear statements around the specific needs of city and rural areas. It identified resources such as GP practices where IAPT would be introduced, and identified a strategy for awareness raising. Key to this was the consultation with service users and patients in order to maximise the effect of any communication approach.

Engaging the public and potential service users

The next step is to engage the public and other stakeholders directly in raising awareness and seeking feedback. The Public Health Practitioner's Public Engagement Toolkit (Wales Centre for Health, 2009) is helpful in that it provides a whole range of methods for use depending on the purpose, the audience to be targeted, and the capacity and constraints of the project/policy being pursued. However, from an ethical perspective, it is important to be clear about what information you are seeking or delivering, what you intend to do with that information and the degree of influence stakeholders have over the policy outcomes. To illustrate this more clearly, the toolkit uses Wilcox's ladder of participation (Table 6.4), which will help you to identify the most appropriate methods to use. For instance, if your intention is to give information and not seek any feedback, this would be level 1 'Informing'. However, if your intention is to work through an issue together and carry through agreed actions, then the 'Acting together' level would be more appropriate.

Problems and concerns arise when an event purports to be an opportunity to influence policy development but is in reality just an information-giving process

Table 6.4 Wilcox Ladder of Participation (Wales Centre for Health 2009)

Informing – giving a message but not requiring feedback or comment

Consultation – allows choice between predetermined options not an opportunity to propose alternatives

Deciding together – views shared, options generated jointly, a course of action agreed upon

Acting together – working with others to make decisions and carry through the action agreed

Supporting local initiatives – supporting groups to develop and implement their own solutions

---

Source: Wales Centre for Health, 2009

with little room for shared decision making. Unfortunately, mishandled events have given public engagement a bad name and led to disillusionment with the process. As public health practitioners we have a responsibility to be open and clear about our intentions in order to avoid misleading participants.

The toolkit provides a list of potential public health applications for the toolkit, such as communicating risk, capacity building and policy making. For the purposes of the mental health initiative the purpose was awareness raising, as well as the opportunity to contribute to the development of the IAPT training programme. As in any policy development and implementation, there were certain constraints imposed by the national delivery team. There were, for example, very strongly prescribed training modules, including specific content, programme structure and assessment methods. This limited freedom to change and negotiate content locally was somewhat counter to the typical philosophical stance around local negotiation and service user participation, but the initial funding available was entirely dependent on delivering the prescribed training programme and so the team was required to comply.

What were we communicating?

It was important to have a clear picture of what we were planning to say at the engagement meetings, and a useful tool in this regard is the Rapid Appraisal Tool for Health Impact Assessment (Ison, 2002). The purpose of this tool is to use the evidence collected to prioritise the potential impact on health of the intended action. In doing this, it would ensure that we were conveying a robust evidence base and that we were emphasising the potential health benefits. Undertaking an appraisal of this nature will assist you in achieving the competence around making a preliminary assessment of the impact of policies and strategies on health and wellbeing.

The tool includes a helpful criteria (Table 6.5) against which judgements can be made about the likely impact of the proposal. This is useful in structuring the communication strategy.

Table 6.5 Prioritisation criteria

- The likelihood of the impact occurring (likely, speculative or unlikely)

- The severity of the impact if it does occur (severe, moderate or minimal)

- The number of people likely to be affected (many, some or few)

- The timescale in which the impact may occur (short, medium or long term)

- Whether the impact will affect some groups within the population more than others (inequalities)

- Whether the issue is a concern to the community

Using this impact criterion, it was evident from the research that the impact would be likely, that the severity of the impact would probably be somewhere between severe and moderate, that many people could potentially be impacted upon, and that the timescales were short to medium. With regards to the distribution of benefit it was evident that access to services had tended to be skewed towards certain postcodes and those who could afford to access private treatment arrangements. This whole project was about providing greater equity of access. Whether this issue was a concern to the community can largely be judged through the lengthy waiting lists to access existing services and the resultant requests for repeated absences from work. There was also discussion with a service user reference group about the importance and benefits of this work.

ACTIVITY 6.5 COMMUNICATION

You want to develop a mental health anti-stigma campaign to encourage health-seeking behaviours among a group of people who do not routinely access public health services. How would you go about developing an effective campaign? Who would you involve in your campaign? How would you seek to maximise the effectiveness of your approach?

Working across boundaries

As indicated earlier in the Marmot Review (2010), any successful new policy initiative is dependent on agencies working together in partnership towards shared strategic goals. This may sound straightforward but different sectors have different expectations, cultures and priorities, which can impact on effective partnership.

In this case there were three aspects to the partnership: first, communicating a shared vision about the delivery of the new service; second, preparing primary

care services for the delivery; and, third, preparing and validating the training programme for the new workers.

The first stage was to bring together representation from the different agencies,
which included the Strategic Health Authority, NHS Trusts, private- and voluntary-
sector providers, Primary Care Trusts, a higher education provider and service users.
The next step was to target key staff in order to provide information and education
about the new initiative in order to allay concerns, begin the process of recruitment
into the new posts and to establish the IAPT services.

Overcoming concerns and challenging misconceptions or misunderstandings
about the benefits of a health campaign is an important public health skill and
is reflected in competency PHP39: Present information and arguments to others
on how policies affect health and wellbeing. There were many stakeholders who
were sceptical about the value of the service, particularly when it meant diverting
scarce resources from one service area towards another new and, in their
eyes, untested service. To address concerns, information on the underpinning
evidence supporting the approach was compiled and presented to individuals and
teams.

The issue of influencing also had a wider imperative, as funding was dependent
on demonstrating the success of the initiative. If the long-term viability of this initiative was to be secured at local level it was important to ensure that those with influence over funding priorities were persuaded of the benefits.

ACTIVITY 6.6 DECISION MAKING

You are required to introduce a policy to improve a community's health, but you are
aware that some doubt and scepticism exist towards the evidence for the approach
being proposed. How would you go about deciding on the approach being taken to influence change? What factors would you address and how would you prioritise your work?

The decision was taken to implement a locality-based communication strategy
that included inter-agency roadshows, newsletters, a 'frequently asked questions'
flyer, and local press releases. The strategy was also supported by articles published
in the national press.

Provide training for the delivery of evidence-based interventions according to the national guidelines and best practice

The second strand of this project was to prepare workers for their new role. The success of this initiative was dependent on practitioners adopting a consistent approach
to the delivery of evidence-based psychological interventions to significant numbers
of individuals in the primary care setting. The training programme was the outcome
of a successful joint bid between two university departments and a number of service
providers. Extensive national and local consultation was undertaken, along with

combining elements of the national programme set down by the Department of Health. It was important to meet the needs of the local service providers who would be delivering the IAPT initiative.

Locally, cross-agency networks were established to support programme roll-out to include representation from primary care, the voluntary and independent sectors, higher education and commissioners.

Following the development and approval of the programme, the university was commissioned by the Strategic Health Authority (SHA) to deliver the training to a set number of practitioners to the level of competence set out in the national curriculum for supporting people with anxiety and depression in primary care. In addition, the SHA commissioned four Local Provider Trusts to deliver IAPT clinical services. Each student is funded by the SHA and is employed by their respective provider to practise.

The underpinning approach is cognitive behaviour therapy (CBT), which is an evidence-based psychological intervention designed to address a range of mental health problems (e.g. anxiety, depression). More recently, evidence has been generated indicating that CBT interventions are useful in increasing the functioning of patients suffering a range of physical health problems (e.g. chronic pain, diabetes, chronic fatigue syndrome).

The government has recently committed to investing £130 million in CBT training as part of the IAPT project. This is designed to train therapists to deliver both 'high'- and 'low'-intensity CBT. This fits within the National Institute for Health and Clinical Excellence (NICE, 2009) model of stepped care for depression, where patients are initially offered self-help for some disorders and then, if they do not improve, they are 'stepped up' to the next level of care, which usually means receiving individual therapy within a primary care service. Low-intensity therapy focuses on self-help and computer-aided CBT, whereas high-intensity therapy may deliver either individual or group therapies. Importantly, the increased investment is the result of an increasingly robust empirical evidence base that supports this approach to common mental health problems.

ACTIVITY 6.7 IMPLEMENTING RESEARCH AND EVIDENCE INTO PRACTICE

The evidence base underpinning some aspects of public health practice may be less robust than for other aspects. Identify any area of work you know in which practice is based on history and routine rather than what you know to be research evidence. What are the barriers that prevent research evidence being used in that situation? What could be done to bring about change?

Determining effectiveness

An important feature of any public health initiative that seeks to develop and implement a policy tackling health and social inequalities is determining effectiveness through benchmarking against other similar services and through robust evaluation of the service. The third key element of the IAPT initiative was to establish networks with other providers and to ensure there were data collection systems in place, in partnership with the service providers, that would achieve effective monitoring and evaluation of the new services.

Benchmarking with other providers

Benchmarking is a useful tool aimed at self-improvement. It allows organisations, services or teams to compare themselves with another similar organisation or initiative in order to identify comparative strengths and weaknesses, and then use this information to make improvements. Strong national IAPT networks have been established for both service providers and higher education institutions, which use these opportunities to benchmark themselves against each other. It is important to consider both the process through which the outcomes are achieved as well as the basic performance data.

Impact of the policy

In demonstrating the impact of this particular policy on the local population, it is important to reflect on the primary aim of the IAPT programme, which was to support the implementation of the NICE guidelines (2009) for people suffering from depression and anxiety disorders. The collection of outcome data includes clinical scores and is an important characteristic of the stepped-care model that shapes the delivery of psychological therapy services. It has been evident from pilot sites that outcome measures have demonstrated benefits in terms of improved health and wellbeing, high levels of satisfaction with the service, improved choice and accessibility and, importantly, helping people to remain in employment and participate in normal activities.

It was very clear from the outset that the intention nationally was to establish data sets that will communicate information about the numbers of people receiving psychological therapies and that will also assure access, consistency, quality and effectiveness. Those delivering the service must provide information on patients, their care pathways and outcome measures, in terms of impact on symptoms. They must also demonstrate equity of access, quality of service, effectiveness and that the model of service delivery provides an appropriate range of interventions across the stepped-care model. A whole range of clinical tools are used to gather this data and information.

Importantly, the collection of population data will allow for a local and national evaluation of the effectiveness of the policy and for recommendations to be made regarding changes to the policy. This ties in closely to the competence PHP40, which requires evaluation and recommending changes to policies to improve health and wellbeing. These are essential skills in an increasingly competitive world in which practitioners will be required to present arguments to commissioners and fund-holders for continued investment in public health activities. Those practitioners who can confidently articulate the proven benefits of a service are more likely to be successful.

Chapter 6 summary

This chapter has considered how the development and implementation of a national policy can address health and social care inequalities at local level. However, it has also demonstrated that the process of translation and implementation can be a complex issue that requires careful planning and partnership with a range of stakeholders.

Despite the challenges, a range of very useful tools are identified that can support you in such an endeavour by determining the policy context and evidence base, assessing the environment and targeting relevant stakeholders. The final, and arguably most important, element is a robust evaluation strategy that demonstrates the level of effectiveness in reducing health and social inequalities.

Targeting local action at populations most in need of services, with the objective of reducing health and social inequalities, demands considerable skill in communication, group work and leadership. However, successful implementation of a policy that brings about greater equity will not only provide wide-ranging benefits to local populations but is a potentially rewarding personal achievement.

GOING FURTHER

Cattan, M and Tilford, S (2006) *Mental Health Promotion*. Berkshire: Open University Press. *A guide to applied mental health promotion across all age groups, demonstrating how both principles and theory can be used to underpin mental health promotion.*

Green, J and Tones, K (2010) *Health Promotion Planning and Strategies*. London: Sage Publications. *This book outlines models for defining 'health promotion' and sets out the factors involved in planning health promotion programmes that work.*

Lloyd, C, Handsley, S, Douglas, J, Earle, S and Spurr, S (2009) *A Reader in Promoting Public Health* (2nd edn). Berkshire: Open University Press. *This book brings together a selection of readings that reflect and challenge current thinking in the field of multidisciplinary public health, addressing issues that are high on the agenda of public health.*

Together, the following three reports provide a comprehensive overview of the issues involved in the causes of health inequalities and dealing with them effectively.

House of Commons Health Committee (2009) *Third Report on Health Inequalities*: www.publications.parliament.uk/pa/cm200809/cmselect/cmhealth/286/28602.htm.

Marmot Review (2010) *Fair Society, Healthy Lives: A Strategic Review of Health Inequalities in England Post-2010*: www.marmotreview.org.

Report from the WHO (2005) Commission on the Social Determinants of Health: www.who.int/social_determinants/thecommission/finalreport/en/index.html.

chapter 7

Social Determinants of Health – Housing: A UK Perspective

Jenny Hacker, David Ormandy and Peter Ambrose

Meeting the Public Health Competences

Core area 3: Policy and strategy development and implementation to improve population health and wellbeing

This chapter will help you to evidence the following competences for public health (Public Health Skills and Career Framework):

- Level 6(d): Knowledge of public service organisation and delivery;
- Level 7(d): Understanding of public service organisation and delivery;
- Level 8(c): Understanding of the political environment in which own organisation is set and how this affects its policy and strategy;
- Level 6(4): Contribute to assessing the potential or actual impact of policies and strategies on health and wellbeing in own area of work;
- Level 8(3): Develop and implement policies and strategies in own area of work.

This chapter will also assist you in demonstrating the following National Occupational Standard(s) for public health:

- PHS14: Assess the impact of policies and shape and influence them to improve health and wellbeing;
- PHS15: Implement strategies for putting policies to improve health and wellbeing into effect.

This chapter should also be useful in demonstrating Standard 10 of the Public Health Practitioner Standards:

Standard 10: Support the implementation of policies and strategies to improve health and wellbeing outcomes – demonstrating:

a. knowledge of the main public health policies and strategies relevant to own area of work and the organisations that are responsible for them;
b. how different policies, strategies and priorities affect own specific work and how to influence their development or implementation in own area of work;
c. critical reflection and constructive suggestions for how policies, strategies and priorities could be improved in terms of improving health and wellbeing and reducing health inequalities in own area of work.

Overview

This chapter explores the links between housing and health, and the evidence that underpins this, as well as some of the research issues involved in housing research. It describes how key aspects of housing affect physical, mental and social health, and the links with health inequalities. Finally, the chapter explores the policy context around housing, and why addressing housing should be a key component of public health work, locally and nationally.

Introduction

Multiple housing deprivation appears to pose a health risk that is of the same magnitude as smoking and, on average, greater than that posed by excessive alcohol consumption.

(British Medical Association, 2003, p1)

While most now accept the role that housing plays as a key determinant of health, public health in recent years has failed to give the same attention to housing as it has to lifestyle issues such as smoking. In his review of health inequalities, Marmot is critical of what he calls the *lifestyle drift*, whereby *attempts to reduce health inequalities have not systematically addressed the background causes of ill health and have relied increasingly on tackling more proximal causes (such as smoking), through behaviour change programmes* (Marmot, 2010, p86). Both smoking and poor housing conditions make a significant contribution to the persistent health inequalities gap we witness in the UK. While not detracting from the significant progress that has been made with major killers such as smoking, with governments across the globe intervening with legislation to tackle smoking, it is regrettable that this focus on behaviour change has not been accompanied in policy terms by efforts to tackle underlying contributors to unhealthy lifestyles, such as housing. Housing remains one of the 'prime prerequisites for health', a term first penned in the seminal Black Report of 1980, widely held responsible for launching the debate on health inequalities in the UK. It has however very much become the 'forgotten' public health issue. This has not always been the case.

Historical development

In the early nineteenth century, the work of the Poor Law Board and key public health figures such as Chadwick, Snow and Southwood Smith highlighted the appalling living conditions of the labouring population. This movement led to a demand for state intervention to tackle the causes of disease, believed at the time to be smells from rubbish and raw sewage, and provide for fresh air and light. Although we know now that the beliefs on which action was based were flawed, the solutions adopted were relatively effective in removing some of the more blatant threats to health.

Table 7.1 Deaths and injuries from accidents at home, at work and on the road (England and Wales)

	Accidental deaths	Injuries	Total accidents
Road (2002)	3,431	299,174	302,605
Work (12 months during 2002/3)	235*	154,430	154,665
Home and garden (2002)	3,000**	2,701,326	2,704,326

Source: data combined from information obtained from the Royal Society for the Prevention of Accidents and the Health and Safety Executive

* 2003/4 figures.
** Official estimate.

As the public health issues of the day have now largely shifted from communicable diseases, such as tuberculosis and cholera, to chronic diseases including asthma, diabetes, heart disease and mental health, housing retains its importance as a key determinant of health. In 2003 it was estimated that poor housing conditions were implicated in up to 50,000 deaths (approximately 1 per 1,000 population) and around 0.5 million injuries and illnesses requiring medical attention (approximately 1 per 100) each year in England (Office of the Deputy Prime Minister, 2003b). Seventeen times as many people are injured in the home or garden each year than at work; nine times as many as on the roads. In terms of actual deaths the number killed in the home or garden is equivalent to those dying on the roads each year (Table 7.1).

Housing-related illness or injury has huge implications for NHS budgets, alongside broader societal costs such as to work and the economy. A recent study in the Netherlands estimated that home injuries cost around €0.66 billion (about £0.45 billion) in healthcare costs alone (Meerding *et al.*, 2006). Another study, from the USA, estimated the total cost to society of accidental home injuries to be at least $217 billion (about £149 billion). In the UK, work by the Building Research Establishment, using data from the English House Condition Survey (EHCS, Department of the Environment, Transport and the regions (DETR), 1998) has estimated that health outcomes from unhealthy housing are currently costing the National Health Service in the region of £600 million every year (Nicol *et al.*, 2010).

From a public health perspective, then, as well as from an economic one, housing cannot and should not be ignored. Public health needs to be at the forefront of new demands for changes to housing policy and for strategic approaches to improving housing locally. For this to happen, practitioners require a clear understanding of health and housing issues, and of the links between housing and health, alongside a clear vision of what needs to happen. This chapter aims to provide both.

What do we mean by 'house' and 'housing'?

This chapter is premised on several assumptions. First, the terms 'house' and 'home' – although often used interchangeably – are not synonymous. A 'house' denotes a physical structure intended for human habitation. The term 'home' goes beyond this, incorporating for example social and cultural aspects of the household. This has implications for any analysis of housing and health: we go beyond the basic need for shelter associated with the bottom of Maslow's hierarchy of needs (Maslow, 1943), with which few would argue, to incorporate a broader perspective of housing. The term 'housing' also goes beyond bricks and mortar and incorporates both the local community and the immediate housing environment, i.e. the local neighbourhood, streets or estate, including shops, places of worship, recreational and green space, and transport.

Finally, it is important to recognise that housing has the potential to have both positive and negative (indeed fatal) impacts upon health. The role of public health should be to maximise the positive and minimise the negative. Neither our dwellings nor our neighbourhoods can be completely hazard free: clearly, we require facilities such as stairs, heating and cooking facilities, and there are also clear hazards within the neighbourhoods in which we live. However, to enable a household to establish a home and enjoy positive health, dwellings should not only ensure that necessary and unavoidable hazards should be as safe as possible, but be designed and constructed to take account of the spectrum of lifestyles and cultures that may typically occupy them. Similarly, neighbourhoods should be designed to minimise harm, encourage community life and promote healthy lifestyles.

Housing and health framework

The links between housing and health are complex. In 2006, the then Housing Corporation called for evidence on housing and health to be produced in *easily digestible chunks . . . in context and preferably related to possible policy options*, adding that *The evidence base needs to be organised and translated in such a way that it speaks to a broader audience of professionals so that they can use the information to inform partnership working more easily* (Housing Corporation, 2006, Part 5). Although time and space prevent a detailed consideration of the barriers to closer engagement between housing and public health in recent decades, professional and language barriers have undoubtedly made a contribution.

ACTIVITY 7.1

List some of the social, professional and language barriers between housing and public health within your area of practice.

Although several frameworks have been produced that aim to summarise the complex relationship between health and housing, none have yet done so from the perspectives of both housing and health professionals. The evidence-based framework developed by the United Kingdom Public Health Association (UKPHA) (2010), and presented in Table 7.2, is an attempt to do this. It presents three main aspects of housing that impact upon health (access to housing, quality of housing and vulnerability of

Table 7.2 UKPHA housing and health framework

Housing perspective	Health perspective
There are three broad aspects of housing that can impact – positively or negatively – on health	There are three broad areas of health upon which aspects of housing can make this impact

1. Access to housing

1. Physical health

- Homelessness and threat of homelessness
- Affordability
- Security of tenure

Housing is associated with increased mortality and morbidity via:

2. Quality of housing

Aspects affecting physiological health, e.g.

- Damp and mould
- Excessive cold or heat
- Asbestos
- Carbon monoxide, lead, radiation

Aspects affecting psychological health, e.g.

- Crowding, light pollution, noise

Aspects associated with infection, e.g.

- Pests, sanitation and drainage
- Water supply

Aspects associated with accidents, e.g.

- Falls, fire, electrical hazards, structural collapse

Quality of the local neighbourhood, e.g.

- Walkability, open and green spaces, community safety, social capital

- Accidents in the home (linked to poor design, bad state of repair, overcrowded conditions)
- Cardiovascular disease (excess cold, smoking in the home)
- Infant mortality (overcrowding)
- Infectious diseases (e.g. TB, influenza, meningitis, linked to crowding, living in temporary accommodation)
- Low immunisation rates (homelessness, living in temporary accommodation)
- Poisoning (carbon monoxide, radon)
- Poor lifestyles (i.e. smoking, poor nutrition, linked to homelessness, living in temporary accommodation)
- Respiratory disease (excess cold, secondhand smoke, damp and mould, infestations)

2. Mental health

Housing is associated with increased stress, depression and anxiety, which can be linked to:

- Homelessness
- Threat of homelessness/insecurity of tenure
- Poor housing conditions, damp, cold
- Overcrowding
- Noise
- Fear of crime
- Anti-social behaviour, litter, graffiti
- Poor social and community networks

3. Vulnerability of residents

The provision of support on housing and health-related issues, including household budgeting, can ameliorate some of the worst effects of poor housing, and improve health:

3. Social health

Housing is linked to poorer social health via:

- Households or individuals on low incomes
- Households or individuals spending much time at home, e.g. older people, younger children, those with a health problem or disability
- Those with drug or alcohol problems
- Those whose situation puts them in urgent housing need, i.e. those experiencing or at risk of domestic violence, care leavers, offenders, asylum seekers and refugees, travellers

- Low educational attainment (linked to living in temporary accommodation, overcrowded conditions)
- Developmental delay (overcrowding)
- Poor employment prospects (stigma of particular estates/addresses)
- Social isolation (cold, damp homes, high-crime estates)

Source: UKPHA (2010)

residents) alongside three categories of health (physical, mental and social), which the evidence indicates are linked to the housing aspects. The framework can be 'flipped', with the user choosing to start with housing issues or health impact, depending on their perspective and profession. Finally, the details beneath the framework account for both the positive and negative potential of housing to impact on health.

Housing and health: the evidence base

The evidence base for the framework will now be presented. Each section concludes with a bulleted, non-exhaustive list highlighting the policy and strategy role for public health. Where possible, this is also evidence based, however it is acknowledged that, while there is a growing body of evidence linking housing to health, the evidence of effective interventions is more limited. However, a recent American journal supplement attempted to address this with a new series of articles summarising recent research in the USA. This concentrates upon the effectiveness of interventions that tackle healthy homes holistically, rather than individual housing issues, or combine different interventions (i.e. smoke alarm installation with meals on wheels services) (*Journal of Public Health Management and Practice*, 2010).

Access to housing

The first and important characteristic of housing for which there is evidence of an impact on health is whether an individual or family has access to housing in the first place. This incorporates three broad but linked issues:

1. homelessness;
2. affordability;
3. security of tenure.

Homelessness

There is a great deal of evidence to demonstrate the adverse impact of homelessness on health (Fitzpatrick *et al.*, 2000). The term 'homelessness' incorporates those who are literally sleeping on the streets (rough sleepers); those living in temporary accommodation such as hostels, bed and breakfasts or other types of accommodation where they are awaiting rehousing; and the 'hidden' homeless, i.e. those who do not have their own tenancies or properties, and are not included in official definitions, but who are nonetheless lodging with friends and relatives. When compared to the general population, physical health problems are found to be at least twice as common among rough sleepers or hostel dwellers, with mental health problems eight times as high among hostel dwellers and 11 times as high in rough sleepers (Joseph Rowntree Foundation, 1994). The street homeless are also around 40 times less likely to be registered with a GP than the general population (Crisis, 2002).

ACTIVITY 7.2

Consider the relationship between health and homelessness. Identify possible issues and suggest ways of addressing these through policy implementation.

The relationship between health and homelessness is complicated by its two-way nature since those with pre-existing health problems are more prone to homelessness, and the street homeless are more likely to suffer from mental health problems and alcohol and drug misuse. Although more longitudinal studies would be needed to categorically prove a direct link, there is no doubt that homelessness – both street homelessness and hostel living – can compound pre-existing drug, alcohol or mental health problems. Studies have less commonly included the impact on social health, however there is a strong association between homelessness and withdrawal from education, employment or training, and from social networks (Quilgars *et al.*, 2008).

Rough sleeping is the extreme end of homelessness. Although street homelessness is far from having been eradicated in the UK, in the decades prior to the 2010 fiscal financial crisis at least there have been major reductions in homelessness. In public health terms, many more individuals and families are without their own home but have been placed in local authority, housing association or voluntary-sector-run temporary accommodation while on the housing waiting list, thus any analysis of the impact of homelessness on health must avoid focusing purely on rough sleeping.

In 2010, there were almost two million people on council waiting lists for social housing and around 70,000 people in temporary accommodation in England (Marmot, 2010). Less easy to quantify are the 'hidden' homeless who are without their own home but lodging with others. Some of the health implications of this (such as overcrowding) will be covered below. However, there is evidence that living in temporary accommodation (particularly bed and breakfast) has adverse outcomes for children, and is linked to increased rates of accidents, infectious diseases, hyperactivity, poor nutrition, dental decay, low immunisation rates and impaired development (Vostanis, 2002).

Affordability

Costs of rents and mortgages relative to income clearly affect a household's ability to access a suitable home. Given the adverse effect that poor housing can have on health outcomes, an inability to afford decent housing that is, for example, in a good state of repair, free from hazards, of an appropriate size for the household, in a desirable location, and so on, whether renting or purchasing, is a serious issue, and one closely linked to health inequalities. People on low incomes, who spend a greater proportion of their wages on rents or mortgages, will clearly find affordability more of a problem. Those on low incomes living in London and the south-east, where rents can be considerably higher than elsewhere in the UK, are doubly disadvantaged.

It is also important to recognise that affordability is not just about rents and mortgages: it needs to incorporate the costs of running and maintaining a home, heating costs and other essential items. Misjudging the cost of home ownership often results in 'new' low-income owner-occupiers finding they cannot afford to maintain their property, or, at worst, cannot meet the repayments, leading to repossession. As the following two case studies show, high housing costs can have a detrimental effect on health by leaving fewer resources for essential items such as food and heating.

Case Study: A natural experiment in rehousing and health

In 1927, researchers compared the health of residents of a poor housing estate, who had been rehoused to modern accommodation, with a control group that remained living in slum housing. This natural experiment in Stockton-on-Tees revealed dramatic changes in the age-standardised death rates of the group that was rehoused. However, this was not in the direction that would have been expected! There was a sharp *increase* in death rates among those rehoused from slum dwellings to better housing. This *unexpected finding was eventually traced back to a deterioration in diet among those re-housed, resulting from a reduction in disposable income, itself caused by the higher rental costs of the newer housing* (Pencheon et al., 2001, p77).

Case Study: The Central Stepney SRB health gain study

As part of the Single Regeneration Budget (SRB) regeneration of parts of Central Stepney in the mid-1990s, a 'health gain' study was commissioned to assess any improvements in self-reported health following housing improvements (Ambrose, 2002). A four-year time interval was allowed before re-surveying residents to enable the rehousing to be carried out and for the residents to avoid any 'honeymoon' effect; only around half of the original households were still in the area in 2000. In 2000 the incidence of illness days was less than one-seventh that of 1996, with a commensurate fall in the use of some NHS resources in both primary and secondary care (Table 7.3).

Table 7.3 Comparison of illness days (1996 and 2000)

Illness Days	1996	2000
Number of people in sample	525	227
Survey period in days	150	75
Person/days	78,750	17,025
Illness days	29,114	926
Illness days per person/day	0.37	0.05

Source: Ambrose (2002)

A subsequent project of the 'before' and 'after' finances of 20 households found that the combined costs of higher rents, council tax and water rates represented a rise of about 27 per cent, or £22.87 per week (Ambrose and Macdonald, 2001). Residents reported that they were spending less on food, recreation, social life and, for some, heating costs. Many respondents were also increasingly worried about the debts they had incurred to help meet living costs. Since all these items and issues have a direct bearing on health, it seems at least plausible that the decreased affordability of their housing following regeneration was working to erode the health gains noted.

Security of tenure

One of the major reasons for loss of tenancies, repossessions and subsequent homelessness is rent or mortgage arrears. Living with the threat of homelessness has been shown to impact upon health. Using data from the 1998 British Household Panel Survey (University of Essex), Nettleton and Burrows (1998) have demonstrated that mortgage arrears were independently associated with self-reported wellbeing for men and women, and with increased visits to general practitioners by men. There may be a similar pattern in terms of rent arrears, but this is not explored here. However, the evidence of the impact on children living in temporary accommodation can be life changing and this is now examined.

> *Eviction puts children's wellbeing at risk, potentially pushing them into overcrowded, poor quality or temporary housing and seriously disrupting their lives.*
>
> (Shelter, 2009, p9)

Shelter highlights that not only do children lose homes, travel out of areas, and lose friends and family, but they are often moved several times, reside in more than one bed and breakfast accommodation and face long periods of instability in their lives. New schools and the pressure of 'fitting in' can lead to periods of stress and insecurity, seriously disrupting their lives.

ACTIVITY 7.3

Consider the 2010 coalition government policy for welfare reforms and identify the positive and negative impacts these could have on access to housing. Compare and contrast particular impacts when examining major cities such as London and Cardiff or sought-after rural settings.

Comment

The policy and strategy role for public health in addressing access to housing suggests the following.

- Homelessness prevention: partnership working to encourage a strategic approach to the prevention of homelessness, using local intelligence to identify the extent and address the main causes of all types of homelessness in the local area, and in particular seeking to identify and prevent repeat homelessness. Ensuring debt counselling and income maximisation services are in place and accessible to those most in need, alongside local strategies to tackle worklessness.
- Support for rough sleepers to mitigate the worst impacts of homelessness – for example, increasing access to health services, screening and immunisations.
- Addressing supply/demand issues: working with planners, council leaders, elected members and others to assess and address local demand for housing and increase the provision of affordable housing in the short and long term; encouraging schemes to maximise the supply of local housing, i.e. voluntary transfer schemes.
- Ensuring that health professionals understand and are able to support local rehousing systems.
- Undertaking health impact assessments of renewal programmes, identifying populations with specific housing needs.
- Illuminating the catastrophic health effects of repossession and ensuring that repossession is an absolute last resort locally.

Quality of housing and local neighbourhoods

As with demonstrating the links between homelessness and health, there are methodological challenges in trying to unravel the potential impact of individual and combinations of housing conditions from other environmental, social and economic factors – not least poverty.

As Marmot (2010) comments, this has become more difficult with the 'residualisation' of social housing and suggests that *While the quality of housing is important for health, part of the health disadvantage relates to the make-up of the population of social housing.*

The report highlights that, with reduced supply of social housing, tenants tend to have higher rates of unemployment, ill health and disability compared with the average for the rest of the population. This is known as the residualisation effect within the social housing tenant population. In addition, it is also noted that poverty rates for this group are double those of the population as a whole, with fewer than half in paid work and only a third in full-time work.

ACTIVITY 7.4

Examine your area of practice and current housing policy, and interpret any available data to determine social housing tenancy structure and possible residualisation effect.

Interest in gathering and strengthening evidence on the relationship between housing and health has grown over the past 20 or so years. Evidence on building conditions and the health of users has been the subject of several revisions (Mant and Muir Gray, 1986; Cox and Sullivan, 1995; Raw and Hamilton, 1995; Raw *et al.*, 2001; Communities and Local Government, 2010) and several reviews on housing and health have been published (e.g. Ranson, 1991; Burridge and Ormandy, 1993; Ineichan, 1993; *American Journal of Public Health*, 2003; British Medical Association, 2003; Howden-Chapman and Carroll, 2004; Reviews on Environmental Health, 2004; *Journal of Public Health Management and Practice*, 2010). During 2003, work was carried out that included analyses of matched databases – a Housing and Population Database and datasets on reported illness, injuries and other health conditions – to provide information on the prevalence of a range of illness, injuries and other health conditions that could be linked to particular housing conditions and features (ODPM, 2003b). Analysis in 2006 identified 29 potential hazards, shown in full in Table 7.4, known as the Housing Health and Safety Rating System (HHSRS).

Table 7.4 Housing Health and Safety Rating System (HHSRS) hazards

Physiological requirements	Protection against infection
Damp and mould growth	Domestic hygiene, pests and refuse
Excessive cold	Food safety
Excessive heat	Personal hygiene, sanitation and drainage
Asbestos, etc.	Water supply
Biocides	

CO and fuel combustion productions
Lead
Radiation
Uncombusted fuel gas
Volatile organic compounds

Psychological requirements

Crowding and space
Entry by intruders
Lighting
Noise

Protection against accidents

Falls associated with baths, etc.
Falling on level surfaces
Falling on stairs, etc.
Falling between levels
Electrical hazards
Fire
Flames, hot surfaces, etc.
Collision and entrapment
Explosions
Position and operability of amenities, etc.
Structural collapse and falling elements

Source: ODPM (2006a)

This chapter cannot do justice to the 29 hazards included in the HHSRS. However, *Excessive cold* will be discussed under 'Housing policy', below, as it has implications for public health due to its association with deaths and illness from heart disease, stroke, respiratory disease and falls; and can also worsen symptoms of arthritis, increase recovery time and lead to social isolation (Howden-Chapman *et al.*, 2007). '*Crowding*' (overcrowding) is also worth highlighting, since it is included in the HHSRS as a factor affecting psychological health, and associated with mental health issues such as anxiety and depression in children and adults (Harker, 2006). Equally, it is also associated with poorer physical and social health, and can have fatal consequences. Children in overcrowded conditions are ten times more likely to contract the potentially life-threatening diseases meningitis and tuberculosis, as well as asthma and wheezing. Overcrowding is also linked to infant mortality, developmental delay and poor educational attainment (Ambrose and Farrell, 2009).

ACTIVITY 7.5

Evaluate your local housing policy and explore ways it could or does address overcrowding. What is your role in this area?

The HHSRS focuses on hazards that, to a greater or lesser extent, are attributable to the condition of the dwelling. It does not include hazards solely attributable to occupier behaviour, so makes no reference to secondhand smoke (SHS), the sidestream smoke from cigarettes, which contains 4,000 chemicals. There is conclusive evidence that exposure to SHS causes cot death, respiratory illnesses, respiratory symptoms, impaired lung function, and middle ear disease (glue ear); there is also substantial evidence that it causes the development of asthma among those previously unaffected and worsens symptoms of cystic fibrosis; a possible link has been suggested (but not proven) between exposure to SHS and cancer, meningitis and cardiovascular disease (BMA Board of Science, 2007). Smoking in the home is linked to death or injury from fire. Exposure to SHS is particularly harmful to children since they breathe faster than adults and have undeveloped immune systems. In the UK, around 17,000 children are admitted to hospital every year because of illnesses caused by secondhand smoke (Royal College of Physicians, 1992).

The earlier discussion set out a central premise of this chapter – that the term 'housing' encompasses not just bricks and mortar, but the local community and neighbourhood. It is important to be aware of the evidence that health can be affected – positively and negatively – by factors associated with local neighbour-hoods. In terms of the negative effects, those that have been particularly highlighted are crime and fear of crime, antisocial behaviour, noise, litter, vandalism, lack of social cohesion, as well as poor access to health services, parks, play areas and healthy food (NICE, 2005; Braubach, 2010; van Kamp et al., 2010). Feeling unsafe increases the likelihood of poor health by 40 per cent, even after controlling for other factors such as tenure, gender and age (Parkes and Kearns, 2004) and is also associ-ated with higher smoking prevalence (Blackman and Harvey, 2001; Davidson, 2010). In addition, for many living on traditional council-built estates in the UK, access to a healthy diet is made extremely difficult.

Thus the fact that poor-quality accommodation is often situated in impoverished surroundings with few local amenities contributes further to poor health outcomes by discouraging healthy lifestyles and making many vulnerable individuals effec-tively housebound. American studies have shown that neighbourhoods that are 'walkable' are associated not only with higher social capital (Leydon, 2003) but with lower levels of obesity (Smith et al., 2008). Good social networks and social capital can also foster good health (Ambrose and Stone, 2010).

With the aforementioned 'residualisation' of housing (Marmot, 2010), social housing estates can often acquire a negative reputation that can lead to the popula-tion becoming labelled: *In the eyes of many people, council estates are little more than holding cages for the feral and the lazy* (Hanley, 2007, p146). Consequently some of the worst estates in Britain not only suffer from poverty and unemployment but are viewed as suffering from a sort of social disease. This in turn is reflected in the way others see residents as being somehow less human, and incapable of acting in a posi-tive manner to change their lives (Hanley, 2007).

ACTIVITY 7.6

Many of these estates are *isolated, cut-off from passers by, car routes, local shops and every class of people except the people who live on them* (Hanley, 2007, p163).

Read Hanley's account of life on a London estate. Can you identify with this scenario in your area of practice and how could you address some of the issues?

Comment

The policy and strategy role for public health in improving the quality of housing suggests the following.

- Ensuring local areas are taking comprehensive enforcement action to deal with HHSRS *hazards* in the private sector and that systems are in place for undertaking or enforcing action to remedy all defects that may be hazardous to health using the Housing Act 2004, landlord licensing and/or tenant accreditation schemes.
- Multi-agency, strategic approaches, to systematically identify and reduce other hazards in the home. Examples include local handyperson services, programmes for fitting smoke detectors, schemes to alleviate crowding, such as empty homes schemes, lateral housing conversions and incentives to release under-occupied housing.
- Ensuring local areas have achieved Decent Homes standards for social housing and for private-sector housing occupied by vulnerable households.
- Ensuring that health professionals understand and are involved in referring patients to Affordable Warmth schemes.
- Identifying properties and residential land affected by radon, and ensuring appropriate mitigation action is taken, e.g. increased under-floor ventilation.
- Addressing homes with defective gas, solid fuel and oil-burning appliances and associated carbon monoxide risk.
- Establishing Smokefree Homes schemes to reduce exposure to secondhand smoke in the home, alongside fire risk.
- Strategic approaches to improving safety in the most deprived areas, e.g. better street lighting, community wardens, community alarm services available to repeat victims and other vulnerable groups.
- Working in partnership to ensure services are in place, and responding quickly and effectively to environmental problems such as litter, graffiti and noise nuisance.
- Ensuring Health Impact Assessments are routinely undertaken during the planning of new housing developments in both public and private sectors; withholding permissions for new schemes not building in provision for health, such as green and recreation space and transport. Encouraging food growing via neighbourhood gardens, allotments or community farms.

Support for potentially vulnerable groups

The final, but important, aspect of the framework concerns those who are or may be particularly vulnerable and in need of support in terms of securing housing, dealing with repairs and tenancy issues, household budgeting, etc. The more vulnerable members of society are more likely to be exposed to the worst and most health-threatening conditions. These have been categorised into those who are vulnerable due to income, amount of time spent at home, drug or alcohol problem, or other vulnerability. Clearly, those on a low income will be most affected by a lack of affordable homes, and therefore by threat of homelessness and insecurity. They are also less likely to benefit from decent housing. The 2003 English House Condition Survey (ODPM, 2006b) reports that households with low income are more likely to live in 'non-decent' homes. Similarly, those on low incomes will also be less able to afford to adequately heat a home. A household is said to be in 'fuel poverty' if it needs to spend more than 10 per cent of its income on fuel to sustain satisfactory heating. In 2005/06, 7 per cent of households were spending more than this, over half of which were single-person households. Fuel poverty rates fluctuate with the price of fuel. In November 2008 the rising price of domestic fuel resulted in over half of single pensioners and two-thirds of workless households being in fuel poverty.

While all of us may spend at least 8–12 hours a day at home, the very young, the elderly, those ill or otherwise not healthy enough to go to work or school, or the unemployed, may spend up to 24 hours a day in and around the dwelling. Any system for regulating housing conditions should be directed to protecting the main users, and if a dwelling is safe for these, the more vulnerable, then it will be safe for all.

Other potentially vulnerable groups include those with a drug or alcohol problem, black and minority ethnic groups – who are ten times more likely to live in overcrowded homes (ODPM, 2006c) – and women, who are more likely to be victims of domestic violence and in need of emergency housing than men, and who may also be more susceptible to the effects of damp than men (Rennie *et al.*, 2005).

ACTIVITY 7.7

Examine your area of practice for areas housing vulnerable groups of people. How do you propose to tackle any public health issues identified?

Comment

The policy and strategy role for public health in supporting vulnerable groups suggests the following.

- Public health's main role here is to seek to identify specific vulnerable groups, and illuminate the nature of the vulnerability and potential impact on physical, mental and social health, both positive and negative, of interventions.
- This will involve both awareness of issues most likely to affect particular groups, and use of techniques such as needs assessment to articulate demand and compare with local provision (for example, in terms of women's refuges).
- Public health also has a role in ensuring that services provided for vulnerable groups are effectively joined up, and that, for example, local areas are taking an integrated approach to addressing homelessness, mental health, drugs and alcohol problems.

Housing policy

How, then, has government policy addressed this relationship between housing and health? For reasons of time and space, the decision has been taken to focus on three aspects of housing policy: affordability, security of tenure, and housing conditions.

Affordability

It was noted earlier in this chapter that notions of affordability need to go beyond the actual cost of housing and incorporate vital additional costs associated with housing, including the costs of heating the property itself. However, much policy discussion about housing is flawed in that not only does it avoid the above, but it uses the concept of affordability without any meaningful definition at all. 'Affordable' is officially taken to mean simply below market price or rent; as a result much of the 'affordable' housing produced when a planning agreement specifies that x per cent of the housing should be 'affordable' often produces homes that are not remotely affordable to many local people.

In early 2008, a London Citizens team was commissioned to calculate the affordable housing figure for a specified household (two adults, and two children aged ten and four) living at a specific address in Stepney. The figure arrived at was £135 per week. Figures can similarly be worked out for any household type living in any specified area. In other words, there is now a method for calculating an evidence-based housing affordability figure. This was termed the Housing Affordability Standard (HAS) and was launched at a hustings meeting for the London Mayoral candidates in April 2008 (see www.humanrightstv.com/london-citizens/a-better-housed-london/305; the definition of 'affordable' was that included in Zacchaeus Trust, 2005).

Part of any approach to affordability is to ensure an adequate supply of social housing. In 2007, the then government's Green Paper, *Homes for the Future* (Department for Communities and Local Government (DCLG), 2007) promised a more affordable, sustainable future. It encouraged authorities to develop their strategic housing role by using the full range of housing and land use planning powers. Local areas were to be working with partners to meet the needs of residents by ensuring the delivery of new and affordable housing while making best use of existing stock, meeting targets to increase the housing supply progressively to 240,000 per year by 2016, delivering around two million additional homes by that time and maintaining that level to deliver approximately three million in total by 2020 – targets that were subsequently dropped following spending cuts.

A second approach to affordability lies in the benefit system. Housing benefit and local housing allowances are designed to make good the difference between what can be afforded for rent and what it is actually necessary to pay. There are widespread and well-documented problems with these allowances. Very often they do not cover the rents that have to be paid, and the shortfall needs to be made good from other means-tested benefits, themselves not adequate to protect health. Often, also, claimants' circumstances change or mistakes occur, and either significant overpayments are made then claimed back or underpayments are made. A final problem is that reliance on benefits and allowances complicates the transition into work since the income required from work must be such as to more than make up for the loss of benefit income. If the income gained from work is only a small amount over the benefit lost it means that the marginal rate of taxation on the earnings may be very high – certainly much higher than the rate of taxation paid by the vast majority of those not reliant on benefits. Following the 2010 election, the new coalition government has been developing new policies for accessing housing benefit that will theoretically revolutionise this structure (Spending Review, October 2010). What evolves remains to be seen.

ACTIVITY 7.8

Analyse the coalition government's proposed housing benefit access. What implications would this have for your area of practice?

Security of tenure

Until the last 15–20 years the vast majority of tenants in both the public and private sectors had reasonable security and could not be lawfully evicted without a court order, granted only for good reason. However, there has been a weakening of the security of tenure with measures designed to 'free up' the private rented sector. In 1989, assured short-hold tenancies were introduced by Part 1 of the 1988 Housing Act. These are now the most common form of tenancies, and are usually granted for a six-month period with no guarantee of renewal. Along with the 'right to buy' policy, whereby public-sector tenants were encouraged to buy their council housing at discounted prices, drastically reducing the availability of council stock to rehouse families and individuals in need, this policy has had dramatic effects. While private landlords have obligations to repair, their lack of security means that tenants are either unlikely to feel secure enough to challenge their landlords, or relatively transient, so unlikely to bother.

Housing conditions

Efforts to improve housing need to include but go beyond investing in new homes. At least 70 per cent of housing for the year 2050 is already built (Sustainable Development Commission, 2006). As renewal of the existing stock is a very gradual process (and at the current rate of replacement, it will take more than 1,000 years), there is a need for controls on existing housing to try to ensure that it is as free as possible from threats to health.

More than half of the English housing stock was built before 1960, and in excess of 20 per cent is more than 100 years old (ODPM, 2006b). Despite major improvements in the conditions of housing, millions of households still live in unacceptable housing conditions. In 2003, of the 21.3 million dwellings in England (ODPM, 2006b), 6.7 million failed to meet the Decent Homes Standard (ODPM, 2004), a standard originally introduced in 1997 for housing to satisfy four requirements:

1. to be free of any unacceptable hazard within the Housing Health and Safety Rating System (HHSRS; Table 7.4);

2. in a reasonable state of repair;

3. have reasonably modern facilities;

4. provide a reasonable degree of thermal comfort.

It was the Labour government's (1997–2010) declared aim that all public-sector housing, plus all private-sector housing occupied by 'vulnerable' individuals, should meet the Decent Homes Standard by 2010 (ODPM, 2005). Current estimates are that this target is unlikely to be met. The HHSRS was adopted in April 2006, replacing the 1990 Housing Fitness Standard (ODPM, 2006a). One of the criticisms of the Fitness Standard was that it did not effectively cover energy efficiency or thermal insulation. Government guidance stated that this requirement could be satisfied by *a suitably located (13 amp minimum) outlet which may reasonably be dedicated solely to [a fixed electric heating] appliance* (Department of the Environment (DoE), 1996, Annex A, para. 7.4). Despite the fact that the Fitness Standard was so minimal, the 2001 English Housing Condition Survey found that 4.2 per cent of the English housing stock failed to meet it, and that, in 2001, over 88,500 dwellings in England did not meet the appallingly low requirement of having a dedicated 13 amp power socket in the living room (ODPM, 2003a).

Excess cold

The energy efficiency of dwellings is covered by the HHSRS, where one of the hazards to be assessed is 'excess cold'. During work on the development of the HHSRS, Moore estimated that there may have been in excess of 6 million dwellings (28 per cent of the total stock) where this hazard was at an unacceptable level (Moore, 2003). He also estimated that, of these, nearly 4.5 million dwellings (that is, over one-fifth of the total stock) were occupied by 'vulnerable' households.

In 2000, responding to pressure from various quarters, the government set up the 'Warm Front' initiative (Department for Environment, Food and Rural Affairs (DEFRA), 2000), directed at tackling so-called 'fuel poverty'. Both Warm Front and the Decent Homes programme are welcome and will go some way towards dealing with cold homes. However, the scale of the problem is such that these two initiatives are really only the starting point.

> ## Chapter 7 summary
>
> In this chapter we began by considering the ways in which housing affects health. The main aspects of housing that affect health (i.e. access to housing, quality of housing and local neighbourhoods, and support to vulnerable groups) were considered in terms of their positive and negative impacts on physical, mental and social health. The limitations of available research techniques were also considered. The policy contexts for several key aspects of housing were then described.

GOING FURTHER

Ambrose, P and Farrell, B (2009) *Housing: Our Future*. London: London Citizens. *This report uncovered the extent of overcrowding among a sample of primary school children.*

Ormandy, D (2009) *Housing and Health in Europe (Housing and Society Series). The WHO LARES Project*. London: Routledge. *This book explains the nature and development of the World Health Organization's study of housing across Europe; the in-depth analysis provides new evidence of links between the health of inhabitants and their housing conditions.*

chapter 8

Social Determinants of Health – Child Poverty: A Northern Ireland Perspective

Deidre Heenan

Meeting the Public Health Competences

Core area 3: Policy and strategy development and implementation to improve population health and wellbeing

This chapter will help you evidence the following competences for public health (Public Health Skills and Career Framework):

- Level 7(1): Interpret and communicate local, regional and national policies and strategies within own area of work;
- Level 7(5): Assess the actual or potential impact of policies and strategies on health and wellbeing;
- Level 8(2): Influence the development of policies and strategies at other levels and/or within own area of work;
- Level 8(4): Identify opportunities for policy development that will improve health and wellbeing and reduce inequalities;
- Level 9(1): Identify where new policies and strategies are needed to improve the population's health and wellbeing.

This chapter will also assist you in demonstrating the following National Occupational Standard(s) for public health:

- PHP35: Advise how health improvement can be promoted in policy;
- PHP37: Evaluate and review the effects of policies on health improvement;
- PHP39: Present information and arguments to others on how policies affect health and wellbeing;
- PHP40: Evaluate and recommend changes to policies to improve health and wellbeing.

This chapter should also be useful in demonstrating Standard 10 of the Public Health Practitioner Standards:

Standard 10: Support the implementation of policies and strategies to improve health and wellbeing outcomes – demonstrating:

a. knowledge of the main public health policies and strategies relevant to own area of work and the organisations that are responsible for them;

b. how different policies, strategies and priorities affect own specific work and how to influence their development or implementation in own area of work;

c. critical reflection and constructive suggestions for how policies, strategies and priorities could be improved in terms of improving health and wellbeing and reducing health inequalities in own area of work.

Overview

This chapter examines the nature and extent of child poverty. It then looks at some of the key policy developments in this area since devolution in 2002, to assess the extent to which the local administration has developed innovative approaches to addressing the blight of poverty.

Introduction

Child poverty in Northern Ireland

Despite the eventual political settlement in Northern Ireland since the signing of the Good Friday (Belfast) Agreement in 1998, and the establishment of the devolved assembly, the province remains deeply divided along class and sectarian lines. Thirty years of political and civil unrest have cast a long shadow over society and the legacy of the conflict remains a significant aspect of life. Poverty is endemic as Northern Ireland remains among the most deprived regions of the United Kingdom. Urban communities in the two main cities, Belfast and Derry, are routinely at the bottom of every index for multiple deprivation. A lack of investment and regeneration, coupled with high levels of unemployment, disability and debt, have resulted in high levels of disadvantage and reliance on social security benefits.

Research published by the Office of the First and Deputy First Minister (Sullivan *et al.*, 2010) noted that the negative impacts of relative disadvantage on the educational, cognitive, behavioural, general health and obesity outcomes for children was measurable at the age of five years. These negative impacts represent significant barriers that many children will struggle to overcome. In later years these hurdles can translate into lower educational achievement and aspirations, increased risk of welfare dependency, chaotic family and personal lifestyles and risk behaviours, and continuing or worsening poorer health.

Historical and political background

Prior to the introduction of devolution in 2002, the direct rule government in Northern Ireland did not produce data on poverty and there was no specific anti-poverty strategy. While local and regional statistics and indicators such as unemployment rates, income levels and mortality rates have invariably confirmed that it is the most deprived or one of the most deprived regions of the UK, there is a dearth of empirical research and reliable information on the nature and extent of poverty. Unlike other regions of the UK, Northern Ireland has no tradition of publishing household income data to allow comparisons with other regions, and it was not included in the Family Resources Survey until 2003 and the Households Below Average Incomes series until 2004. Commenting on this, an Economic and Social Research Council (ESRC) report (2005) noted that one irony of poverty in Northern Ireland was the poverty of research and reliable statistics. The first ever large-scale survey of poverty and social exclusion in Northern Ireland, *Bare Necessities*, was undertaken in 2002–03 (Democratic Dialogue, 2003). Until this study there was no detailed data on poverty, reliable information was difficult to obtain and consequently rigorous analysis of need was virtually impossible (Dignam, 2003).

The findings in *Bare Necessities* were based around two measures: low income and being unable to afford items that most people regarded as necessities. After extensive consultation, the study came up with 29 basic necessities and these were then used as indicators of disadvantage in a survey of almost 2,000 households. The key findings of the study highlighted a deeply fractured society where income was unevenly distributed:

- 37.4 per cent of Northern Ireland children are growing up in poor households;

- 67 per cent of lone parents are in poverty;

- 29 per cent of women, but only 25 per cent of men, are in poor households;

- 56 per cent of households containing one or more disabled people are in poverty;

- Catholics are 1.4 times as likely as Protestants to live in poor households;

- the richest 40 per cent of households together possess 67 per cent of the total household income;

- the poorest 40 per cent of households have 17 per cent of total household income.

This study concluded that rates of poverty were higher in Northern Ireland than in either the Republic of Ireland or Great Britain. Overall measures revealed that, in Northern Ireland, 30.6 per cent of people were in poor households, compared to 28.2 per cent in the Republic of Ireland and 25 per cent in Great Britain. The authors of the survey described Northern Ireland as one of the most unequal societies in the developed world.

ACTIVITY 8.1

Measuring poverty can be fraught with difficulties, and different methods of measurement often make comparisons problematic. What do you think are the key issues when measuring poverty? With the election in 1997 of the Labour government, the term 'social exclusion' entered the lexicon of social policy in the UK. While low income was central to this idea, it also included other factors relating to severe and chronic disadvantage. What do you think are the advantages and disadvantages of the term social exclusion?

Comment

At this stage it may be useful to draw up a glossary to remind you of the key terms used in the measurement of poverty, including:

- absolute poverty;
- relative poverty;
- social exclusion.

The Joseph Rowntree Foundation (JRF) has produced a number of detailed reports designed to monitor poverty and social exclusion in Northern Ireland. In reaction to the ongoing debate about the terminology, its publications and website generally uses the term 'poverty and social exclusion' throughout, without differentiating between them. These studies draw on a wide range of existing sources, including government statistics and health trust data. The information used is considered to be the most robust and reliable available (Kenway *et al.*, 2006). In 2006, its first report revealed that, on a range of indictors, Northern Ireland compared unfavourably with all of the nine English regions, as well as Scotland and Wales. These indicators include income poverty, benefit receipt, workless households, homelessness, child health and childcare, levels of mental ill health and fuel poverty. This work also highlighted the inequalities that existed within Northern Ireland, with significantly higher levels of disadvantage in western districts. In terms of costs, two particular areas – childcare and fuel – were singled out for attention. The areas where Northern Ireland stood out compared to Great Britain were:

- high numbers receiving out-of-work benefits;

- high numbers of disabled people;

- the extent of low pay among full-time employees;

- high numbers without paid work;

- a very high fuel poverty rate;

- a rise in numbers presenting as homeless;

- a high proportion of 16 year olds failing to reach basic education standards.

These statistics were updated in a further monitoring round in 2009 (Joseph Rowntree Foundation, 2009), which concluded that the overall picture had remained more or less static. However, it was surmised that proposed changes to the welfare system designed to move people off incapacity benefits and on to the actively seeking work register would have a disproportionate impact in the region, given the relatively high levels of dependency on disability benefits.

Child poverty

With the election of the New Labour government, tackling child poverty moved to centre stage. The main reasons for this were twofold: morally it was considered unacceptable, and it was also considered central to addressing adult disadvantage. A significant body of evidence illustrated the detrimental impact of childhood poverty on long-term life chances and opportunities. The continued existence of child poverty in a modern, civilised and progressive society was considered unacceptable. In the annual Beveridge lecture in March 1999, Tony Blair set out his historic aim to end child poverty for ever by 2020. In an impassioned speech, he set out his objectives in this area: *We need to break the cycle of disadvantage so that children born into poverty are not condemned to social exclusion and deprivation* (Blair, 1999, p16).

This declaration radically altered the policy landscape of the UK. Not only was the existence of poverty acknowledged, there was also a commitment to tackle the problem. Unsurprisingly, perhaps, given the levels of poverty, inequality and exclusion, child poverty emerged as major cause for concern in Northern Ireland as studies revealed the extent and nature of the problem. An ESRC report (2005) on income distribution in Northern Ireland provided a particularly damning assessment of child poverty when it noted that *nowhere in the UK is child poverty more entrenched, reaches greater depths, or in many places is more concentrated* (ESRC, 2005, p2).

Until the mid-1990s there had been a lack of reliable statistics and information on the nature and depth of child poverty; consequently analysis tended to be limited and largely descriptive. Prior to the publication of *Britain's Poorest Children* (Adelman *et al.*, 2003) child poverty was generally calculated solely on household income. The most severely poor were children residing in households in the lowest deciles. Adelman and her colleagues contended that this was a flawed system of measurement that did not take account of the nature of poverty. They investigated poverty using three measures: low level of household income, child deprivation and parental deprivation. They concluded that a more effective system of measuring severe child poverty would use all three indicators. The approach was adopted by Monteith and McLaughlin (2004) in research commissioned by Save the Children, and they found that roughly the same proportion of children in Northern Ireland and Great Britain were living in severe poverty: 10 per cent in 2004/05 and 8 per cent in 2005/06, but increasing to 10 per cent in Northern Ireland in 2007/08. Significantly, though, half of all children in Northern Ireland were considered poor using at least one measure, compared to 45 per cent of children in Great Britain. The research also revealed that, while the same proportion of children were in severe poverty, children in Northern Ireland were much more likely to go without three meals a day.

In a subsequent Save the Children study, Monteith *et al.* (2008) compared types of child poverty and concluded that Northern Ireland had double the levels of persistent child poverty in comparison to Great Britain, with one in five children living in persistent poverty. The entrenched and persistent nature of child poverty was again confirmed in a Joseph Rowntree-sponsored report on poverty in 2009 (Horgan and Monteith, 2009). It referred to the data from the first longitudinal analysis of four years of the Northern Ireland Household Panel Survey (NIHPS), which revealed that at some stage in this four-year period 48 per cent of children were living in poverty (before housing costs) and 21 per cent were in persistent poverty – that is, in poverty for at least three of the four years. Therefore, the proportion of children in Northern Ireland who were poor at some point (48 per cent) was considerably higher than the comparable figure for Great Britain (38 per cent). Even more alarming, the rate of persistent poverty in Northern Ireland (21 per cent) was over twice that of Great Britain (9 per cent). Consequently, over half of children in Northern Ireland are likely to experience poverty at some point in their lives, while a fifth will spend a considerable period of their childhood in poverty. On the other hand, when using the after housing costs measure, the Northern Ireland position is not as bad as that of either England or Wales (Northern Ireland Assembly (NIA), 2008a). This can be explained by the fact that the level of housing costs (chiefly rent, mortgage interest, buildings insurance and water charges) are, at present, much lower in Northern Ireland than in any Great Britain region.

Recent research has identified fuel poverty as a particular issue for low-income families in Northern Ireland. Fuel poverty rates among children in Northern Ireland are more than twice the UK average, with children there having one of the highest rates of prolonged exposure to the effects of fuel poverty of any group in the developed world (Liddell, 2008). Living in accommodation that is poorly insulated and heated impacts on children's physical and mental wellbeing, and can severely diminish childhood experiences.

ACTIVITY 8.2

In relation to the nature and extent of child poverty, Northern Ireland compares unfavourably with almost all of the nine English regions, as well as with Scotland and Wales. The level of persistent poverty is over twice as high as the GB average. How do you think persistent poverty impacts on child health and wellbeing? Identify a local policy or intervention that could be designed to address this issue.

Ending child poverty is described as a key challenge for Northern Ireland given the high proportion of children in persistent poverty and the nature of a society emerging from over 30 years of conflict. Monteith *et al.* (2008) contended that, in order to reduce child poverty in the region, the Northern Ireland Assembly needed to address the barriers to working and increase opportunities. It outlined a number of interventions that could be adopted by the Assembly to address this issue. These were:

- working with employers to provide better jobs;
- helping people in work to gain qualifications;
- addressing the lack of childcare;
- ensuring school budgets can provide for all the costs of education;
- providing better access to leisure and social activities for young people in poverty;
- increasing educational attainment for disengaged young people.

A further Northern Ireland Assembly report (NIA, 2008b) focused on the causes of and the difficulties in tackling severe childhood poverty. A number of short- and long-term actions to alleviate the problem are listed, but no commitment is given to adopting any of these. The lack of progress in reducing levels across the UK was highlighted in 2010; while there was little change in levels reported in Northern Ireland and Scotland, the numbers in Wales have actually increased, as has the UK average. It was concluded that government policy and support is clearly not reaching the children that need help the most (Save the Children, 2010).

Policy responses to poverty

Having set out this profile of severe and entrenched disadvantage, it is instructive to examine the scope and impact of policy developments aimed at alleviating key aspects of disadvantage. It should be noted that the tax and benefits system is of fundamental importance in addressing poverty, which is, in practice, the responsibility of the UK government and, therefore, uniform throughout Northern Ireland and Great Britain. This leaves the question as to what extent devolved powers and/or the devolved administration during Direct Rule were used to deal with poverty and disadvantage. Responsibility for early years education and childcare resides with the devolved administrations.

Despite the high levels of child poverty and the lack of access to childcare in Northern Ireland, many of the initiatives introduced in England have not been adopted and there is less public funding for childcare than in any other region of the UK. Spending on Sure Start, introduced in 2001, is also much lower in Northern Ireland. In 2007/08, expenditure per child was £80, which compares unfavourably with the rest of the UK, where it was nearly £600 per child in England, £380 in Scotland, and between £270 and £350 per child in Wales. Even with the caveat that the Sure Start programme started later in Northern Ireland than in the rest of the UK, it is still a huge differential. In 2006, the Northern Ireland Pre-School Playgroup Association (NIPPA) estimated that, at this level of funding, Sure Start could deliver services to only 20 per cent of children aged 0–4 (NIPPA, 2006). Sure Start children's centres were designed to provide a holistic range of services to pre-school children and their families and these were earmarked for significant expansion. In 2000, there were 800 in England, and the target of 3,500 was achieved in April 2010. The former education secretary, Ruth Kelly, claimed children's centres were at the heart of the government's plans to eradicate child poverty. Their role in supporting families and addressing child poverty has been widely acknowledged by children's charities and advocacy groups. In Northern Ireland the government plans were to develop four such centres. To date, these centres have not yet materialised and, even though a partnership working together to improve social and economic conditions in Northern Ireland has described it as 'vital' that government addresses the issue of childcare quality and provision (Concordia, 2007, p27), this inadequate provision and neglect appears set to continue.

Further evidence of the under-funding of children's services in Northern Ireland was provided in 2010 by the voluntary group Early Years in an election manifesto. It noted that, in this region, each child gets 12.5 hours of pre-school education per year, compared to England and Wales, where each child gets 20 hours of government-funded pre-school education per week for two years. In Northern Ireland there is no training and development strategy for working with young children despite a commitment in 2006 by the Department of Education to the publication of an Early Years Strategy, whereas £200 million has been allocated for this type of training in England and Wales. The Department of Education now tends to define early years provision as pre-school, not including early years social care. The review recommends that there should be a reshaping of the childcare vision for Northern Ireland, including the allocation of mainstream funding to the childcare strategy. It also recommends that there should be clearer accountability for action relating to the implementation of childcare policy, and that more robust leadership structures are required to drive forward an integrated childcare and early years service. Northern Ireland has seen an almost complete absence of extended schools and children's centres.

In Northern Ireland, the Executive has not yet agreed lead responsibility for childcare, which underscores the importance of developing a robust childcare strategy and implementation plan. Currently, four government departments – the Department for Health, Social Services and Public Safety; the Department for Employment and Learning; the Department for Social Development; and the Department of Education – share responsibility for childcare. Northern Ireland does not have a children's minister – since 2007 the responsibility has been shared between two junior ministers in the Office of the First Minister and Deputy First Minister (OFMDFM). Speaking at an Assembly debate on child poverty in November 2010, one of the junior ministers, Mr Newton, acknowledged the failings of the devolved government in this policy area (NIA, 2010):

> We are all aware of the difficulties that exist because of the fractured way in which childcare has been managed in the past and because no single Department has responsibility for it. Indeed, no Department currently accepts policy responsibility for school-age childcare. That, in itself, has created a gap.
>
> (www.niassembly.gov.uk/record/committees2010/
> OFMDFM/101124_ChildPovertyChildcare.htm)

Different approaches were adopted by different government departments, with limited co-ordination of policies and strategies. The result was a disjointed approach to child poverty that led to gaps and duplications in provision. No one body had oversight of issues affecting children and, despite the rhetoric, there was little evidence of meaningful engagement with children and young people. The particular economic and social circumstances in Northern Ireland did not inform the development of bespoke policies, relying instead on policy transfer from England.

In 1999, the Northern Ireland childcare strategy was set out in *Children First* (Department of Health and Social Services and Public Safety (DHSSPS), 1999). *Children First* envisaged an integrated approach to early childhood education and care in Northern Ireland, and identified three main challenges for childcare: variable quality, affordability and limited access. This strategy, however, did not have a clear implementation plan with agreed funding, targets and timescales, and to a large extent was simply a paper exercise.

The availability of childcare is a core component of any child poverty strategy, and the lack of childcare facilities, affordable childcare and safe and secure play areas in Northern Ireland has been repeatedly highlighted in studies of early years provision (OFMDFM, 2006; Fawcett, 2009; Horgan and Monteith, 2009). According to the National Children's Bureau, Northern Ireland has one of the lowest levels of childcare provision in Europe, with provision for disabled children particularly poor (NCB, 2007). A comparative study of childcare across the UK and the Republic of Ireland painted a damning indictment of provision in Northern Ireland, describing it as *woefully inadequate* (NIA, 2008c, p1). There is great variation in provision across the country, with rural areas poorly served, and lone-parent families and families with a disabled child particularly disadvantaged. The lack of high-quality affordable childcare is frequently cited as the key barrier to women accessing paid employment. While, in England and Wales, the 2006 Childcare Act created a statutory duty on local authorities to meet the local demand for childcare, there is no corresponding duty in Northern Ireland. Childcare in Northern Ireland is not only relatively scarce, but, outside of London, is also the most expensive in the UK (Horgan and Monteith, 2009).

Save the Children (2009) produced an assessment of the extent to which public spending on primary and secondary education is weighted towards the poorest children in the UK, and whether or not there is a case for strengthening this poverty-focused link. It revealed that spending per pupil in Northern Ireland's primary and post-primary schools is the lowest in the UK: in 2006/07, spending ranged from less than £4,000 in Northern Ireland to nearly £6,000 in Scotland, with the average UK spend at just over £4,700. Since 2002/03, spend per pupil has grown slightly faster in England (29 per cent in real terms) than in Scotland (27 per cent), Wales (23 per cent) and Northern Ireland (just 9 per cent).

This research also commented on spending on personal social services, focusing on children's and families' services. Spending was £311 per child in Northern Ireland in 2004/05, which was 30 per cent below the UK average. Spending is highest in Wales (£544 per child in 2006/07), with spending in Scotland at £539 per child and £455 in England. The relatively low levels of spending associated with children's and families' services in Northern Ireland were described as striking. The authors commented that, in the context of enduring levels of poverty, it was difficult to avoid the conclusion that children's services appear to be a relatively low priority. The policy responses to levels of disadvantage and deprivation in Northern Ireland have not been very effective or innovative in reducing many of the key aspects of poverty. This is indicated in little overall change in the high levels of deprivation in Northern Ireland or reducing comparative disadvantage with England, Scotland and Wales. A strategy for tackling poverty, social exclusion and areas of deprivation was to be one of the priorities for the newly restored devolved government after the St Andrews Agreement in 2006, but to date progress on reaching consensus on a strategy document has been extremely slow.

Case study: Child poverty

Joanne is a lone parent living in Derry. She has five children aged between 2 and 16, and is solely dependent on income from benefits, which is £60 below the government's poverty line. Joanne is determined to return to work in order to improve her family's chances. She has recently started an IT course, but received little support from government. Her parents paid the £120 for the course and look after her children while she attends classes. Without financial, practical and emotional support from her family she would be unable to undertake this training. Childcare costs for her youngest child mean even part-time work is currently impossible. She wants to get qualified, work, be able to save, go on family holidays and treat the children: *I want to get off this hamster wheel of constantly worrying about money and the future. It is not as if I don't want to work, I don't want handouts but the system seems designed to keep me where I am.*

Joanne is concerned about the short-term implications of poverty on her children. They cannot afford school trips and activities, warm winter clothes, are unable to go swimming or the cinema, have friends round for tea or celebrate their birthdays. However it is the long-term issues that cause her most concern, most particularly the extent to which they will be able to break out of this poverty. Will her poverty be transmitted to her children?

A strategy for children and young people

The year 2006 also witnessed the publication of *Our Children and Young People – Our Pledge*, a ten-year strategy for children and young people in Northern Ireland produced by the OFMDFM. This report proclaimed that partnership working was essential to transform the lives of children, and this could solely be the concern of government. Child poverty and the impact of the conflict on the lives of children were identified as core issues. This document included eight pledges designed to transform children's services. The focus here was on a holistic, preventative approach informed by the UN Convention on the Rights of the Child. It has long been accepted that services for vulnerable children should be planned alongside services for all children. To this end, the four existing Health and Social Services Boards in Northern Ireland were required to create Area Children's and Young People's Committees (ACYPCs), to ensure Children's Service Plans were developed and implemented in an integrated, collaborative manner. These committees are made up of senior representatives from the statutory, voluntary and community sectors, and they recommended the production of a regional Northern Ireland Children's Services Plan 2008–11, based on the themes identified in the OFMDFM strategy for children and young people. The plan was published in November 2008 (ACYPC, 2008), and priority themes included safeguarding children and addressing the needs of young carers.

In 2006, the Northern Ireland Executive signed up to the UK-wide target of ending child poverty by 2020. To this end, it pledged to halve the proportion of children living in relative poverty by 2010/11. This initial milestone involved lifting 67,000 children out of poverty. In its progress report on Lifetime Opportunities, the OFM-DFM commented on progress in meeting targets. It noted that child relative income poverty rates had fallen from 29 per cent in the baseline year (1998/99) to 25 per cent in 2008/09. Progress has, as with the UK as a whole, not maintained the earlier momentum seen between 1998/99 and 2004/05. On the basis of current trends it is unlikely that the Northern Ireland Public Service Agreement target to halve child relative income poverty by 2010/11 – that is, to achieve a child relative income poverty rate of around 15 per cent – will be achieved (OFMDFM, 2010a). However, action to promote this agenda has been dependent mainly on benefit uptake campaigns, improving deprived areas through neighbourhood renewal and the work of the Child Support Agency. There is little evidence of major initiatives in Northern Ireland to change significantly the persistence of child poverty. The key factors of benefit and work lie outside devolved powers, while government action on improved education, skills and childcare is negligible (Hirsch, 2008).

The anti-poverty strategy and social inclusion 'Lifetime Opportunities' was published during the period of Direct Rule in 2006 but was not endorsed by the Northern Ireland Executive until December 2008. The strategy replaced the New Targeting Social Need (TSN), which was the previous high-level strategy for tackling need. It retained the principle of targeting resources towards those who needed them most, and adopting a partnership approach to addressing the needs of vulnerable individuals and groups. The strategy adopted a lifecycle approach that focused on the different priority needs at key stages in the life cycle. The strategic aims were to:

- work towards eliminating poverty and social exclusion by 2020;

- end child poverty by 2020.

Like its predecessor, New TSN, Lifetime Opportunities does not have a specific budget of earmarked resources, but instead requires government departments to target resources and efforts towards those in most need. In October 2010, the government published its monitoring report on Lifetime Opportunities, which stated that targets for both absolute and relative poverty were unlikely to be achieved (OFM-DFM, 2010b).

The Child Poverty Act 2010, enacted on 25 March, places a statutory obligation on the Executive to develop a child poverty strategy and lay it before the assembly by 25 March 2011. In December 2010 a draft strategy for consultation was launched by the OFMDFM, which set out the key areas identified by government as crucial in addressing the causes and consequences of child poverty and in meeting the obligations as detailed in the 2010 Act (OFMDFM, 2010a). This draft document also outlines the strategic direction for the eradication of child poverty In Northern Ireland, and is intended to bring focus to the issue and promote a common aim across government departments. Two key strands of work are identified as central to the causes and the consequences of child poverty:

1. reducing worklessness among adults with children;

2. promoting longer-term outcomes through child-based interventions that are designed to tackle the cyclical nature of child poverty.

This is expanded upon in Table 8.1.

Table 8.1 A timeline of political developments

Mar 1999	Tony Blair's commitment to eradicate child poverty by 2020	Jun 2008	Report of Inquiry into Child Poverty by the Committee for the OFMDFM
Apr 2004	Secretary of State for Northern Ireland commits to develop an anti-poverty strategy	Oct 2008	UN Committee on the Rights of the Child, while recognising the commitment to ending child poverty, raises concern at lack of progress in lifting children out of poverty
Jun 2006	Strategy for Children and Young People published; includes an objective on economic and environmental wellbeing		
		Jan 2009	UK government states its intention to introduce a Child Poverty Bill to enshrine its targets in legislation
Nov 2006	Lifetime Opportunities published by Secretary of State; children (0–16) are a key focus of the strategy	May 2009	UK government states publicly that it is unlikely to meet its 2010 target
Mar 2007	Devolution restored; Executive states that child poverty is one of five priorities for children	Mar 2010	Child Poverty Act places statutory obligation on NI Executive to develop a child poverty strategy
Dec 2007	Programme for Government signs up to the commitment to halve child poverty by 2010 and eradicate it by 2020; it also establishes a target to eradicate severe child poverty by 2012	Dec 2010	Draft Child Poverty Strategy released by OFMDFM for consultation

While the key areas identified in strand one are adult focused, centred on supporting parents into work, those relevant to strand two address the cyclical nature of child poverty by increasing the future prospects for the child. Interestingly, it is worth noting that notwithstanding the fact that the Executive states its commitment to this strategy, financial uncertainties mean that it is based around existing current priorities and commitments, with no new delivery vehicle.

Chapter 8 summary

Poverty is multi-dimensional and deep rooted, and there is a need to tackle its causes and symptoms. There is no silver bullet – the complex experience of disadvantage highlights the need for a mix of policy responses to combat poverty across both the medium and long term. This must be a priority for both the Westminster government and the Northern Ireland Executive if it is to have any impact. While the current financial crises in the public sector may mean that some would contend that we cannot afford to address the issue, given that the economic and social disadvantages faced during childhood are strongly associated with the subsequent economic success or failure of young adults, it can be argued that we cannot afford not to. Children caught in a cycle of poverty and disadvantage are learning to be poor, and this poverty of aspiration is threatening their future and the future of society. Innovative strategies to ameliorate the impact of the developmental and social consequences of poverty are urgently required. Increasing polarisation between the 'haves' and the 'have nots' is worrying and should be considered as a top priority for a devolved government attempting to build a successful, dynamic region underpinned by equality, integration and cohesion.

GOING FURTHER

Alcock, P (2006) *Understanding Poverty* (3rd edn) Basingstoke: Palgrave Macmillan. *This book is a comprehensive and accessible introduction to the analysis of poverty and social exclusion, covering the definition, measurement, distribution and causes of poverty, and the policies developed to combat it.*

Birrell, D (2009) *The Impact of Devolution on Social Policy*. Bristol: Policy Press. *This book provides a study and assessment of devolved developments in the major areas of social policy, with a full comparison between Scotland, Wales and Northern Ireland.*

Morris, K, Barnes, M and Mason, P (2009) *Children, Families and Social Exclusion, New Approaches to Prevention*. Bristol: Policy Press. *This book considers new approaches to understanding the complexities of prevention, and how these new understandings can inform policy and practice.*

The following sites provide useful further information on the subject.

ARK: www.ark.ac.uk. *ARK is a resource providing access to social and political material on Northern Ireland that informs social and political debate in the region, and raises the profile of social science research.*

Barnardo's, Northern Ireland: www.barnardos.org.uk/northernireland.htm. *This site includes publications, policy briefings and campaign news.*

Joseph Rowntree Foundation: www.jrf.org.uk.

Northern Ireland Assembly: www.niassembly.gov.uk. This site includes a link to the publications of the NIA.

Northern Ireland Research and Statistics Agency (NISRA): www.nisra.gov.uk.

Poverty Site, the: www.poverty.org.uk. This site monitors what is happening to poverty and social exclusion in the UK. The material is organised around 100 statistical indicators covering all aspects of the subject, from income and work to health and education.

chapter 9

Development and Implementation of Policy – Children and Young People: A Welsh Perspective

Marianne Cowpe and Linda Mages

Meeting the Public Health Competences

Core area 3: Policy and strategy development and implementation to improve population health and wellbeing

This chapter will help you evidence the following competences for public health (Public Health Skills and Career Framework):

- Level 6(1): Contribute to the interpretation and application of policies and strategies to own area of work;
- Level 6(3): Appraise draft policies and strategies and recommend changes to improve their development;
- Level 6(4): Contribute to assessing the potential or actual impact of policies and strategies on health and wellbeing in own area of work.

This chapter will also assist you in demonstrating the following National Occupational Standard(s) for public health:

- PHP30: Work in partnership with others to plan how to put strategies for improving health and wellbeing into effect;
- PHP34: Work in partnership with others to undertake a full assessment of the impact of policies and strategies on health and wellbeing;
- PHP38: Monitor trends and developments in policies for their impact on health and wellbeing;
- PHP39: Present information and arguments to others on how policies affect health and wellbeing;
- PHP40: Evaluate and recommend changes to policies to improve health and wellbeing.

This chapter should also be useful in demonstrating Standard 10 of the Public Health Practitioner Standards:

Standard 10: Support the implementation of policies and strategies to improve health and wellbeing outcomes – demonstrating:

a. knowledge of the main public health policies and strategies relevant to own area of work and the organisations that are responsible for them;
b. how different policies, strategies and priorities affect own specific work and how to influence their development or implementation in own area of work;
c. critical reflection and constructive suggestions for how policies, strategies

and priorities could be improved in terms of improving health and wellbeing and reducing health inequalities in own area of work.

Overview

This chapter comprises three sections: 'Policy development in Wales', 'Interpretation and appraisal of policy', and 'Implementation and impact of policy in Wales'. Each section will examine policy in relation to improving the health and wellbeing of children and young people in Wales. It will support your learning by using local examples and challenge your thinking through practice-based activities. The chapter provides an opportunity to look at equivalent examples or strategies being adopted or already implemented in your own geographical area, thereby gaining insight into the complexity of policy development and implementation.

Introduction

The chapter will use Welsh Assembly Government (WAG) and National Assembly of Wales (NAW) policy examples concerning children and young people to facilitate your understanding of the development and implementation of policy generally, as well as to provide insight into policy made in Wales for Wales. In the words of Rhodri Morgan (former First Minister for Wales), policy that aims to *match the core beliefs of the people of Wales* (WAG, 2007a, p3).

Policy development in Wales

This first section guides your exploration of policy development in Wales by taking you on a journey that is directly linked to the public health competence 'Development and implementation of policy – children and young people: a Welsh perspective', as illustrated in Figure 9.1. It is designed to highlight only the main

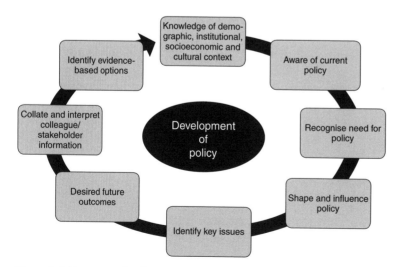

Figure 9.1 Features of policy development identified by public health competences

148

features of the complex iterative process of policy development through the use of local examples and the provision of activities that support self-directed or group enquiry. This section will start by examining key aspects of the policy development context in relation to children and young people in Wales.

Key demographics on Wales

Demographic data provide statistical information on human populations. These data are crucial to responsible policy development by national and local government or institutions, as well as to the co-ordination of policy implementation, not least because demography is a dynamic determinant that is constantly changing. For example, demographic data contribute to the assessment of population needs and enable the identification of key policy issues. They support the monitoring and projection of future trends concerning the geographical location, gender and socio-economic composition, growth and size of affected populations, and the impact of policy in relation to specific needs or issues. Difficult prioritisation of identified issues and policy-related decision making on the distribution of finite resources is underpinned by demographic data. It is important therefore that these data are accurate, timely and in a form that can be accessed and utilised by decision makers. In particular, demographic data can be used to identify health and socioeconomic inequalities between populations at different levels – for example, within a city at a *micro* level, within a country at a *meso* level and between countries on a *macro* level (WHO, 2003; UNICEF, 2009; Marmot, 2010).

The data in Table 9.1 provide a basic insight into the demographic characteristics of Wales compared to the other countries making up the United Kingdom. They also provide statistical information on the demographic structure of Wales in relation to age and gender, changes in population distribution, projected growth of the population, and the life expectancy for males and females. The Health Boards and Local Health Authorities are described. They plan in partnership to provide services that contribute to the protection and improvement of health and wellbeing needs of their respective populations.

Table 9.1 Demographic structure of Wales

Population 2008 (in thousands)

Wales 2,990 Scotland 5,169 Northern Ireland 1,775 England 51,460 UK 61,393
Wales, a small nation that is diverse with a rural population making up one-third of the total.

Wales Children and Young People, 2001 Census:

Males: **Age Range 0–4:** 86,042 **5–9:** 94,750 **10–14:** 100,975 **15–19:** 93,175 **20–24:** 84,382
Females: **Age Range 0–4:** 81,861 **5–9:** 90,575 **10–14:** 95,001 **15–19:** 91,529 **20–24:** 85,111

Life Expectancy 2006–2008 (in years)

Males: Wales 76.9 Scotland 75 Northern Ireland 76.3 England 77.7 UK 77.4
Females: Wales 81.2 Scotland 79.9 Northern Ireland 81.2 England 81.9 UK 81.6

In Wales, the number of people over 85 years of age has increased fivefold from 1951–2001. Adults reporting a life-limiting illness: Wales 23%, Scotland 20%, N Ireland 20%, England 18%. In Wales, 23% of the work-age population report having a work-limiting disability.

Population for areas of Wales in 2001 and 2006, showing population change as a percentage

	2001 population (in thousands)	2006 population (in thousands)	Population change (as a percentage)
North-west Wales	294.3	299.1	*1.6*
North-east Wales	479.9	491.2	*2.3*
Central Wales	362.8	376.2	*3.7*
Pembrokeshire Haven	150.7	155.8	*3.4*
Swansea Bay	548.7	561.9	*2.4*
South-east Wales	1,399.3	1,428.8	*2.1*

Population projections for 2018: England and N Ireland 7% increase; Wales 5% increase.

7 Health Boards: Abertawe Bro Morgannwg University Health Board; Aneurin Bevan Health Board; Betsi Cadwaladr University Health Board; Cardiff & Vale University Health Board; Cwm Taf Health Board; Hywel Dda Health Board; Powys Teaching Health Board.

22 Local Authorities providing services that include trading standards; libraries, leisure and tourism; environmental health, refuse and recycling; transport and highways; housing; social work.

ACTIVITY 9.1 INEQUALITIES IN HEALTH DEMOGRAPHIC ACTIVITY

- Examine the table, 'Age specific mortality rates by local authority 2007', on page 26 of Statistics for Wales (2009) – see full details under 'Useful sources' below. Identify the two local authorities with the highest and lowest mortality rates in each age range for males and females. Put forward possible reasons for these differences.
- Would you expect these reasons to impact positively or negatively on the health and wellbeing of the children and young people living in the identified local authorities? Explain your answers by referring to the existing evidence base.
- Identify and discuss what the key issues would be if you were drafting a national policy to address them. Refer to the local authority website for information to support your answer: http://wales.gov.uk/topics/localgovernment/localauthorities/?lang=en.
- Look for equivalent sources and data from your own geographical area and compare and contrast the key issues raised.

Useful sources

Poverty Site, the (www.poverty.org.uk/summary/wales.htm) monitors what is happening to poverty and social exclusion in the UK, with specific sections for

Scotland, Wales and Northern Ireland, using around 100 statistical indicators covering areas from income and work to health and education.

Save the Children (2008) *Children in Severe Poverty in Wales: An Agenda for Action.* Cardiff: The Wales Programme of Save the Children: www.savethechildren.org. uk/en/docs/wales_poverty_report_08_eng.pdf.

Statistics for Wales (2009) *Wales's Population: A Demographic Overview 2009.* Cardiff: Welsh Assembly Government: http://wales.gov.uk/docs/statistics/ 2009/090326walespop09en.pdf.

Tudor-Smith, C, Head of Health Improvement, WAG: *Tackling Health Inequalities in Wales*, PowerPoint presentation: www.dur.ac.uk/resources/wolfson.institute/ Neil_Riley.pdf.

WAG (2005) *Inequalities in Health: The Welsh Dimension 2002–2005*: http:// wales.gov.uk/dhss/publications/health/reports/inequalitieshealth/inequali- tieshealthe.pdf;jsessionid=Xh4HMVTF311ryZFKc51v1d3FZ4fbLMcRCwxb2 2pxK53TRG0JhV2K!-42672990?lang=en.

The devolved policy-making institutions of Wales

Devolution is defined as, *the process of devolving power from the centre to sub-national units* (Leeke *et al.*, 2003, p7). In theory, it is reversible as under parliamentary sovereignty the devolved institutions are subordinate to the UK Parliament. A referendum on devolution was held in Wales on 18 September 1997, in which the 'yes' campaign won by the narrow majority of 0.6 per cent with only 50.3 per cent of people voting yes. The Government of Wales Act (GOWA) (1998) provided the legislative framework that established the National Assembly for Wales as a single corporate body invested with legislative and executive functions. To enable the transfer of devolved powers, as listed in Table 9.2, from the Secretary of State for Wales to the Assembly for Wales, the 1998 Act also created the National Assembly for Wales (Transfer of Functions) Order 1999. Powers within the fields listed in Table 9.3 are not devolved and the UK Parliament retains control.

The Government of Wales Act of 2006 formally separated the National Assembly for Wales (NAW) and the Welsh Assembly Government (WAG) on 3 May 2007. WAG retained its executive powers and NAW was given Legislative Competence. This allowed NAW to create secondary legislation, defined as new laws in relation to matters listed under Section 5 of the 2006 Government of Wales Act. To create laws on matters that are not listed under Section 5, known as primary legislation, NAW must obtain a Legislative Competence Order (LCO) that must be approved by the NAW, the Secretary of State for Wales, the Houses of Parliament and the Queen.

Table 9.2 Devolved fields

Field 01: Agriculture, fisheries, forestry, rural development
Field 02: Ancient monuments and historical buildings
Field 03: Culture
Field 04: Economic development
Field 05: Education and training
Field 06: Environment
Field 07: Fire and rescue services
Field 08: Food
Field 09: Health and health services
Field 10: Highways and transport
Field 11: Housing
Field 12: Local government
Field 13: National Assembly for Wales
Field 14: Public administration
Field 15: Social welfare
Field 16: Sport and recreation
Field 17: Tourism
Field 18: Town and country planning
Field 19: Water and flood defences
Field 20: Welsh language

Table 9.3 Non-devolved powers

- Defence
- Foreign policy
- Economic, fiscal and monetary policy
- Corporate law and regulation
- Employment and equality legislation
- Social security
- Transport safety and regulation
- Nuclear safety
- Film, video and broadcasting
- The Ordnance Survey
- Assisted area designation
- The National Lottery
- Abortion, human fertilisation, embryology
- Control and safety of medicines
- Vivisection

It is NAW that makes laws and develops policy for Wales on devolved matters, votes on the budget and holds the WAG to account. Sixty politicians, known as Assembly Members (AMs), are democratically elected to NAW to represent the interests of the people of Wales in the assembly building known as the *Senedd*. WAG is a maximum size of 14 ministers, including the First Minister, Cabinet Ministers and the Counsel General, who is the chief legal adviser for the Welsh Government (GOWA, 1998; 2006).

How is Welsh policy distinctive?

It is argued that the system of asymmetrical devolution characteristic of the UK has successfully supported the distinctive identities of each of the devolved countries (Curtice, 2006). Williams (2007) presents a sociological view that devolution has engaged policy makers in socially reconstructing the national identity of Wales, while Day (2002) suggests that contemporary ideas of Wales and Welshness are constructed on multiple understandings and stereotypical images such as traditional, rural, cohesive and working class. Policy cannot be regarded as a neutral and value-free activity.

The ideologies of political parties uphold assumptions on the responsibilities and roles of the individual, society and government. They involve debate on the duty of governments to limit personal liberty in order to protect versus the right of individuals to make choices that may be harmful. The political actors who shape and influence the ideological constructions underpinning policy development hold a diverse range of views, values and ideas as to what the key issues are, their relative importance, how policy should address them, who is 'deserving' or 'undeserving', and how scarce resources should be distributed. Currently, the relationship between political ideology, material interests, political decision making, content based on strong scientific evidence, and the timing of policy is not fully understood. This picture is further complicated by ideological change as political actors face interpretation of new challenges in the context of changing interests, constraints and knowledge.

In Wales, policy can be described as pragmatic, needs specific, ideological on public service delivery and communicating a sense of national identity (Williams, 2007). The principles of social justice, working together, sustainability, regeneration, inclusivity, community cohesion, a right to learn, and promotion of the Welsh language are at the heart of social policy in Wales (WAG, 2007b). For Rhodri Morgan, political ideology embodied fundamental beliefs on how society in Wales should be organised, and on the important role of government in providing publicly provided and delivered services. Meeting need in a fair way through the timely redistribution of wealth and opportunity between children, young people, families and geographical areas are central to Welsh policy. In summary, the 'Clear red waters' speech of Rhodri Morgan, former First Minister for Wales, captures the ideological position of policy development in Wales:

> *The actions of the Welsh Assembly Government clearly owe more to the traditions of Titmuss, Tawney, Beveridge and Bevan rather than Hayek and Friedman. The creation of a new set of citizenship rights has been a key theme in the first four years of the Assembly – and a set of rights which [are] as far as possible: free at point of use, universal and unconditional.*
>
> (www.sochealth.co.uk/Regions/Wales/redwater.htm, accessed January 2011)

ACTIVITY 9.2 POLITICAL POSITIONS ON EQUALITY AND EQUITY

The quotations and further reading below help to provide insight into different ideological positions and their possible influence on policy development and implementation; prioritisation and difficult decision making on the distribution of available resources; and the public- or private-sector emphasis of service delivery. You can identify and explore in depth those that Rhodri Morgan mentioned in his 'Clear red waters' speech.

Beveridge Report (1942) *Social Insurance and Allied Services* (Cmd 6404). London: HMSO: www.sochealth.co.uk/history/beveridge.htm.

Dahrendorf, RG (1969) The nature and types of social inequality, in Beteille, A, *Social Inequality*. Middlesex: Penguin Books (page 21). *The very existence of social inequality . . . is an impetus towards liberty, because it guarantees a society's on-going, dynamic, historical quality. The idea of a perfectly egalitarian society is not only unrealistic, it is terrible.*

Friedman, MA (1962) *Freedom and Capitalism*. Chicago: University of Chicago Press.

Hayek, FA (1944) *The Road to Serfdom*. Chicago: University of Chicago Press.

Tawney, RH (1931) *Equality*. Allen & Unwin (page 47). Equality is viewed as theoretically unattainable but should be *sincerely sought*.

Tawney, RH (1931) *Equality*. Allen & Unwin (page 12). Inequality is described as *A perpetual misdirection of limited resources . . . the human energies which are the source of wealth are, in the case of the majority of the population, systematically under-developed from birth to maturity.*

Titmuss, RM (1970) *The Gift Relationship. From Human Blood to Social Policy*. New York: The New Press. . . . *the study is about the role of altruism in modern society. It attempts to fuse the politics of welfare and the morality of individual wills* (page 59).

YouTube (2008) *NHS at 60. A Look at Bevan and Tredegar*. BBC: www.youtube.com/watch?v=2lLBRs-sT6o&feature=related.

ACTIVITY 9.3 THE POLITICAL INFLUENCES OF WELSH POLICY

- Compare the similarities and differences that characterise the constitutions and policies of the four main political parties represented in the National Assembly for Wales:

  1. Plaid Cymru – www.plaidcymru.org
  2. Welsh Conservative Party – www.welshconservatives.com
  3. Welsh Labour Party – www.welshlabour.org.uk
  4. Welsh Liberal Democrats – http://welshlibdems.org.uk

- Consider how their political ideologies would influence policy development for children and young people in Wales.

The Welsh language and promoting bilingualism

One Wales clearly stated its goal to ensure *that Wales uses its two national languages to their full potential* (WAG, 2007a, p34), as legislated in the Welsh Language Act (1993), which put Welsh and English on an equal footing in public life. An earlier policy review on the Welsh language, conducted by the Culture Committee and Education and Lifelong Learning Committee, stated:

> *In a truly bilingual Wales both Welsh and English will flourish and will be treated as equal. A bilingual Wales means a country where people can choose to live their lives through the medium of either or both languages; a country where the presence of two national languages and cultures is a source of pride and strength to us all.*
>
> (WAG, 2002, p6)

On March 2010 a new measure seeking enhanced legislative competence on the Welsh language was proposed to achieve three key objectives (WAG, 2010g). First, the measure would declare official national status for the Welsh language in Wales. Second, it would approve the appointment of a Welsh Language Commissioner and, last, it would uphold the freedom to speak Welsh by establishing linguistic rights for Welsh speakers in relation to the provision of services. Paul Davies (Conservative Assembly Member) responded to concerns that the proposed legislation may adversely affect businesses and lead to discrimination against non-Welsh speakers, stating:

> *We are determined to ensure this new legislation does not erect barriers to businesses in Wales which would damage investment and competitiveness . . . nor must it discriminate against English speakers.*
>
> (Paul Davies, Conservative AM, March 2004,
> http://news.bbc.co.uk/1/hi/wales/wales_politics/8548279.stm)

The Welsh language is viewed by people living in Wales as a symbol of Welsh identity (Economic and Research Council, 2004). *One Wales* upheld that the Welsh language *belongs to everyone in Wales as part of our common national heritage, identity and public good* (WAG, 2007a, p34).

Challenges arise due to the concentration of Welsh speakers in particular areas, the differences in Welsh language capability between generations and the partisan connotations of the language (Economic and Research Council, 2004). Aitchison and Carter (2004) also reported that the 2001 population census showed possible socioeconomic divisions between Welsh speakers, indicating that they were less likely than the rest of the population to be long-term unemployed or employed in routine or semi-routine occupations. In addition, the 2001 population census also indicated that there appeared to be a marked lack of parental transmission of the Welsh language to their children, particularly when only one parent was a Welsh speaker. Should this situation be allowed to continue, it would certainly threaten the future survival of the Welsh language. Relatively little is known about the complex acquisition and socialisation factors that influence the transfer of the Welsh language.

Table 9.4 presents the views of people in Wales on a number of Welsh language options that might shape policy development and implementation. The survey found that the majority of people living in Wales accept that more Welsh language speakers need be trained to occupy new posts, which would support an increased bilingual capacity of public service delivery. However, there is opposition to certain jobs being reserved for bilingual speakers and a controversial proposal to restrict immigrants buying property in Welsh-speaking areas (Economic and Research Council, 2004, p5).

Table 9.4 Attitudes to the Welsh language

	Strongly agree (%)	*Agree (%)*	*Disagree (%)*	*Strongly disagree (%)*	*Don't know (%)*
The Welsh language is an important part of Welsh identity	37	47	13	2	1
We need to train more people who speak Welsh to take up posts in the public sector	16	51	22	6	5
Certain jobs in Wales should be reserved for bilingual speakers	7	39	39	12	3
There should be restrictions on immigrants buying property in mainly Welsh-speaking areas	8	16	48	21	7

Source: Economic and Research Council (2004, p5)

Drivers and inhibitors of policy for children and young people in Wales

Policy drivers can be viewed from two opposing positions. They can be viewed negatively as broadly defining the problem, or positively as describing a desired outcome of policy. For example, access to healthcare provision or enhancing the skills of young people can be viewed from both the problem and outcome positions. Understanding policy drivers provides insight into the issues that are impacting on public need, expectation and opinion. They instigate the policy-making process because they require governments, both national and local, to prioritise issues and make difficult decisions on aims and objectives, ethical issues that arise, resource allocation and target population group. Inevitably, policy decisions will benefit some members of society but not others, producing winners and losers. A range of factors will drive or inhibit policy outcomes, and this is illustrated in Figure 9.2.

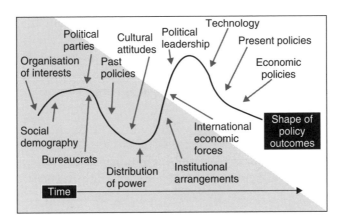

Figure 9.2 Factors influencing policy outcomes over time

Source: Parsons (1996, p509)

The policy responses engendered will reflect the influence of the ideological position of government, as discussed earlier in the chapter. They will also reflect the differential power, authority, priorities and value positions of a range of interest groups to changing global and national factors, including demographic, socioeconomic, cultural, environmental and lifestyle trends. Meier (1991) distinguishes between state-centred and society-centred groups, as shown in Figure 9.3.

The policy case study on *One Wales* (WAG, 2007a) will now be incorporated into the chapter in order to highlight important policy drivers in Welsh policy.

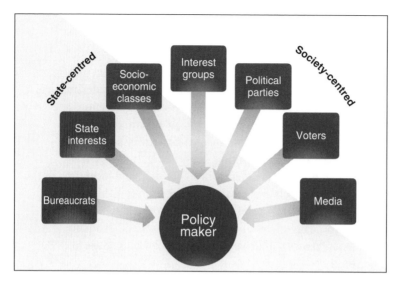

Figure 9.3 Interest groups, power and authority

Source: adapted from Meier (1991)

One Wales: A Progressive Agenda for the Government of Wales. An Agreement between the Labour and Plaid Cymru Groups in the National Assembly (WAG, 2007b)

This document presents a progressive agenda for improving the quality of life for the people of Wales. Driving the policy agenda is a commitment by Labour and Plaid Cymru to uphold the principles of social justice, sustainability and inclusivity. Policy drivers identified encompass the geographical, social, linguistic and cultural diversity of Wales, and are comprehensive in their coverage, including health, society, communities, learning, environment and culture.

Policy drivers for children include:

- ensuring access to healthcare;
- improving patient experience;
- supporting social care;
- creating jobs across Wales;
- enhancing skills for jobs;
- establishing a right to learning;
- ensuring the best start for young children;
- creating twenty-first-century schools;
- tackling child poverty and inequalities;
- ensuring an effective youth and criminal justice system.

For example, the Welsh Assembly Government identified a number of key barriers to the provision of mental health services for children and young people in Wales during a review conducted by the Healthcare Inspectorate Wales (HIW) and the Wales Audit Office, published in November 2009. The case study next goes on to examine the review's findings in relation to inhibitors identified by the 2001 *Children and Adolescent Mental Health Services (CAMHS) Strategy, Everybody's Business* (National Assembly of Wales (NAW), 2001).

Everybody's Business (NAW, 2001) identified the following concerns on the provision of CAMHS:

- services based on historical patterns, not the needs of children and young people;

- poorly developed multi-agency collaboration on planning and delivery of services;

- inadequately trained staff to deal with mental health issues;

- inadequately trained staff to safeguard children and young people;

- staff were uncertain of their role in dealing with mental health issues;

- a lack of education and training opportunities for staff;

- distribution, focus, role and volume of specialised services needed rethinking.

Services for Children and Young People with Emotional Needs (WAG, 2009) found that, although improvements had been achieved since *Everybody's Business*, there were a number of key barriers to overcome:

- a lack of clarity on the role and responsibilities of different agencies, resulting in

  - areas of service provision remaining underdeveloped – for example, those targeting children and young people at risk of mental health issues

  - unacceptable variation in availability, access and quality of services for children over 5 years and no services for children under 5 years of age;

- inadequate co-ordination of services – for example, at transition from child to adult mental health services or between educational psychology and CAMHS, and information sharing;

- difficulty professionals have in understanding the different roles of other professionals and agencies involved;

- the complexity and range of services presents a challenge for coherent, consistent leadership, planning and commissioning;

- Children and Young People Partnership Plans agreed by the Local Health Boards and Local Authorities are not providing clear strategic direction for CAMHS.

Children and young people as actors in policy

The United Nations Convention on the Rights of the Child (1989) guides policy development by the WAG on children and young people. *Children and Young People: Rights to Action* clearly states that *Children and young people should be seen as citizens, with rights and opinions to be taken into account now. They are not a species apart, to be alternately demonised and sentimentalised, nor trainee adults who do not yet have a full place in society* (WAG, 2004b, p4). The Participation Unit of Save the Children in Wales has developed the National Children and Young People's Participation Standards which aim to improve children's participation in services that affect them. *Children in Wales* (WAG, 2007c) supported the position held by many children, young people and their advocates that lowering the voting age from 18 to 16 years may help to politically empower children and give due recognition to the economic contribution that many young people of this age make to Wales. It identified the promotion of children and young people as *Citizens of their Community* for immediate action (WAG, 2007c, p12). The WAG consultation document, *Proposals for a Rights of Children and Young Persons (Wales) Measure* (2010d) gives comprehensive recognition to the important contribution that children and young people can make to improving communities in Wales. If agreed by the National Assembly for Wales it will make Wales the first country in the United Kingdom, and one of the few in Europe, to commit to integrating the Convention on the Rights of the Child (UN, 1989) into law.

ACTIVITY 9.4 EXPLORING THE VOICE OF CHILDREN IN WALES

Explore the following websites so that you are familiar with their aim and content:

- Pupil Voice Wales – www.pupilvoicewales.org.uk
- Funky Dragon – www.funkydragon.org
- Children and Young People's Partnerships – for example, the Cardiff Children and Young People's Plan: Partners Working Together to Improve Services for Children and Young People in Cardiff – www.ifanc.org.uk
- Children in Wales, web page for access to all Children and Young People's Plans across Wales – www.childreninwales.org.uk/index.html
- British Youth Council, UK Young Ambassadors give young people a voice in Europe – www.byc.org.uk/Represent-the-UK-Young-Ambassadors
- UK Youth Parliament – www.ukyouthparliament.org.uk

Look for equivalent sources in your own geographical area.

Interpretation and appraisal of policy

Aspects of interpretation and appraisal of policy require an in-depth baseline knowledge of contemporary demographic and socioeconomic trends and the impact of recent policy. The process of appraisal will involve the identification of the key issues, focus and desired outcomes of the policy, including their relation to the existing evidence base, demographic, socioeconomic and service trends. Drawing on the appraisal findings, changes may be recommended that need to be supported by the presentation of relevant information and coherent evidence-based arguments. This process is illustrated in Figure 9.4.

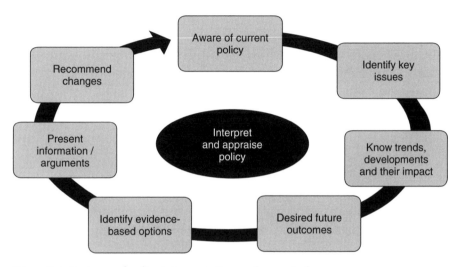

Figure 9.4 Features of policy interpretation and appraisal

Interpretation and appraisal of policy involves understanding the issues that are driving it. These by may be local, concerned with need or opinion – for example, the *Children and Young People's Partnership Plans* that Health Boards and local authorities are required to produce; national, such as social justice and equity upheld in *One Wales* (WAG, 2007b) setting out an agenda for the government of Wales by Labour and Plaid Cymru; or, international – for example, economic, security, climate change, and the rights of children and young people. Scrutiny of the policy intentions and objectives will involve asking an array of questions: Is it redistributive? How is it redistributive? Is it integrative? How is it integrative? Does it positively discriminate in favour of certain population groups? How does it do this? How does it address socioeconomic inequalities? Who benefits and how? Who loses out and how? Does it aim to drive specific service delivery approaches like inter-professional and multi-agency working?

Extending Entitlement: Supporting Young People in Wales (NAW, 2000)

This report was produced to inform the development of the Assembly's policies for young people aged 11 to 25 years. The scope of the report was to outline the principles underpinning the development of policies for young people, improve connections between policies and suggest priorities for action. It took full account of the Assembly's commitment to the UN Convention on the Rights of the Child. Importantly, it began a process of policy development that promoted a more holistic and universal entitlement to quality services, a central tenet of the youth service. It also recognised the need to tackle the gaps in services for young people, and to prevent and reduce social exclusion. By embracing a partnership multi-disciplinary model of service delivery, its target was to provide a comprehensive service that aimed to promote inclusion, offer opportunity and motivate young people to engage on a voluntary participation basis.

ACTIVITY 9.5 PAIRED INTERPRETATION AND APPRAISAL

Extending Entitlement (NAW, 2000) acknowledges the strong links between the health and social welfare of young people.

- What are the policy aims?
- What political agenda do you think has influenced the policy aims?
- Outline how this policy will achieve its aims.
- Which professionals and groups of people are most likely to be involved in this?
- How will this policy affect the way a range of professionals work?
- Decide whether you agree or not with the key principles outlined in this document, and justify your position.

Appraisal will also involve examining the administration, funding and decision making evidenced by the policy, and linking these to political ideology, prioritisation, ethical issues that arise and the evidence base. Examination of non-decision making is as important as scrutiny of decisions agreed. Ham and Hill (1993) understand policy development as a dynamic process involving a complex web of decisions by a network of diverse decision makers extending over a long period of time to support or constrain government action.

ACTIVITY 9.6 APPRAISING CHILDREN IN WALES

Children in Wales is the national children's organisation umbrella in Wales. See: www.childreninwales.org.uk/index.html.

- What are its aims and objectives? How do these sit with the political ideology of Wales?
- How does it influence and support new and existing policy initiatives?
- What equivalents are there in England, Northern Ireland, Scotland, Europe and worldwide?
- What similarities and differences can you identify between the organisations in the positions they hold on policy for children and young people?
- What explanations would you give for the similarities and differences you have identified?

Features of modern policy making

Bullock *et al.* (2001, p14) identified nine features of modern policy making, as shown in Table 9.5, which can be used as benchmarks against which policy can be appraised. They view the policy-making process as highly complex for three main reasons. First, the policy-making context is often dynamic and unpredictable over time. Second, this context involves changing interdependent factors that interact at local, national, UK, European and global levels. Last, the issues instigating the need for policy are multi-faceted and unstable, rarely sitting within the remit of a single agency or professional (Hunter and Ritchie, 2008). The importance of listening, learning, reviewing, evaluating and responding to what is current is emphasised. To achieve this requires the utilisation of contemporary research evidence; learning lessons from other countries, through prior experience and by sharing good practice; consultation with stakeholders, professionals and service users, including children and young people; and the embedding of review and evaluation in the policy-making process.

Table 9.5 Nine features of modern policy making

Looking forward	*Evidence based*	*Review*
• Clear outcomes identified early in the policy-making process • Contingency planning that recognises the dynamic and complex nature of the policy-making context • Includes consideration of the long-term view based on statistical forecasting of future socioeconomic and demographic trends	• Decision making is based on a review of existing research early in the policy-making process • Commissions new research to support the decision-making process, prioritisation and targeting of population groups • Is consultative and gives consideration to a range of experts, stakeholder and service user views, including children and young people • Policy options are rigorously costed and evaluated for their benefits and disadvantages	• Ongoing review against measurable outcomes to ensure the policy is successfully tackling the issues it was designed to address • Provide opportunities for stakeholders and service users, including children and young people, to feed back on the impact of the policy from their perspectives • Appropriate changes made in the light of information obtained from review. Changes may include minor modification of existing policy strategy, agreeing a number of new additional outcomes, to abandoning a failing policy
Outward looking	*Inclusive*	*Evaluation*
• Considers the national, UK, European and global context, including possible influences on Wales	• Consults and seeks feedback from those responsible for service delivery and therefore the	• Systematic evaluation is ensured by the identification of appropriate evaluation points during the policy-

- Learns from how other countries deal with the issues identified for policy
- Recognises variations within Wales
- Plans how the policy will be communicated to the public

implementation of the policy
- Consults and seeks feedback from service users, including children and young people, who will be on the receiving end of policy implementation
- Assesses the impact of policy implementation on target populations

making process – that is, evaluation is viewed as an integral part of the policy-making process and is therefore built in to the policy-making process from the start
- Identification of success criteria; these criteria will embrace qualitative or quantitative evidence of changes that demonstrate the achievement of the policy outcomes
- Use of pilots to support difficult decision making

Innovative and flexible	*Joined up*	*Learning approach*
<ul><li>The process is open to the ideas and perspectives of stakeholders, professionals and service users, including children and young people</li><li>The process is open to non-traditional innovative ideas and methods of policy making</li><li>The policy-making process identifies, assesses and manages any risks</li><li>Effectively brings people from the outside into the policy-making team</li></ul>	<ul><li>Collaborative working arrangements are clearly identified and roles defined based on an understanding of the respective legal, ethical and professional positions of the agencies and professionals involved</li><li>Barriers to effective joined-up working are identified, and strategies put in place to minimise their impact or overcome them</li><li>To understand the rationale for joined-up working, which will include the need for a holistic approach to tackle complex and unpredictable issues</li></ul>	<ul><li>A learning approach to policy development is used</li><li>This requires that lessons are learned from prior experience through utilisation of the evidence base, consultation, evaluation and review processes</li><li>Distinguishing between failure of the policy to address the problem and operational difficulties of implementation</li><li>Dissemination and sharing of good practice</li></ul>

Source: adapted from Bullock *et al*. (2001, p14)

Implementation and impact of policy in Wales

Implementation can be defined as action that mobilises identified resources to carry out planned actions directed at achieving the agreed outcomes within the planned costs over the agreed timescale. Two schools of thought have evolved that describe the process of implementation as *top down (downstream)* or *bottom up* (upstream). *Top-down* models of policy implementation include academic advocacy such as think-tanks, research institutes and universities; governments, government and non-government organisations. *Bottom-up* models of policy implementation include community-based participatory and capacity-building approaches.

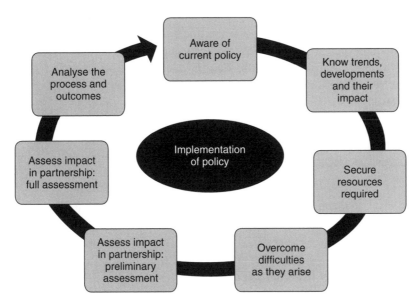

Figure 9.5   Features of policy implementation

Translating policy into action for children and young people in Wales

Since devolution, the Welsh Assembly Government has introduced initiatives that have made a real difference to the everyday lives of children and young people. These initiatives emanate from policy developments that reflect national and local priorities, such as tackling lifestyle issues and obesity (WAG, 2004a). Their scope, focus, aims, approach and desired outcomes reflect the political ideology of the government, intrinsically influencing the identification and prioritisation of issues as well as decision making on resource allocation and target population group. The initiatives below illustrate policy translation into action that increasingly has emphasis on multidisciplinary, multi-agency, preventative and early intervention solutions.

- The Primary School Free Breakfast Initiative aims to give a flying start to the youngest children by increasing their capacity to learn and achieve by improving their health and concentration through provision of healthy nutrition (WAG, 2007d; 2008).

- The Welsh Network of Healthy School Schemes (WNHSS) was established to promote local healthy schools schemes within a national framework by providing guidance and facilitating the sharing of information on local schemes through supporting networking between professionals, schools and at network events (WAG, 2008a).

- Free Swimming for Children and Young People Initiative for those aged 16 and under improves access to local authority leisure services at specific times in order to increase participation in physical activity and improve health and wellbeing (WAG, 2010c).

- The Cooking Bus was launched in 2006 and is funded by WAG. It is part of the Food and Fitness Implementation Plan (WAG, 2007d) to improve the health and wellbeing of children and young people in Wales by targeting its visits to schools in the Welsh Network of Healthy Schools Scheme and those located in Communities First Areas (WAG, 2008b).

- The Foundation Phase is the curriculum for 3–7 year olds in Wales. It is based on the principle of learning by doing through play, with greater emphasis on achieving understanding and developing problem solving (WAG, 2010f).

- Eco-Schools uses a whole-school approach, reaching out to parents and the community, to promote environmental awareness across the curriculum and to support schools towards more sustainable operations (WAG, 2010a).

Investigating the evidence base of policy

Evidence-based policy making (EBP) gained momentum under Tony Blair's 1997 New Labour government. EBP advocates a more systematic, rational approach to informing the policy-making process, claiming to achieve a movement away from political ideological opinion-based influences. Underpinning its rationale is a view that policy and practice based on the best available evidence will produce better outcomes. However, different forms of evidence do not have equal standing or relevance. The problem that arises is how to determine what constitutes good evidence, and this has led to the hierarchical ranking of evidence to justify the choice of evidence (Evans, 2003). This has, in turn, led to an emphasis on empirical data, often referred to as 'hard evidence', at the expense of tacit forms of practice-based knowledge. Increasingly, there is a view that a wide range of evidential sources should be used to inform policy making, including the voices of ordinary people, children and young people.

ACTIVITY 9.7

- Choose one of the initiatives outlined earlier in the chapter and locate or download relevant information from the internet.
- By searching for literature using appropriate databases, find published literature that could support the aims and objectives of your chosen initiative.
- Find information on hierarchies of evidence – for example, the paper written by David Evans (see below) – and identify the type of evidence you have found.

Discuss how it is relevant and appropriate to use as supporting evidence for your chosen initiative.
- Now use this approach to look at an initiative in your own area of practice

Useful sources

Bullock, H, Mountford, J and Stanley, R (2001) *Better Policy-Making*. London: Centre for Management and Policy Studies, Cabinet Office. Online at: www.civilservant.org.uk/betterpolicymaking.pdf.

Evans, D (2003) Hierarchy of evidence: a framework for ranking evidence evaluating healthcare interventions. *Journal of Clinical Nursing*, 12: 77–84.

Sutcliffe, S and Court, J (2006) *A Toolkit for Progressive Policymakers in Developing Countries*. London: Overseas Development Institute.

Assessing impact: ensuring the survival of the Welsh language

Impact assessment asks 'What has happened?' and enables greater understanding of what works, what does not and what is relevant to the effective implementation of policy. It also provides a tool that can support good decision making and a means of accountability on progress towards achieving policy outcomes.

Twf is a Welsh Language Board project sponsored by the Welsh Assembly Government, set up to increase the transmission of the Welsh language from the target group, mixed-language-speaking parents, to their children. Research on the revitalisation of minority languages identifies the crucial role played by the home and family in transmitting language from one generation to the next. It was launched under the name of Twf in March 2002 following a successful pilot in Carmarthenshire. It aims to raise awareness of the benefits of bilingualism with parents and prospective parents; midwives and health visitors working with families; the public at large; and to change the spoken language patterns of mixed-language families so that greater numbers of children speak Welsh at home.

ACTIVITY 9.8

Download the Twf report using the details below:

Edwards, VK and Newcombe, LM (2003) *Evaluation of the Efficiency and Effectiveness of the Twf Project, Which Encourages Parents to Transmit the Language to Their Children*. University of Reading. Online at: www.byig-wlb.org.uk/Pages/Hafan.aspx.

- How was the Twf project's impact, efficacy and effectiveness evaluated?
- What insights to the project did you gain from this analysis?

Chapter 9 summary

This chapter identified the competences for public health in relation to the development and implementation of policy on children and young people in Wales. The chapter sections provided activities to support your learning on policy development, appraisal, implementation and impact assessment.

GOING FURTHER

Davies, J (2007) *A History of Wales*. Harmondsworth: Penguin Books. *This is a history of Wales, from the earliest times to the late twentieth century.*

Day, G, Dunkerley, D and Thompson, A (eds) (2006) *Civil Society in Wales: Policy, Politics and People* (Politics and Society in Wales Series). University of Wales Press. *This book provides a critical evaluation of some of the main themes and points of contention in debates on civil society, past and present, with particular reflection on the consequences of devolution for civil society in Wales.*

Royles, E (2007) *Revitalising Democracy: Devolution and Civil Society in Wales* (Politics and Society in Wales). University of Wales Press. *This study examines the impact of devolution on civil society during the Welsh Assembly's first term, with a particular focus on civil society's contribution to enhancing democracy, and the interrelationship between civil society and national identity.*

The following resources provide a wealth of further reading on Wales and its public policies and statistics following devolution.

Institute of Welsh Politics: www.aber.ac.uk/interpol/ (all the reports can be downloaded free at www.aber.ac.uk/interpol/en/research/IWP/template_for_gwenan.html).

National Centre for Public Policy: www.swansea.ac.uk/ncpp

Statistics for Wales (2009) *Wales's Population – A Demographic Overview, 2009.* Cardiff: Welsh Assembly Government. Online at: www.wales.gov.uk/docs/statistics/2009/090326walespop09en.pdf.

Welsh Legislation Online: www.wales-legislation.org.uk

chapter 10

Communities and Health: A Scottish Perspective

Jean Cowie and Linda Mages

Meeting the Public Health Competences

Core area 3: Policy and strategy development and implementation to improve population health and wellbeing

This chapter will help you evidence the following competences for public health (Public Health Skills and Career Framework):

- Level 6(4): Contribute to assessing the potential or actual impact of policies and strategies on health and wellbeing in own area of work;
- Level 7(1): Interpret and communicate local, regional and national policies and strategies within own area of work;
- Level 7(2): Work with a range of people and agencies to implement policies and strategies in interventions, programmes and services;
- Level 7(3): Contribute to the development of policies and strategies beyond own area of work;
- Level 7(5): Assess the actual or potential impact of policies and strategies on health and wellbeing;
- Level 7(7): Alert the relevant people to issues and gaps in policies and strategies that are affecting health and wellbeing.

This chapter will also assist you in demonstrating the following National Occupational Standard(s) for public health:

- PHP31: Work in partnership with others to implement strategies for improving health and wellbeing;
- PHP34: Work in partnership with others to undertake a full assessment of the impact of policies and strategies on health and wellbeing;
- PHP35: Advise how health improvement can be promoted in policy;
- PHP37: Evaluate and review the effects of policies on health improvement.

This chapter should also be useful in demonstrating Standard 10 of the Public Health Practitioner Standards:

Standard 10: Support the implementation of policies and strategies to improve health and wellbeing outcomes – demonstrating:

a. knowledge of the main public health policies and strategies relevant to own area of work and the organisations that are responsible for them;

b. how different policies, strategies and priorities affect own specific work and how to influence their development or implementation in own area of work;

c. critical reflection and constructive suggestions for how policies, strategies and priorities could be improved in terms of improving health and wellbeing and reducing health inequalities in own area of work.

Overview

This chapter will examine the development and implementation of policy within communities, taking a Scottish perspective. First, a brief overview of Scotland with reference to relevant policy will be provided to set the chapter in context. Then the concept of community will be defined prior to exploration of the different approaches to working with communities. This will be followed by examples of strategies and initiatives from both urban and rural and remote areas of Scotland, to address inequalities in health at a local level, and to improve the effectiveness of the NHS systems in terms of resources and access to services.

Introduction

Public health practitioners can work in many different ways to enable them to work towards National Occupational Standards for public health, and to improve national and local services as identified in the Knowledge and Skills Framework (Skills for Health, 2009). Strengthening community action, as identified in the Ottawa Charter (World Health Organization (WHO), 1986), is one significant way to improve public health, taking both a top-down and bottom-up approach.

Scotland: an overview

To understand the differing health and social care needs in Scotland as compared to the rest of the UK, it is necessary to have an understanding of the geography of Scotland as well as the demography. Scotland covers a land mass area of approximately 78,772 square kilometres and has a population of approximately 5,165,000, while the population of England is estimated to be 61,792,000 and the land mass 130,410 square kilometres. Indeed more people live in London, which has a population of 7.5 million, than live in Scotland as a whole. The population density of Scotland is 64 people per square kilometre, compared to 395 people per square kilometre in England and over 10,000 per square kilometre in London. Similar to other western countries, the demographics are changing, with an increasingly ageing population, a particular growth in the number of people over 75 and a decline in the birth rate over the past 20 years (General Register Office, 2009).

With regard to healthcare provision and access to services, the geography of Scotland creates many challenges. It has many mountain ranges that separate populations and make distances that would be short as the crow flies very long and arduous journeys. In addition to the challenges on the mainland, Scotland also has 800 islands, of which 130 are inhabited; again this poses challenges for access to health services. From Figure 10.1 you will see that only four cities in Scotland have a population density greater than 1,000 people per square kilometre and that the greater density of people live in central Scotland, in and around the two largest cities, Glasgow and Edinburgh. The majority of Scotland has a population density of 10–99 people per square kilometre or, as in the Highland Region, 0–9 people per square kilometre. It is said (Scottish Government, 2008a) that one in five people in Scotland live in a remote and rural area. Everyone in Scotland, however, should have an equal right to access good-quality and appropriate healthcare. The geography of Scotland, therefore, can lead to an inequality in access to healthcare services for communities and people living in remote and rural areas. With the challenge of providing healthcare in remote and rural areas comes the issue of professionals maintaining their skills and practice. Potentially, this could impact on the quality of care that communities and people living in remote and rural areas could expect to receive, again leading to an inequality in service provision. Consequently this has led to increasing use of technology, such as telemedicine, and also role development and overlap between health professionals in an attempt to provide the same standard of healthcare in remote and rural areas as one would expect in an urban area.

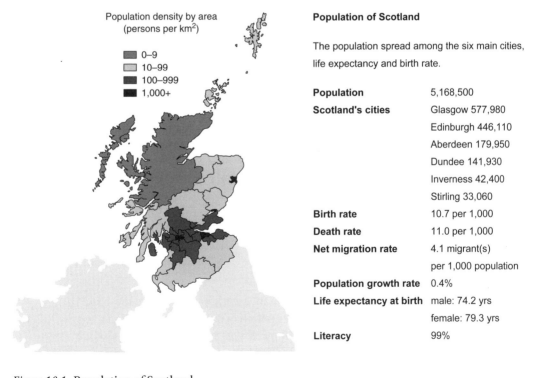

Figure 10.1 Population of Scotland

Source: reproduced courtesy of Scottish Government, 2010 (www.scotland.org/facts/population, accessed 11 November 2010)

Policy context in Scotland

Although on the whole Scotland's health is improving, tackling inequalities in health continues to be a key challenge that remains high on the political agenda. For example, the Scottish Government (2008b) highlighted a ten-year difference in healthy life expectancy between men living in the most deprived areas of Scotland (57.3 years) and the average for men in Scotland (67.9 years). Furthermore, those living in the most deprived areas of Scotland were reported to have a suicide risk that was twice the Scottish average, while people striving on a low income and in poverty had poorer mental health and wellbeing than their wealthier peers (Scottish Government, 2008b). Nevertheless the government in Scotland has acknowledged that life circumstances – that is, housing, education and employment – can have a major impact on health and wellbeing, as can a person's age, gender, disability, race and religion (Scottish Government, 2008b). Living in poverty therefore isn't just about surviving on a low income, it is also intrinsically linked with poor access to resources and services, lack of opportunity and, ultimately, low aspirations. Consequently, since devolution in 1999 the government in Scotland has pledged to address inequalities in health and life circumstances, and to promote social justice (Scottish Office, 1999). Health improvement, therefore, as advocated by the World Health Organization (WHO, 1986) is not the sole remit of the health service – it involves working in partnership with local authorities, and statutory and voluntary agencies, and this is reflected in the ensuing policies and strategies concerned with health improvement. Following the publication of the White Paper *Partnerships for Care* (Scottish Executive, 2003a), Community Health Partnerships were established throughout Scotland.

The general aim of Community Health Partnerships (Scottish Executive, 2004) is to promote partnership working between health services, local authorities, voluntary sectors and other stakeholders (e.g. social work, housing, education and regeneration); to actively involve the public, patients and carers in decisions that affect the planning and delivery of healthcare and health services for their communities; with the ultimate goal of promoting and supporting health improvement in local communities, as well as improving services for the local people.

The work and activities of Community Health Partnerships, therefore, focus on the following three key policy areas:

1. shifting the balance of care to more local settings;

2. reducing inequalities in health;

3. improving the health of local people.

Multi-professional and multi-agency collaborative working is central to the success of Community Health Partnerships. The notion of partnership working, however, was further strengthened in *Delivering for Health* (Scottish Executive, 2005); *Better Health: Better Care* (Scottish Government, 2007b) and, more recently, in the *Scottish Community Empowerment Action Plan* (Scottish Government, 2009a). In tandem with the emphasis on partnership working, key themes central to all these policies included the concepts of participation and empowerment, as well as a focus on communities. This emphasis on partnership and multi-agency working, therefore,

---

ACTIVITY 10.1

Given that many policies within Scotland, and indeed the UK, are influenced by the World Health Organization, you may find it useful to:

- review relevant local and national policy documents, and examine the commonalities;
- consider the influence of the WHO on the strategies and recommendations within these national and local policies, and how they impact on the health of communities.

---

has led to a convergence on community-based and community development-focused health improvement interventions.

Community working

Defining community

The concept of the term 'community' appears difficult to define in that it can mean different things to different people. For example, 'community' can be used to refer to a geographical area or neighbourhood. However, living together within a geographical area does not necessarily equate to commonality of interest or community spirit. Alternatively, the term can be used with regard to groups of people that share characteristics or interests, such as the 'gay community', homeless people or other ethnic or religious groups. These groups of people may, or may not, live within a defined geographical area. Nevertheless when using the word 'community' it is important to clarify its meaning within the context in which it is used. Laverack (2009) identified the following key characteristics of 'community' that may be useful in defining the concept in practice:

- spatial dimension referring to place or location;

- non-spatial dimension – that is, heterogeneous groups of people that share interests, issues or identities;

- social interactions that are often powerful in nature, and tie people into relationships or strong bonds with each other;

- sharing of needs and concerns that can be addressed by collective and collaborative actions.

Community-led approach to health improvement

The Scottish Executive (2003b) highlighted that, for health improvement to be effective, it needed to be community led. Within this context a community-led approach to health improvement recognised that disadvantaged and vulnerable people need to have a voice, and to be heard. For social injustice and inequalities to be tackled in earnest, the disadvantaged in society need to be given the opportunity to express the challenges they face and to identify their needs as they see them, and also to be involved in identifying and addressing actual and potential solutions. A community-led approach to health improvement therefore is a bottom-up approach to health improvement that should influence local strategy and top-down approaches for health improvement (Dailly and Barr, 2008). This approach to health improvement also acknowledges that top-down strategies on their own are ineffective in truly addressing the complexity of factors influencing and often reinforcing disadvantage and inequality.

Community development

Community development as an approach to health promotion has attracted increasing attention in recent years. However, the concept is not new and, according to Wills (2009), can be traced back to colonialism in the nineteenth century, where it was used as a means of social control. More recently, in the 1970s and 1980s, community development tended to be associated with activities to address issues related to inequalities (Wills, 2009). Dalziel (2000) indicates that community development is an approach that aims to involve vulnerable and socially excluded people in decision-making processes. In other words, it aims to promote and foster empowerment at both an individual and a community level. The National Occupational Standards in Community Development Work (Lifelong Learning UK, 2009) state that the key purpose of community development work is collectively to *bring about social change and justice, by working with communities to:*

- *identify their needs, opportunities, rights and responsibilities*

- *plan, organise and take action*

- *evaluate the effectiveness and impact of the action in ways which challenge oppressions and tackle inequalities.*

Community development therefore is concerned with equality and equity of opportunity, and strives to include the vulnerable and socially excluded, by fostering empowerment, participation and partnership working with people in the communities in which they work, live and play. The National Occupational Standards for Community Development Work (Lifelong Learning UK, 2009) identify the following five key values and principles that support and underpin community development work:

1. equality and anti-discrimination;

2. social justice;

3. collective action;

4. community empowerment;

5. working and learning together.

Community development should not, however, be confused with community-based health improvement work. Community-based work, although addressing the needs of, and actively engaged in, communities tends to have a top-down approach and to be professional or agency driven, and operating within the confines of local or national agendas (Gilchrist, 2007; Wills, 2009). Community development, on the other hand, utilises a community-led approach to health improvement. It aims to actively engage with the people in the community and empower them to identify their own needs and priorities, as well as to work in partnership with them to effectively address these. A key difference between the two approaches, therefore, is in the balance of power. With community-based health improvement strategies, the professionals retain the power, whereas power is more equally shared with the participants and the community in community development work. The professionals in community development work act as facilitators and attempt to shift the balance of power by giving the participants and the community greater power in the decision-making processes. A useful differentiation between the two approaches is shown in Table 10.1.

Table 10.1 Comparison of community-based and community development work

Community-based health improvement	*Community development*
Professional led in that needs, targets and actions are set by the professional or sponsor	Community led in that needs, targets and actions are identified by the community
Emphasis on imparting knowledge; usually facilitated by a professional	Local and individual knowledge and expertise valued equally with that of the professional
Community seen as medium, venue or setting for intervention	Focus on capacity building and empowerment within the community
Generally concerned with individuals within a defined geographical area	Concerned with community structures and services that can impact on the health of the community
Actions and interventions generally health orientated	Interventions and activities more broad based and take account of the wider influences on health, with related concepts such as social capital and empowerment also considered
Decision making processes and power unequally shared. Professional has more power	Efforts made to ensure that decision making processes and power shared more equally with those in the community

Source: adapted from Sines *et al*. (2009, p 53); Cowley (2008, p114)

Case studies demonstrating community development and community-based health improvement in Scotland are shown later in this chapter

Social capital

A key tenet that can be considered an outcome of community development work, as well as a factor that can influence the success of community development work, is the concept of social capital. Essentially, social capital refers to the networks among people, and the benefits and shared values that arise from these networks. It is also concerned with citizenship, neighbourliness and civic participation, as well as social networks. Key factors identified by the Office for National Statistics (Economic and Social Data Service, 2010) that underpin the notion of social capital include:

- views of the local area and satisfaction with living in the area;

- civic participation, and the ability to take action on local and national issues;

- social networks and support such as contact with friends and relatives;

- social participation and involvement in local groups and/or voluntary activities;

- trust, mutual agreement and 'give and take'.

These factors are also integrated within community development work. There has been an increasing interest in the concept of social capital in recent years, particularly following the government focus on social inclusion in 1999 (Scottish Office, 1999). Evidence is also available to suggest that health outcomes are improved in instances where the social capital is high (Putman *et al.*, 1993). Cognisance of the role and value of social capital in promoting optimum health and wellbeing should be central within all community development work.

ACTIVITY 10.2

Compare the principles and values of community development with the principles of health promotion (WHO, 1986). You will be aware that equity, empowerment, participation and partnership working are all key elements of community development work. However, adopting and incorporating these approaches into practice can, in some instances, prove quite challenging. In order to develop your understanding of communities and community development work, you may find it useful to undertake a 'community walk' or 'neighbourhood study' to learn about the services, resources and dynamics within a given area. For some of you this will be a different way of working and learning. This can prove invaluable in learning about a community and its needs, and to build networks and links with the local residents, as well as other professionals and agencies working within that environment or geographical patch.

Community initiatives

Remote and rural healthcare

The national agenda in Scotland, as well as in the rest of the UK, has committed itself to supporting people within their own homes and local communities. A major challenge in Scotland is the provision of health to those living in remote and rural areas. Government statistics indicate that an ageing population live in the more remote and rural areas. Coupled with the increase in people suffering from long-term conditions this creates an additional burden on an already stretched National Health Service (NHS). In addition to this in Scotland, rural areas tend to experience more road traffic collisions. This is particularly relevant in the more northern parts of Scotland where the road structure is not as developed as in central Scotland. Again this leads to extra demand on the health service and great pressure on health professionals to be competent in dealing with a wide range of health conditions, and also varying degrees of seriousness and emergency of presenting health issues. In addition to this, the geographical nature of Scotland can create difficulties for emergency services in gaining access to communities and individuals in the remote and rural areas, and conversely for such patients to access specialist services. This creates an enormous challenge, especially as the Scottish Government (2008a) states that everyone in Scotland should have equal access to the NHS regardless of where they live. Consequently, to try to overcome this problem, there has been an increasing interest in the role of community hospitals and also in the use of technology in healthcare provision in Scotland. Several policy documents link technology as a way to address inequalities in health and the demands on service provision resulting from demographic changes (Scottish Executive, 2005; Scottish Government, 2007b).

There has been a lack of consistency around the terms to support this increasing use of technology to address health needs. NHS Scotland and the Scottish Executive Health Department (2007) use the term eHealth within this context and suggest it is an umbrella term with a wide scope, and includes:

- internet or intranet to access health information by patients and healthcare professionals;
- eLibrary to support access to literature and information;
- teleconferencing, videoconferencing and computer-based learning applications to support education and clinical networks;
- the use of mobile technology such as mobile phones and portable devices to record, view and communicate information;
- e-mail or other messaging devices to support communication;
- telehealth to monitor, consult, diagnose, or treat remotely;
- the electronic health record;
- software applications that support the management of health service resources.

Within the broad term eHealth, there are some other key terms such as health informatics, nursing informatics, information communication technology, telemedicine, telenursing and telecare. The eHealth strategy is about supporting the political agenda and focusing on national priorities in a co-ordinated and collaborative way. It is not about technology, but about improving outcomes, the safety of care and the efficiency with which care is provided (NHS Scotland and the Scottish Executive Health Department, 2007). The following case studies give examples of how technology has been used within communities in Scotland to address identified needs and to contribute to the implementation of health policy.

Case study: eHealth, telecare, a community development, community-based health improvement using eHealth – Aberdeenshire Council Telecare Project

Telecare is defined as the use of communications technology to provide health and social care direct to the patient (Barlow *et al.*, 2007). In 2006 the Scottish Executive made £8.35 million available to ensure that telecare becomes an integral part of community care service provision. The principal aims were to shift the balance of care and address:

- delayed discharges from hospital;
- unplanned hospital admissions;
- avoidance of admission to care homes;
- promotion of independent living;
- change in use of existing support/care resources;
- locally identified outcomes.

This resulted in several projects across Scotland being developed, one being the Aberdeenshire Council Telecare Project, which was granted £316,248 over a two-year period (Sergeant, 2008).

Aberdeenshire, like much of Scotland, is a diverse area, with many towns and villages as well as widespread rural communities. It also has a significant growing elderly population, resulting in increased demand on services. Therefore the initial focus of the Aberdeenshire Telecare Project was on services for older people. To address this focus, the Aberdeenshire partnership membership consisted of Aberdeenshire Council, NHS Grampian, Robert Gordon University, Alzheimer's Scotland, Age Concern Scotland, Scottish Centre for Telehealth and Regional Communication Centre. It was viewed that the theoretical membership of the partnership represented all interested parties, with the voluntary agencies representing users and carers (Sergeant, 2008). This supports the principles of participation and the formation of partnerships (Table 10.2). However, considering Arnstien's level of participation it may be viewed that it is a token participation by users and carers rather than that they have control over the setting of the priorities (Naidoo and Wills, 2009). Sergeant (2008) does acknowledge the challenges in the partnership and not always having true representation at all times. However, this is stated from a management perspective rather than that of a user, as many of the managers were not able to attend meetings due to other pressures.

The partnership agreed to initially focus on a sheltered housing complex with tenants representing most client groups. The partnership aimed to provide:

- a central focus for the implementation of telecare equipment;
- the opportunity to explore connectivity;
- individual support and address care needs;
- a potential hub for application of virtual care.

Twenty-three tenants were assessed regarding their suitability for telecare and environmental control systems to aid independent living. It was agreed that the Single Shared Assessment was the most appropriate tool to identify initial need. From that, 15 were identified as having a need and this resulted in 14 tenants being provided with equipment. The tenant that did not receive equipment had her need met through the provision of a more traditional day care placement. The next element of the project was for it to become community based, where community care and occupational therapy team leaders identified and referred users from their caseloads that would benefit from enhanced telecare. During the period January–June 2008, 36 assessments were performed. The equipment provided ranged from a dispersed alarm system to fall detectors and bed sensors, with the reasons for this identified in Table 10.2 (Sergeant, 2008). The whole process of assessment and installation was complex due to difficulties in engagement with front-line staff, ownership of processes to integrate telecare in current practice, geographical issues linked to responder provision, installation and maintenance, and the need for ongoing research and development in a rapidly moving marketplace.

Table 10.2 Reason for receiving telecare

Reason for receiving telecare	Main reason	Secondary reason	Anticipated long-term benefit
Minimise client risk	23	22	11
Promote client independence	17	30	10
Prevent long-term admission to residential care	4	2	20
Prevent/reduce unplanned hospital admission		2	
Facilitate hospital discharge	2		
Monitor client to assess longer-term needs		4	5
Intermediate care			
Carer support	2	36	2

Training was an important element of the project. Throughout the project, advice relating to individual service users' needs, and potential solutions, have been provided to social work and healthcare staff on request. Additionally, a number of activities were undertaken to provide basic telecare awareness training, and more intensive training aimed at operational staff supporting users of telecare.

The evaluation of this project identified clear benefits, although it is difficult to fully quantify. In particular, risks were able to be managed that allowed users to stay in their homes rather than consider residential care, or to come home earlier from hospital. This resulted in significant financial savings, as Table 10.3 illustrates (Sergeant, 2008), with a shifting balance of care as directed by the Scottish Executive. Within the evaluation phase, further areas for development were identified, such as development of effective partnerships with health colleagues and continued development of linkages with neighbouring partnerships.

Table 10.3 Financial savings

Hospital days saved	£23,190
Reduction in care home days	£301,600
Reduction in sleepover nights	£4,260
Total	£329,050

ACTIVITY 10.3

Considering the principles of community development and community-based work discussed in this chapter, appraise the Aberdeenshire Council telecare project or a similar project in your area.

- What is the purpose of the initiative?
- Who is involved and to what extent?
- Are those involved representative of the community?
- What is the balance of power between the participants?
- How important is the approach taken to the outcome?

Case study: Telehealth, a community development, community-based health improvement using eHealth

Another key element within eHealth is telehealth. *Better Health, Better Care* (Scottish Government, 2007b) recognised that telehealth offers the opportunity to monitor, consult, diagnose or treat remotely via telephone, mobile phone and broadband. This has an important role in improving access to quality and effective care, as well as maintaining services to remote and rural areas (NHS Scotland and the Scottish Executive Health Department, 2007). Within Scotland these developments are supported by the Scottish Centre for Telehealth and there are several initiatives within this field.

One such example is within Grampian. Aberdeen Royal Infirmary is the largest teaching hospital north of Glasgow and Edinburgh. It is situated in Aberdeen, which is on the coast and in the east of the Grampian region. Transport to Aberdeen from rural areas can be lengthy and, for elderly patients or young children, a long and tiring journey. In an attempt to meet the Scottish Government directive that care should be accessible and delivered as close to communities as possible, the 14 community hospitals in Grampian are linked to each other and to Aberdeen Royal Infirmary by telemedicine facilities. In practice this means, for example, that an elderly person who falls and sustains a wrist injury can be seen at the local hospital by a minor injury nurse. The minor injury nurse can request a second opinion using the telemedicine link if needed. The patient will then be seen in line with other patients presenting to Accident & Emergency but via the medium of telemedicine rather than in person. X-rays and ECGs can all be read and interpreted at a distance as required. Advice regarding the management of the patient, as well as follow-up care of the patient can all be delivered using the telemedicine service. Not only is this more convenient for the patient, it can often prevent long and unnecessary visits to the A&E department.

It is essential in any telehealth initiative such as this that a collaborative approach is adopted to develop the policy and organisational arrangements. This promotes the establishment of an infrastructure that will contribute to health improvement and ensure that the initiative is not driven by technology (NHS Scotland and the Scottish Executive Health Department, 2007).

Case study: Urban areas, a community development, community-based health improvement

As seen in Figure 10.1, as well as Scotland having large areas that are remote and rural, there are also areas of population density, particularly across the central belt. In the north-east there is also a more densely populated area within Aberdeen city. Aberdeen is a city of international significance and has been strongly influenced by the gas industry in recent years. This has helped to raise living standards for many, however this is variable across the city, and in among the areas of affluence there are areas of significance deprivation. The 2009 Scottish Index of Multiple Deprivation (Scottish Government, 2009b) reports that 10.5 per cent of Aberdeen's city data zones were found in the 15 per cent most deprived data zones in Scotland.

The Middlefield project

Middlefield is a residential area on the north side of Aberdeen, which consists of 940 houses, 70 per cent of which are council rented properties, while a further 19 per cent are owner occupied; 65 per cent of the population live in blocks of flats (Aberdeen City Council, 2009). Middlefield continues to be identified as the area that suffers from the most acute deprivation within Aberdeen city (Scottish Government, 2009b) and has been the target of an evolving project since 1991; it is now managed by Aberdeen Council's Regeneration Strategy.

Middlefield, however, continues to suffer deprivation when measured against a range of factors, but despite this it has a strong sense of community. In 1997 the local people expressed concern about the lack of facilities in their area and in particular the lack of provision to health services. Several general practitioners covered the area at that time but none was located within it. As a result, local residents established the Middlefield community project, including a:

- food co-op;
- welfare rights service;
- health promotion worker jointly funded by the Health Board and the local council.

The following year, after lobbying by the local community, there was a decision to establish a 'new' type of healthcare service for Middlefield, to focus on health improvement strategies and shift the emphasis from the treatment of ill health to its prevention. This was the birth of a nurse-led service: 'the healthy hoose'. This service has continued to develop over the past ten years to meet the local population's needs.

Over the years, further services have been developed, such as part-time nurseries and crèches, adult groups, a youth flat that provides a drop-in service for young people with facilities for pool and internet access, as well as providing educational and employment support.

The community planning process continues to address Middlefield's issues to improve residents' quality of life (Aberdeen City Council, 2009). As part of this process a Neighbourhood Network has been established, which is an informal network of key stakeholders within Middlefield, including community representatives. This network identifies neighbourhood priorities and ways to address them to bring about positive changes to Middlefield. Engaging with communities to identify needs, priorities and to plan is essential in health improvement (Wills, 2009).

It is acknowledged that, despite these developments within Middlefield to reduce inequalities, it remains an area of significant deprivation. This could question the value of such community work. However, as the work is on so many levels and considers socioeconomics and environmental determinants it can be difficult to evaluate. What is clear is that a long-term strategy is required in order to address inequalities of health as indicated in government policy (Scottish Government, 2008b) and it may be several years before conclusions can be drawn.

ACTIVITY 10.4

Identify a public health issue within your local community that would benefit from community development work and consider the following questions.

- What key elements would need to be considered?
- What would be the challenges?
- What would be the opportunities?
- How would you support empowerment?
- How would you incorporate the principles of community development?
- What is the underpinning evidence base for the development?
- What factors would be considered in the evaluation?

Chapter 10 summary

This chapter provided a brief overview of the geography and demographics of Scotland prior to examining some of the theoretical concepts underpinning working with communities. Community-based health improvement work and community development is explored and it is recognised that, although it is an integral part of national policy, applying these principles in practice can be a challenge. Although in theory they are different, in the real world things are not always as clear-cut as theories suggest. This is illustrated within selected examples of public health work in Scotland discussed in this chapter. What is key to recognise is that true community work does require people involvement, however the benefits are not necessarily immediate.

GOING FURTHER

Cowley, S (ed.) (2008) *Community Public Health in Policy and Practice* (2nd edn). Edinburgh: Bailliere Tindall. *This second edition places positive emphasis on developing and describing public services in relation to their purpose, emphasising multi-disciplinarity and service focus rather than individual professions.*

Green, J and Tones, K (2010) *Health Promotion, Planning and Strategies* (2nd edn). London: Sage. *This second edition outlines models for defining 'health promotion' and sets out the factors involved in planning health promotion programmes that work.*

Macdowell, W, Bonell, C and Davies, M (2006) *Health Promotion Practice.* Maidenhead: Open University Press. *This book considers the key steps in the practical application of health promotion, showing how it is first necessary to determine the needs of a population and to review the scientific evidence to justify intervening.*

Scottish Government: Community Engagement 10 January 2011. Online at: www.scotland.gov.uk/Topics/Built-Environment/planning/National-Planning-Policy/themes/communities. *The Scottish administration's principles of community engagement in various public sectors.*

chapter 11

Lifestyle Factors – Nutrition: An English Perspective

Penny Nestel and Samantha Greene

Meeting the Public Health Competences

Core area 3: Policy and strategy development and implementation to improve population health and wellbeing

This chapter will help you evidence the following competences for public health (Public Health Skills and Career Framework):

- Level 7(1): Work with a range of people and agencies to implement policies and strategies in interventions, programmes and services;
- Level 7(6): Provide specialist input to policies and strategies that are under development;
- Level 8(1): Interpret and apply local, regional and national policies and strategies;
- Level 9(2): Lead on the development and implementation of policy and strategy to improve the population's health and wellbeing;
- Level 9(3): Lead on assessing the impact of policies and strategies on the population's health and wellbeing.

This chapter will also assist you in demonstrating the following National Occupational Standard(s) for public health:

- PHP29: Work in partnership with others to develop and agree priorities and targets for improving health and wellbeing;
- PHP32: Work in partnership with others to monitor and review strategies for improving health and wellbeing;
- PHP34: Work in partnership with others to undertake a full assessment of the impact of policies and strategies on health and wellbeing;
- PHS14: Assess the impact of policies and shape and influence them to improve health and wellbeing and reduce inequalities.

This chapter should also be useful in demonstrating Standard 10 of the Public Health Practitioner Standards:

Standard 10: Support the implementation of policies and strategies to improve health and wellbeing outcomes – demonstrating:

a. knowledge of the main public health policies and strategies relevant to own area of work and the organisations that are responsible for them;
b. how different policies, strategies and priorities affect own specific work and how to influence their development or implementation in own area of work;
c. critical reflection and constructive suggestions for how policies, strategies and priorities could be improved in terms of improving health and wellbeing and reducing health inequalities in own area of work.

Overview

Understanding how policy is developed and implemented is a key competency for public health practitioners. This chapter will guide you through the process of identifying the causal pathway for the development of obesity policy in England as an example of a lifestyle-related health policy.

Policy defines the direction and guiding principles of an organisation towards meeting a specific goal. The development of health policy is a means to identify and address obstacles in health promotion through both health and non-health sectors (DoH, 1992). Lifestyle refers to areas of choice that people have that can impact upon health outcomes – for example, dietary patterns, doing physical activity, smoking or consuming alcohol.

Over the past 20 years 'over-nutrition', manifested as overweight and obesity, has become increasingly prevalent in England and is now occurring at a younger age. This has huge cost implications for both the National Health Service (NHS) and the economy as a whole, and has been the major driver for policy development.

This chapter reviews the development of obesity policy in England. It then guides you through a critique of the key documents that were instrumental in developing obesity policy in England, and shows the causal pathway for obesity policy development. The Southampton obesity strategy is used as a case study to illustrate how obesity policy has been translated to a local level.

You are encouraged to use this chapter as an example of how policy can be reviewed. Activities and case studies will be used to encourage engagement with the process of policy development for different lifestyle factors.

The problem

Overweight and obesity have become increasingly prevalent in England (NHS Information Centre, 2009). Between 1993 and 2008, overweight remained constant among women and declined among men, but obesity levels in both genders increased between 35 per cent and 45 per cent (Table 11.1).

Table 11.1 Body mass index (BMI) in 1993 and 2008 for adults over 16 years old in England, by gender

BMI (kg/m2)	Men		Women		All adults	
	1993	*2008*	*1993*	*2008*	*1993*	*2008*
Underweight (< 18.5)	1.4	1.6	1.9	2.0	1.6	1.8
Normal (18.5–24.9)	41.0	32.5	49.5	41.1	45.5	36.8
Overweight (25–29.9)	44.4	41.8	32.2	32.0	38.0	36.9
Obese (30+)	13.2	24.1	16.4	24.9	14.9	24.5
Morbidly obese (40+)	0.2	1.1	1.4	2.8	0.8	2.0
Overweight including obese	57.6	65.9	48.6	56.9	52.9	61.4

Source: NHS Information Centre (2009)

Importantly, the onset of both overweight and obesity is now occurring at a younger age. Among children age 2 to 15 years the prevalence of obesity increased from 12 per cent to 16 per cent between 1995 and 2008, more so among 11–15 year olds than 2–10 year olds, while that for overweight increased slightly from 13 per cent to 14 per cent (Table 11.2).

Table 11.2 Body mass index (BMI) for age in 1995 and 2008 for children age 2 to 15 years old in England

	2–10 years		11–15 years		2–15 years	
BMI for age	1995	2008	1995	2008	1995	2008
Overweight	12.9	13.4	14.1	15.7	13.3	14.3
Obese	10.1	13.9	14.7	19.5	11.7	16.0
Overweight including obese	23.1	27.3	28.8	35.2	25.0	30.3

Source: NHS Information Centre (2009)

The short- and long-term consequences of obesity on individuals are diverse, and range from psychosocial to pathological, as shown in Table 11.3. This has huge cost implications for the NHS – currently estimated at £4.2 billion per year and forecast to increase more than twofold by 2050 unless checked (Foresight, 2007) – and the economy as a whole due to, for example, productivity losses due to absences from work as a result of sickness. Indeed, the Foresight report estimated that obesity costs the nation £16 billion annually, and it forecast it to rise to £50 billion per year by 2050 if no action is taken.

Table 11.3 Health risks associated with obesity

Childhood	Adult

Emotional and psychological effects:
  – Low self-esteem
  – Anxiety
  – Depression
  – Teasing from peers
  – Lower quality of life
Fatigue
Disturbed sleep
Type 2 diabetes
Early puberty
Eating disorders:
  – Anorexia nervosa
  – Bulimia
Skin infections
Asthma and other respiratory problems
Musculoskeletal disorders:
  – Slipped capital femoral epiphysis
  – Blount disease
	Respiratory problems:
	  – Asthma
	  – Sleep apnoea
	Disability
	Premature mortality
	Hypertension
	Cardiovascular disease:
	  – Coronary artery disease
	  – Stroke
	  – Deep vein thrombosis
	  – Pulmonary embolism
	Raised cholesterol and dyslipidaemia
	Metabolic syndrome
	Osteoarthritis
	Type 2 diabetes
	Malignancy:
	  – Endometrial
	  – Breast

- Colon

Stress incontinence in women

Menstrual abnormalities, polycystic ovarian syndrome and infertility in women

Erectile dysfunction

Gastrointestinal and liver disease:
- Non-alcoholic fatty liver disease
- Gastro-oesophageal reflux
- Gallstones

Psychological and social problems:
- Stress
- Low self-esteem
- Social disadvantage
- Depression
- Reduced libido

Source: National Obesity Observatory (2010a; 2010b)

A model for organisational policy creation

A realistic model for the organisation of policy development in government is that of 'Institutional Politics' (Baggott, 2000). In this model, health policy development is the product of the interactions between political institutions. The latter may include international institutions such as the World Health Organization (WHO) and the European Commission, national institutions including central government and government agencies (e.g. the National Institute for Health and Clinical Excellence (NICE)), sub-national institutions, such as Strategic Health Authorities (SHAs), and local institutions such as Primary Care Trusts (PCTs). The model states that networking and interrelationships between agencies and organisations influence the way in which policy formation and policy implementation is processed on a backdrop of agenda promotion. The interdependency and relationship context between these organisations and agencies influences the process of policy development over time.

In health policy development the political agenda can be described as a means to ensure choices are made to meet targets. Healthcare policy development exists within an 'open system', interacting with changes in the environment and population demographics (Baggott, 2000). The development of policy is affected not only by objective neutral activities, but by the political agenda, ideological and economic interests (WHO, 2005b). Legislation and budgetary process are essential elements in ensuring policy and politics work together to implement change (Baggott, 2000).

The 2004 Public Service Agreement (PSA) for obesity (DoH, 2004d) between the Department of Health (DoH), Department for Children, Schools and Families (DCSF) – now the Department of Education, Skills and Culture (DESC) – and the Department of Culture, Media and Sport (DCMS) illustrates institutional politics, in which government departments used a joined-up approach to set a health agenda and develop health policy. However, in this case the DoH was responsible for this health agenda while working with two other departments for whom health was not their focus. The DoH policy could, therefore, be said to be weakened by 'issue networks' whereby the relationships between the organisations were unequal (Baggott, 2000).

Historical context and critique

To understand the causal pathway of lifestyle-related obesity policy development, the chronological context in the policy formation stages will be considered.

Lalonde Report (1974)

The Lalonde Report (1974) recognised that lifestyle factors contributed to the burden of ill health in populations. This led to the concept that behavioural risk factors need to be incorporated in policies aimed at reducing risk factors associated with non-communicable diseases. Lalonde also highlighted the role of health promotion in reducing health service costs through disease prevention and holistic care for the individual. In the UK, the concept of disease prevention was considered with the publication of *Prevention and Health: Everybody's Business* (Hunter, 2003). This report aimed to increase awareness of health promotion as a concept, and shifted some of the emphasis on health from hospital-based medicine to a broader, community setting for preventing ill health. Although it did not make recommendations as to how policy might be formulated, it played a role in problem identification. Importantly, the shift in public health approach was recognised internationally.

The Black Report (1980)

The significance of the Black Report (1980) is that it identified inequalities as a key determinant of health, with class difference having a substantial impact on morbidity and premature death despite a decrease in the prevalence of infectious disease. Moreover, lifestyle factors were identified as determinants of health:

> *People unwittingly harm themselves or their children by the excessive consumption of harmful commodities, refined foods, tobacco, alcohol or by lack of exercise.*
> (Black, 1980, para. 6.28)

The concept of environment and health was also highlighted, and Black argued that environment affects health through a *culture of poverty* that, in turn, affects lifestyle choice. At this time, however, the aetiology of non-communicable diseases with regards to lifestyle choice was not fully understood. However, the report did positively identify the influence of a modern environment in which consumption of refined foods had increased while work and leisure activities had become increasingly sedentary.

The Health of the Nation (1992)

The creation and evolution of a specific lifestyle-related obesity policy in England began in 1992 with the White Paper, *The Health of the Nation* (DoH, 1992), which set out a strategy for health in England and how it might be improved. National objectives were outlined, along with actions required to meet identified targets that included a framework for monitoring, development and review. The strategy focused on five key areas, namely: cancer, mental illness, HIV/AIDS and sexual health, accidents, and finally coronary heart disease and stroke where obesity and smoking are main contributors to ill health. Specific targets for diet and nutrition were identified and included a reduction in food energy from saturated fatty acids and from fat, obesity among men and women, and alcohol intake.

The Health of the Nation also recognised the importance of populations making informed lifestyle choices with regard to their own health. It noted that lifestyle choices can have *profound effects on subsequent health*. Consequently, health promotion became a key intervention in its own right in programmes that considered lifestyle as a determinant of health.

The environment in which people live with respect to access to physical activity, sport and healthy foods, was emphasised as an area in which the public had little control, but which the government had a responsibility to influence through policy creation. This became a greater part of the health agenda after the introduction of the WHO (1999) *Charter on Transport, Environment and Health*. The evaluation of the *Health of the Nation* White Paper (DoH *et al.*, 1998) noted that, while it had a symbolic role in promoting inter-sectoral working for the promotion of health improvement, it was an initiative without cross-governmental commitment and ownership. Moreover, health authorities suggested that the decentralisation of lifestyle policy was a barrier to implementation and cohesion, that a stronger central role was needed to avoid conflicts between policies.

On a positive note, the evaluation found that the White Paper enabled health promotion efforts to be prioritised and co-ordinated. Although not specifically linked to the obesity targets, 'diet and nutrition' was identified as a health determinant, and the recognition for identifying targets was introduced. Despite this, the White Paper did not result in health authorities increasing or prioritising their long-term investment priorities in health promotion, and there was a negligible effect on local policy making. Through the identification of nutrition and diet in a wider context of health, the White Paper had played an important role in the identification of lifestyle factors as a part of a health agenda. It also identified the environment as an area in which government policy could impact upon the future health of the nation. Thus the *Health of the Nation* White Paper played an instrumental role in problem identification and contributed to the beginnings of lifestyle policy formation.

Acheson Report (1998)

In 1997 the new Labour government came into power, motivated by a climate for social change. The Minister for Public Health signalled a change in the agenda by commissioning an independent review to identify areas for policy development to reduce health inequalities. The outcome was the *Independent Inquiry into Inequalities in Health Report*, also known as the Acheson Report (1998). The report reviewed the evidence for inequalities and health, and identified key areas that were thought to play an important role in shaping lifestyle policy in England and thus its development. Early life experience as a determinant of health behaviour, including the social and economic environment, was identified as being complex and related to health inequalities. The report stressed that both policy 'upstream' and individual 'downstream' interventions designed to influence behavioural determinants of health were long term and may take time to have measurable outcomes. The recommendations for lifestyle policy from the Acheson Inquiry are shown in Table 11.4.

Table 11.4 Recommendations for health-related lifestyle factors from the Acheson Report

Health-related behaviour	*Recommendation for policy development*
General lifestyle	• Policies to promote healthier lifestyles, particularly those relating to strong social gradients in prevalence and consequence
Diet and nutrition	• Improve nutrition in schools: provision of school food policies, free school meals, and free fruit in schools; restrict availability of less healthy foods
	• Increase availability and accessibility of food for an adequate diet
	• Provide food to those who are disadvantaged, from retailers
	• Reduce the sodium content of processed foods
	• Eliminate food poverty
	• Prevent and reduce obesity
	• Improve health and nutrition for women of child-bearing age and their children
	• Increase prevalence of breastfeeding
Physical activity	• Develop measures to encourage walking and cycling, including environmental modification
	• Promote moderate-intensity exercise

Source: Acheson (1998)

The Acheson Report was instrumental in shaping policies related to lifestyle. Indeed, largely as a result of this report, the following actions have been taken (Wanless, 2004; Naidoo and Willis, 2005):

- Welfare Food Scheme reformed;

- Sure Start targets set;

- Healthy Schools programmes implemented;

- National School Fruit Scheme implemented;

- 'five-a-day' programme implemented;

- *Smoking Kills* White Paper published.

Although the Acheson Report was instrumental in highlighting lifestyle issues and inequalities for policy development, it did not comprehensively address the requirement for a more joined-up, cross-governmental approach, nor did it propose mechanisms to ensure progress was maintained (Exworthy *et al.*, 2003; Wanless, 2004).

NHS Plan for England (DoH, 2000)

The 2000 *NHS Plan for England* was created in response to the increase in health spending, indicating a need to reprioritise funding. The document focused primarily on increasing NHS staff numbers and facilities as well as clinical priorities. Nutrition, physical activity, alcohol and smoking, as lifestyle factors, were confined to a section on improving health and inequality directly related to disease prevention. Although playing a role in lifestyle policy formation, this document provided little suggestion or input for public health approaches to improving health outcomes. Moreover, recognition of the role of primary prevention in its objectives to improve health outcomes was lacking (Naidoo and Willis, 2005).

Wanless Report (HM Treasury, 2002)

Prior to the 2002 spending review, Derek Wanless was commissioned to examine future health trends, and to identify the determinants of the long-term financial and resource needs of the NHS. His report (HM Treasury, 2002; Wanless, 2004) identified the increasing demands on the health service from rising expectations from the public and patients, delivering a 'world class' service, the changing health needs of the population, and technological development and medical advances. Scenarios of the service delivery engagement that would be needed to meet the growing demands on the health service were used to model how life expectancy and health could be influenced. The expected health service outcomes identified for different scenarios of public engagement – slow uptake, solid progress and fully engaged – are shown in Table 11.5.

Table 11.5 Scenario modelling for service engagement in delivering high-quality health services

Scenario	Engagement	Outcome
Slow uptake	• No change in public engagement levels • Relatively unresponsive health service • Low health service productivity • Low rates of technological uptake in health service	• Lowest rise in life expectancy of the three scenarios • Population health status maintained at constant level or deteriorates • Projected spending on health expected to increase the most in terms of gross domestic product (GDP)
Solid progress	• Greater engagement of population in relation to their health	• Primary care services gain higher level of population confidence

	• Increased responsiveness of the health service	• More appropriate use of primary care services
	• Higher rates of technological uptake in the health service	• Considerable increase in life expectancy
	• More efficient use of resources in the health service	
Fully engaged	• High levels of public engagement in relation to health	• Increase in life expectancy beyond current forecasts
	• Health service is responsive	• Dramatic improvement in health status
	• High rates of technological uptake in health service	• Population demand high-quality care from health service
	• High rates of technological uptake regarding disease prevention	• Population confident in healthcare system
	• Efficient use of resources	• Life expectancy 2.9 years higher for men, 2.5 years higher for women
	• Need to increase capacity of health service in the long term	• Least expensive scenario
		• More costs associated with people living longer
		• Greater gains in reduction of ill health in older age groups, and in public health and prevention

Source: HM Treasury (2002)

Wanless also identified that the growing public concern regarding obesity, children's diet and smoking signalled a movement towards public engagement with health. He identified services that would need to be *fully engaged* in actively making positive health decisions for optimal health outcomes. Barriers to full engagement, such as engrained behaviour, lack of information and socioeconomic inequalities, needed to be addressed from an individual to local and national governmental level. Although the short-term funding needs would be similar for all three scenarios, Wanless identified that the difference between *fully engaged* and *slow uptake* in services, health expenditure and outcomes would be £30 billion by 2022/23.

Because Wanless showed that chronic conditions such as diabetes and cardiovascular disease were increasing, the focus on prevention through lifestyle choices began to increase in profile as a component of a wider health agenda. Influencing personal behaviours such as healthy eating, exercise promotion and smoking cessation became a focus for improving population health. At the same time the need to consider personal liberty in choice, while directly facilitating healthy behaviours, was deemed important.

Chief Medical Officer's Annual Report (DoH, 2002)

Driven by National Audit Office data which showed that the prevalence of overweight and obese children had increased, the 2002 *Chief Medical Officer's (CMO)*

Annual Report (DoH, 2002) stated that obesity was a *time bomb*. He recommended action through a multi-layered multi-agency approach. However, because the CMO's role is to recommend and highlight areas that require attention, rather than to develop or implement policy, he did not provide a functional or practical plan of action to work to implement the recommendations.

Food Standards Agency Review (2003)

In view of the concern about children's food choices, the Food Standards Agency (FSA) published a review (Hastings *et al.*, 2003) indicating that food marketing influenced children's preferences, purchasing power and consumption. This swayed the government to have a cross-departmental approach to tackle obesity, and a more responsible approach to food marketing to children. The Department of Health expressed an interest in using a variety of activities in both the public health and voluntary sectors to influence lifestyle and diet as a means to promote children's health. Importantly, in a retrospective review of actions taken, the Department of Health indicated that restrictive legislation on food advertising would be created if the industry was not seen to have reacted appropriately by 2007 (House of Commons Committee of Public Accounts, 2007).

Choosing Health: Making Healthy Choices Easier (DoH, 2004b)

The next key publication was the government's White Paper titled *Choosing Health: Making Healthy Choices Easier* (DoH, 2004b), which outlined the principles for public support aimed at increasing informed healthier choices in the population. The ethos was that this would enable the government to promote fairness and equality in health. It was proposed that environmental barriers to healthier choices would be shaped through commercial and cultural action. This was reflected in the Prime Minister's Foreword:

> *We are clear that Government cannot – and should not – pretend it can 'make' the population healthy. But it can – and should – support people in making better choices for their health and the health of their families.*
>
> (DoH, 2004b, Foreword)

The balance between creating an environment in which healthier choices can be made easier was emphasised as needing to also account for the importance of personal choice and freedoms. The government stressed the need for personal choice to be at the centre of health improvement, alongside interventions to create the right environment.

The shift from public health prevention of communicable diseases to tackling the growing trend of chronic disease associated with lifestyle factors drew on a large public consultation. The key lifestyle issues raised are shown in Table 11.6.

Table 11.6 Results of the Choosing Health consultation

Area	Main issues raised by consultation
Diet and nutrition	• Restrict advertising to children, and increase information and nutrition messages on food labels • Reintroduce home economics at school • Deliver stronger positive media messages • Provide obesity and nutrition services and primary care interventions • Tax foods high in sugar, salt and fat • Provide breastfeeding support and training of healthcare staff • Subsidise fresh fruit and vegetable purchases for low-income families • Focus on the role of the food industry • Create Healthy Schools and healthy food in schools • Encourage employer action to provide healthy options in workplace canteens
Physical activity	Improve access to leisure facilities for physical activity. Areas included: • Reduce cost, travel and childcare barriers • Increase information provided on facilities within local area • Discourage use of cars and encourage public transport • Improve facilities for walking and cycling • Encourage children's play and school-based physical activity
Health inequalities	• Target high-risk groups

Source: DoH (2004b)

Obesity was highlighted as a condition that was expected to have huge implications for both the health service and the health of the population. Its impact on the prevalence of chronic diseases such as type 2 diabetes, heart disease and life expectancy was emphasised. Indeed, of the lifestyle factors commented on in the consultation submissions, smoking, diet and nutrition were the two areas with the greatest response.

Public Service Agreement (DoH, 2004)

In 2004 a PSA was created between the DoH, DESF and DCMS in response to a noted increase in childhood obesity from 1995–2004 (DoH, 2004d). Specifically, it was to *[h]alt the year-on-year rise in obesity among children under 11 by 2010 (from the 2002–04 baseline) in the context of a broader strategy to tackle obesity in the population as a whole.*

Because obesity was known to be a risk factor for non-communicable disease, and was estimated to cost the NHS £1 billion a year, the PSA aimed to provide a holistic approach to controlling childhood obesity by addressing environmental and lifestyle factors. The three departments responsible for the obesity PSA identified four main strategies to address diet and lifestyle factors in children, which followed directly from the Acheson Report (Acheson, 1998), namely school meals, school sports, Healthy Schools and the Children's Play Initiative. Performance was to be measured against the annual *Health Survey for England*. Measuring the weights and heights of reception and Year 6 school children as surveillance was introduced in 2006.

Choosing a Better Diet: The Food and Health Action Plan, and Choosing Activity: A Physical Activity Action Plan (DoH, 2005a)

The *Choosing a Better Diet* plan (DoH, 2005a) followed the *Choosing Health* White Paper and outlined key actions related to diet and nutrition that the government would take over the next three years (Table 11.7).

Table 11.7 Aims and objectives of *Choosing a Better Diet*

Choosing a better diet aims and objectives	Proposed mechanisms to meet aims
Improve health	• 'Health Direct' will link to motivational lifestyle improvement programmes and services • Social marketing through the National Consumer Council to build on campaigns such as five-a-day, and extend to obesity, healthy eating and physical activity
Reduce the prevalence of diet-related disease	• Develop the Food and Health Action Plan through co-ordinated action between local communities, private, public and voluntary organisations, regional government and policy makers • Implement the Strategy for Sustainable Farming and Food
Reduce obesity in England by improving the nutritional balance of the average diet	• Increase consumer awareness of what constitutes a healthy diet and encourage self-efficacy • Develop cross-government campaign to increase awareness of health risks associated with obesity, and how to prevent it. • Develop healthy eating messages; five-a-day • DoH to collaborate with creative media and stakeholders to create a simple set of clear health messages • Obesity education campaign 'across the public sector and beyond' • Collaborate with food industry to promote positive health information
Reduce health inequalities by 10% by 2010	• Healthy Start • Five-a-day focusing on groups of consumers with the lowest fruit and vegetable intakes • Frontline support aimed at addressing the problems of specific communities and individuals • The Food and Health Action Plan

Reduce mortality rates from cardiovascular disease by at least 40% and to reduce inequalities	
Reduce mortality rates from cancer by 2010 (20% in under 75 years) and reduce inequalities by 6% in areas of high deprivation (PSA target)	
Halt the year-on-year increase in obesity among children under 1 years by 2010	• Tackle obesity in the population as a whole • Social marketing • DoH to collaborate with creative media and stakeholders to create a simple set of clear health messages • Obesity education campaign 'across the public sector and beyond' • Collaborate with food industry to promote positive health information, and reduce levels of salt, fat and added sugars in foods • Simplify nutritional labelling • Work with OFCOM to consult on proposals to restrict advertising of food and drink to children; work with food industries to promote messages positive for health • Monitor these measures

Promotion of a healthy balanced diet	• Base promotion of a healthy diet on recommendations of the Committee on Medical Aspects of Food and Nutrition Policy, Scientific Advisory Committee on Nutrition and the WHO
	
	  • Increase consumption of fruit and vegetables to at least five portions per day
	  • Increase average intake of dietary fibre to 18 grams per day
	  • Reduce average salt intake to 6 grams per day by 2010
	  • Reduce average intake of saturated fat to 11% of total food energy
	  • Maintain intakes of fat at 35% of total food energy
	  • Reduce average intake of added sugars to 11% of food energy
	
	• Implement Strategy for Sustainable Farming and Food
	• Develop Personal Health Guides

Source: DoH (2005a)

The key priority was to create an action plan that enabled obesity, particularly in children, to be tackled effectively. This priority was linked to the *Choosing Activity* plan. Inequalities in access to healthier food options and the link between nutrition and health were clearly emphasised at the beginning of the document. Obesity was shown to be increasing in prevalence in both children and adults, and was recognised as a major player in the development of cardiovascular disease, type 2 diabetes and premature death. It was also estimated to cost the NHS £4 billion each year, which was clearly a motivator to intervene in order to reverse current trends.

The *Choosing Activity* plan (DoH, 2005b) was created concurrently because the majority of adults (67 per cent of men and 76 per cent of women) were doing less physical activity than was recommended by the CMO. As with the *Choosing a Better Diet* plan, the *Choosing Activity* plan also aimed to decrease inequalities. Physical activity was linked to maintenance of health, and reducing mortality and morbidity, which was estimated to cost the NHS £8.2 billion annually. In addition to this, the wider cost implications of physical inactivity related to obesity were thought to be between £6.6 and £7.4 billion per year. Once again, cost was a driving force in developing the plan.

Choosing Activity was the first co-ordinated government action plan that aimed to bring together the commitments made in *Choosing Health* to increase physical activity. The target of 70 per cent of adults to achieve the recommended levels of activity each week fell under the 2004 PSA umbrella for halting the year-on-year increases in child obesity. Using the scenarios developed by Wanless (HM Treasury, 2002) the plan noted that a *medium-term* scenario that enabled physical activity to be built in to people's lives was needed to meet the physical activity targets set by the CMO.

Tackling Childhood Obesity: First Steps (2007)

The House of Commons Committee of Public Accounts (2007) session was convened to review progress being made on implementing the services to meet the 2004 PSA target (DoH, 2004d). This Committee Report highlighted the complex delivery chain for the government departments responsible for the PSA, and noted that the removal of advertising of foods high in salt, fat and sugar from television before 9 p.m. had not been put in place by the Office of Communications (OFCOM). In response, OFCOM (2008) announced restrictions on the advertising of foods and drinks high in salt, fat and sugar before 9 p.m.

Foresight Report (2007)

The Foresight Report (2007), commissioned by David King, the Chief Scientific Advisor to the government, aimed to investigate how a sustainable response could be made to the increasing problem of obesity. Driven by the substantial economic costs arising from the rising tide of obesity, and the rapid increase in obesity prevalence, the report examined potential avenues for action. The need for greater prioritisation of obesity as a public health concern was emphasised, with encouragement to create clearer leadership, and accountable structures and strategies between government departments and the NHS. Analysis of issues relating to obesity was designed to be based upon a scientific approach to assessing the evidence base.

A long-term (30 years), *whole-system* approach to public engagement in health was recommended to sustainably increase public engagement and environmental barriers to *passive obesity*. This approach would require integrated policies engaging all sectors and society as a whole. The greatest opportunity to address obesity was a scenario of a *socially responsible and prevention-focused* service and population. This approach mirrors that of the Acheson Report (Acheson, 1998) in which a fully engaged scenario provided the environment for producing the best health outcomes. The Foresight Report noted that current interventions were not operating at a sufficient depth to successfully create a population shift in the distribution of obesity.

Core principles were recommended for tackling obesity, creating challenges for government policy in medicine, public health and governance. These principles included:

- a system-wide approach, redefining the nation's health as a societal and economic issue;

- higher priority for the prevention of the health problems, with clearer leadership, accountability, strategy and management structures;

- engagement of stakeholders within and outside government;

- long-term sustained interventions;

- ongoing evaluation and a focus on continual improvement;

- creation of a comprehensive portfolio of interventions.

The Foresight Report was clearly a key driver for the creation of the *Healthy Weight, Healthy Lives* White Paper (DoH, 2008b) that followed. Being non-political, the paper highlighted the need for policies that promote greater engagement with the environmental determinants of obesity.

Healthy Weight, Healthy Lives (DoH, 2008b)

In 2008 the government released the *Healthy Weight, Health Lives* strategy, outlining its commitment to addressing obesity, and set out its aims and objectives for reducing obesity in England (Table 11.8).

Table 11.8 Aims and objectives of *Healthy Weight, Healthy Lives*

Aims	Immediate objectives
For children to have healthy growth and a healthy weight	Identify at-risk families in order to promote breastfeeding Provide better parental information on children's health, and provide results from the Child Measurement Programme Increase investment so all schools are 'Healthy Schools' Healthy lunchbox policies encouraged in schools Increase participation of obese and overweight pupils in sport and PE through development of tailored programmes Invest £75 million for evidence-based marketing to enable parents to make positive changes to their child's diet and levels of physical activity

	Invest in cycling infrastructure and skills in areas identified for child obesity; this was to be part of the £140 million announced to further Cycling England
Promote healthier food choices	Finalise healthy Food Code of Good Practice in partnership with the food and drink industry Enable local authorities to manage fast-food outlet proliferation through promotion of planning regulation flexibilities Request the bringing forward of advertising restrictions for unhealthy foods by OFCOM
Build physical activity into lifestyle	Invest in 'Walking into Health' campaign Invest £30 million in 'Healthy Towns' to improve walking infrastructure Increase collaboration and set up working group with entertainment industry to enable parents to manage the time their children spend in sedentary play Review approach to physical activity and create new programmes to encourage more activity
Create incentive for better health	Work to promote wellness through employers and employer organisations Launch wellbeing assessments through NHS in 2008 Pilot and evaluate approaches to using personal financial incentives to encourage healthy living
Personalised advice and support	Develop NHS Choices website, with information on healthy weights Provide extra funding to support the commissioning of weight management services
Research	Invest in research to identify causes and consequences of obesity and overweight Increase evidence base for prevention and treatment of obesity and excessive weight Establish Obesity Observatory

Source: DoH (2008b)

The strategy was a response to the continued upward trend in obesity in England, and based on the causal evidence provided by NICE. It addressed environmental barriers to increasing the prevalence of healthy weights in the population, built on previous initiatives, and continued to focus on children as a key target group for reducing obesity. Importantly, the strategy indicated that the government pledged to invest £372 million between 2008 and 2011. This strategy was published by the DoH and the DCSF, with a Foreword written by the Prime Minister, which noted that obesity, part of the modern lifestyle epidemics, was *one of the biggest threats to our health and that of our families* (DoH, 2008b, piii).

This report signalled a change in government strategy to one of enabling the whole population to see progress in reducing the prevalence of obesity. This was to be achieved by ensuring access to opportunities to make healthy choices is available, and this would be done by government and wider society. The responsibility of the individual in maintaining a healthy weight was emphasised. Part of the policy for child health and wellbeing was:

> To be the first major nation to reverse the rising tide of obesity and overweight in the population by ensuring that everyone is able to achieve and maintain a healthy weight. Our initial focus will be on children: by 2020, we aim to reduce the proportion of overweight and obese children to 2000 levels.

However, although this confirmed a renewed commitment to reducing levels of obesity, in reality this could be described as simply a resetting of the goalposts given that the 2004 PSA (DoH, 2004d) had not been achieved.

Determinants of lifestyle policy creation

In reviewing the above key policy papers it is possible to see how the development of lifestyle-related obesity policy has moved through the cycle of policy development shown in Figure 11.1.

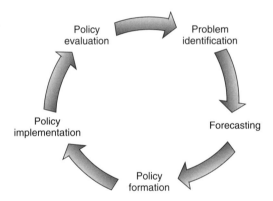

Figure 11.1 The cycle of policy development

The evolution of the obesity-specific policy in *Healthy Weight, Healthy Lives* (DoH, 2008b) effectively occurred over 40 years, and this is described below in terms of the policy creation cycle. This section discusses how the papers reviewed fit in to the model shown in Figure 11.1.

ACTIVITY 11.1

- Reflect on what you've read so far.
- Identify the two most influential reports. Why have you chosen these?
- Identify where each paper identified above fits in to the policy cycle shown in Figure 11.1. Why?

Problem identification and forecasting

The identification of lifestyle as a determinant of health started with the Lalonde Report (Lalonde, 1974; 1977). Some 20 years later, a White Paper (DoH, 1992) was issued, in which obesity was flagged as a key issue. Over the next five to ten years, inequalities in health were highlighted as an important determinant of obesity (Acheson, 1998). This led to the Wanless Report (2004), which provided scenarios of health service spending and demonstrated the cost benefits of public engagement in health. Subsequently, the Foresight Report (2007) forecast the financial and health impacts of obesity on the nation and the economy. The existing and potential future economic costs, linked to the increasing prevalence of obesity, were the major drivers for the development of policy that progressed rapidly after the publication of the Foresight Report.

Policy formation

The aetiology of obesity means any policy needs to envelope its broader context in terms of the environment, i.e. transport provision, the food industry, attitudes and awareness of healthy food messages at an individual and societal level, and so forth. These complexities have meant that the approaches to tackling obesity have required collaboration between many facets of society, but this has not been done in a timely way. The Acheson Report (1998), which identified health and behaviour as a product of the environment and early life experience, recommended school food policies be introduced, such as Healthy Schools, five-a-day and Sure Start targets, and broader campaigns be developed, such as the FSA salt initiative and the reformation of the welfare food scheme. This was reinforced by *Choosing Health* (DoH, 2004b), which proposed that environmental barriers to tackling obesity were within the jurisdiction for governmental policy development.

In 2004 the PSA for childhood obesity (DoH, 2004d) was announced, and cross-government department targets for controlling obesity were set. Recognition was given to obesity's complex aetiology. The PSA to *halt the year-on-year increase in childhood obesity by 2010* reflected a change in policy and approach to acknowledging that obesity was a huge public health concern. In other words, this was the first signal of a greater emphasis on obesity in the public health agenda.

Policy implementation

Recommendations for policy implementation were identified in the Acheson Report (1998), which reviewed key areas for development in health and lifestyle choices. These included the need for improved food provision in schools and campaigns to address the nutritional quality of food. However, at this stage, a joined-up across-government approach to obesity policy development had not yet been recommended. The 2001 National Audit Report on Obesity (NAO, 2001) identified an explicit need for this, and moved for a clarification of responsibilities between government departments. In 2004 this was identified in *Choosing Health* (DoH, 2004b), which stated that the environmental impacts on lifestyle factors were within the jurisdiction of government policy. Diet and health was identified as an area of interest by the public, thus providing a driver for intervention. A year later, *Choosing a Better Diet* (DoH, 2005a) was published as a government action plan to tackle childhood obesity. A driver for this was the financial burden on the NHS of the increasing prevalence of chronic disease. The DoH was to collaborate with stakeholders and creative media to provide simple health messages for the public, alongside the National Consumer Council and the Department for Environment, Food and Rural Affairs (DEFRA). The commitment to tackle obesity was furthered in the development of the NICE guidelines for the assessment and management of overweight and obesity (NICE, 2006).

In 2006 a parliamentary session met to monitor and account for progress (House of Commons Committee of Public Accounts, 2007) in meeting the 2004 PSA obesity targets. Although designed to have a holistic approach to obesity, the report acknowledged the complex delivery chain to implement the programmes that arose out of the PSA, and that this in itself was a potential barrier to the effective implementation of policy. The *Healthy Weight, Healthy Lives* White Paper (DoH, 2008b) aimed to define obesity-related policy and its application through measures that addressed the obesogenic environment and health promotion strategies. A re-acknowledgement of the need for a multi-sectored approach to reducing obesity was noted in this paper, based on the background of the political agenda for reversing obesity trends.

Policy evaluation

The evaluation of how existing policy has impacted upon obesity rates was challenged by the 2006 Parliamentary Committee report on *Tackling Childhood Obesity* (House of Commons Committee of Public Accounts, 2007). Questions were asked about previous methods for monitoring children's weight and surveillance methods, suggesting that the Committee was concerned about the school child measuring programme and a need to improve it. The surveillance of children in reception and Year 6 in primary schools allows for a trend in nutritional status – based on anthropometric measurements – to be observed, but it does not allow for changes in nutrition status through specific interventions to be assessed because the same children are not measured twice. The ethical dilemma of surveillance versus monitoring and informing parents about over-nourished children limited the potential for measured individuals to benefit from the evaluation, as those at risk of developing obesity or its complications were not informed. Subsequently, changes were made in the disclosure of indicators for obesity and parents are now informed.

The Foresight Report (2007) provided a broad evaluation of public engagement with the issue of obesity and found that a full engagement of public services was the approach with the greatest potential for benefit. At current costs there would be a sevenfold increase in NHS costs by 2050. As described above, *Healthy Weight, Healthy Lives* (DoH, 2008b) was the national government's response to this evaluation. It indicated that the policy cycle had been completed and was back at the problem identification stage, forecasting a continued increase in the prevalence and costs of obesity at current levels of government commitment.

Drivers and barriers for the development of lifestyle policy

Drivers and barriers influence how policy makers develop a lifestyle strategy at national and/or local level. The key drivers are shown in Table 11.9 and the barriers in Table 11.10.

Table 11.9 Drivers of lifestyle policy development

Potential driver	Influencing factor	Critique
Financial	Long-term cost implications for the health service and economy	The long-term financial benefits of policy creation for obesity-related lifestyle factors are huge
	'Fully engaged' public strategy on obesity projected to save £30 billion by 2050 (Foresight, 2007)	The potential for increasing costs from the burden of obesity-associated ill health is a driver for national and local government to create policies and implement effective strategies
Structure for policy implementation	Delegation of responsibility to organisations	Smaller organisations may benefit from the delegation of lifestyle-related policy tasks in terms of funding
	Local structures and mechanisms through Local Strategic Partnerships and Children's Trusts (NAO, 2006)	This decentralisation of policy implementation allows centralised responsibility for government departments meeting targets to be buffered
Stakeholders	Public Health professionals NHS PCTs DoH Chief Medical Officer Schools Regulatory bodies (e.g. OFSTED)	An increase in public interest in lifestyle determinants of health influences political agendas and health to motivate policy evolution and implementation Increased pressure on health services within hospitals and primary care from lifestyle-related health determinants, such as obesity, may increase pressure on policy makers Published advice from healthcare professionals and yearly CMO reports on the nation's health create pressure for policy creation; they may also increase the profile of issues such as rapidly increasing rates of obesity, thereby creating increased political pressure

Media	Jamie Oliver Newspaper and other media coverage of obesity	Using food in schools to control childhood obesity became more high profile after the launch of *Jamie's School Dinners*
Evidence base	The aetiology of obesity is complex and multifaceted The modern environment is obesogenic, making it harder for people to maintain a healthy weight (Foresight, 2007; DoH 2008b) Foresight (2007) recommended government attention on promoting healthy food, promoting child health, building physical activity into everyday lives, supporting initiatives aimed at widely promoting health, and providing services for people who are already overweight or obese	

Table 11.10 Barriers in the development of obesity policy

Potential barrier	Influencing factor	Critique
Time course	Health benefits related to lifestyle choices may not be evident at the population level in the short term (HM Treasury, 2002)	Policy related to lifestyle can be implemented, but the implications for population health are long-term and may not be seen for many years. Unless the long term benefits of change are persuasive enough, policy makers may not be pushed into creating stringent environmental changes
Financial	Funding in DoH for public health Available funding for social marketing	The current economy is not conducive to public health department funding Funding for social marketing is considerably less than corporate companies' budgets – how can it effectively compete for attention? The transference of funding provision to the private sector has been looked at suspiciously in terms of future development and interests, e.g. fit-4-life
Structure for policy implementation	Three government departments were to co-ordinate their action – over-delegation, but	For cross-departmental policies to be created, a joint recognition of responsibility for policy creation is needed; the 2004 PSA showed cross-departmental acknowledgement of targets and

	dilution of responsibility, i.e. leadership and alignment of activities, did not ensure progress towards meeting the 2004 PSA	overriding policy to reduce obesity prevalence, however initial responses of OFCOM did not reinforce the PSA
	Complex delivery chains and lack of clarity for regional leadership (NAO, 2006) Governmental delegation for funding through local authorities (British Medical Association Board of Science, 2005), e.g. school meals via education authorities	From government department level, policy to reduce obesity through delegation to other organisations may cause confusion on the part of local governmental policy Complex delivery chains may dilute responsibility for meeting PSA targets and therefore fail to advise local health policy effectively
Stakeholders	Food industry Government departments Political party in power Public European law makers	Restrictions from government policy may not be optimal for food companies; their influence in the economy will be under consideration Differing ethos between political parties will impact upon their involvement in lifestyle-related policy creation; inequality became an area for policy development under the New Labour government in 1998, indicating the influence of political party on public policy The consultation for *Choosing Health* indicated that the public wanted to maintain control over their diet and nutrition choices; until there is a strong enough push for policy change or government intervention, individual choice needs to be respected by policy makers The smoking ban in public places indicates that policies related to restrictions in lifestyle can be imposed when backing from the public is strong enough, however it is important that personal liberties remain intact; this balance needs to be considered before creating stringent public health policy, e.g. imposing 'fat taxes' on food
Evidence base	A multi-faceted approach to controlling childhood obesity is needed, however programmes and initiatives have not	Without sufficient evidence that interventions are effective in preventing or controlling obesity, it will be difficult for funding to be secured for these initiatives; it is also important that interventions are effective; interventions

demonstrated that they are sufficient to achieve government targets for reductions in population obesity (HM Treasury, 2002; NAO, 2006)	need to be monitored and evaluated to provide an evidence base for the future
Need for reliable baseline data through nationally compatible data sets on obesity (DoH 2008b; NAO, 2006)	There is a need for robust surveillance in addition to that for reception and Year 6 primary school children

---

ACTIVITY 11.2

- Identify which three barriers or drivers had the greatest impact upon obesity policy development.
- Why do you think this is?
- Outline further potential drivers or barriers that have not been mentioned – how could you build an evidence base for these?

Case study: How does national policy translate to local strategy?

The effective translation of national policy to local strategy is essential for the lifestyle determinants of health to be addressed. The application of the national obesity policy to a local policy and strategy is considered below using the Southampton obesity strategy as a case study.

Fit-4-Life Southampton obesity strategy (Southampton City, 2008)

The Fit-4-Life strategy for tackling obesity in Southampton was created in response to the *Choosing Health: Making Healthy Choices Easier* (DoH, 2004b) policy, and evolved from the previous local policy and strategy on obesity (Southampton City PCT and Southampton City Council, 2003). It also fits into the wider agenda for health in Southampton, set out in the *Southampton Health and Wellbeing Strategic Plan (2009/12)* (Southampton Partnership, 2009), which was created in response to local priorities highlighted by the city's Joint Strategic Needs Assessment (JSNA) in 2008 (Southampton City NHS PCT and Southampton City Council, 2008). The aim of the Fit-4-Life Strategy is: *To promote and improve the health and wellbeing of the people of Southampton; by identifying, implementing and evaluating effective programs of work through a partnership approach to enable people to be Fit-4-Life.*

Determinants of local policy development

The context and drivers for the development of the Southampton Fit-4-Life Strategy are explored here in terms of the national and local implications of obesity. The parallels between the national and local drivers for obesity strategy development are shown in Table 11.11.

Table 11.11 Parallels between national and local influences on obesity policy development

Influential factors in policy development	National	Local
Other policies/ strategies that acted as drivers in the development of obesity policy	• *Choosing Health: Making Healthy Choices Easier* (DoH, 2004b) • *Healthy Weight, Healthy Lives: A Cross-Government Strategy for England* (DoH, 2008b) • *Tackling Inequalities: A Programme for Action* (DoH, 2003) • *Saving Lives: Our Healthier Nation* (DoH, 1999b) • *Reducing Inequalities: An Action Report* (DoH, 1999d) • *Independent Inquiry into Inequalities in Health* (Acheson, 1998)	• *Southampton Obesity Strategy 2003–2008* (Southampton City PCT and Southampton City Council, 2003) • *Health and Wellbeing Strategy* (Southampton Partnership, 2009) • *Southampton's Children and Young People's Plan* (Davies, 2010) • *Active Southampton: Action Plan 2009/10* (Davies, 2010) • *Fit-4-Life Strategy* (Southampton City, 2008) • *The South East England Health Strategy* (South East England Health Strategy, 2008)

Financial drivers for obesity policy development	• The House of Commons Health Committee (2004) estimates the annual cost of obesity and overweight in England was ~£7 billion • The NAO (2006) reports that obesity costs the NHS ~£1 billion per year in direct costs and a further £2.3–£2.6 billion in indirect costs • Foresight (2007) estimates that the cost of obesity and overweight to society could be £45.5 billion by 2050	
Health statistics as drivers for policy development	• 24% of adults in England were obese in 2006 – a 15% increase since 1993 (NHS Information Centre, 2009) • Foresight (2007) estimates that ~60% of males and 50% of females could be obese by 2050 • In 2006 only 28% men and 32% women consumed five or more portions of fruit and vegetables daily (NHS Information Centre, 2009)	• 26.2% adults obese in Southampton in 2006–07 • 11.1% 4–5 year olds overweight, with 9.2% obese in 2006–07 (Southampton City, 2008) • 13% 10–11 year olds overweight with 16.9% obese in 2006–07 (Southampton City, 2008) • 2008 JSNA (Southampton City NHS Primary Care Trust, Southampton City Council, 2008) identified need for environmental interventions to address diet, obesity and physical activity, and Southampton to be 'fully engaged' in health

		• and wellbeing; lifestyle choices such as diet and exercise to be addressed • Physical activity levels in Southampton are particularly low in areas of greatest socioeconomic deprivation • 45% respondents to Southampton's Health and Lifestyle Survey reported consuming >5 portions of fruit and vegetables per day (Southampton City, 2008)
Evidence of the need for holistic obesity strategies	Complex relationship between obesity and its causes means isolated initiatives will be largely ineffective in creating a population level shift in obesity	• Limited evidence for effectiveness of actions to prevent, treat and manage obesity; interventions need to create a population-level shift through changes to the obesogenic environment • NICE (2006) guidance used to inform and guide the development of action plans
The influence of a multi-agency holistic approach to obesity prevention	PSA 2004 to encourage cross-departmental working	• Used in Fit-4-Life strategy (Southampton City, 2008) through Steering Group creation • Intention to identify other organisations and leads for cross-departmental working

Challenges to policy makers	• Distinction between prevention and obesity treatment • NICE (2006) guidance developed for best practice of the treatment of obesity	• Distinction between prevention and treatment of obesity • NICE (2006) guidelines to be used as a basis for evidence of best practice for treating obesity
Approach and objectives of existent policies	1. School Meals 2. School Sport Strategy 3. Health Schools Programme 4. Play 5. Obesity Campaign 6. Sure Start 7. Better-designed funding arrangements 8. Controlling administration costs 9. Effective collaborative working 10. Clear measures of progress 11. Making better use of assets	Six key objectives (Southampton City, 2008): 1. Healthy growth and healthy weight for children 2. Enabling people to keep active and eat well 3. Incentives for better health 4. Providing personalised support for individuals who are overweight or obese 5. Preventing obesity through addressing the obesogenic environment 6. Monitoring and evaluation mechanisms effectively in place

---

ACTIVITY 11.3

• Why do you think there are parallels between national and local policy development?
• What is the difference between drivers and barriers at national and local level? Why?
• Which are the most significant differences? Parallels?

The development of policy at local level is dependent upon the national objectives and local requirements. Southampton's JSNA (Southampton City PCT and Southampton City Council, 2008) and the data profiling by the Association of Public Health Observatories (APHO) indicated that the city was performing below the England average for several indicators (APHO, 2010). Indicators for adult obesity showed that Southampton was worse than England's average, although not significantly different from the mean for obesity and physical activity for adults. The proportion of adults reported to be eating healthily in Southampton was significantly better than the England average, however binge drinking and smoking prevalence were significantly worse. Deaths from heart disease, stroke and early cancer were also significantly worse than the England average. Additionally, indicators for physical activity and children's tooth decay were significantly worse. The JSNA identified diet and physical activity as lifestyle factors that increase the risk of poorer health, and forecast increases in the prevalence of diabetes and overweight and obesity in children unless measures were put in place to prevent this. This forecasting and problem identification led to the need for a *whole systems approach* to promote *healthy diets* and *redesigning the built environment to promote walking ... and shifts in cultural and societal values around physical activity.*

ACTIVITY 11.4

Imagine you are working as the obesity lead for the Southampton PCT and have just received the JSNA data.

- How would you go about identifying your priorities? What actions would you take?
- How could the *Healthy Weight, Health Lives* strategy be translated effectively to meet the needs of Southampton?

The JSNA outlined areas for action based on the identified problem areas. However, it is unclear how the strategies outlined in the Southampton obesity policy will be implemented by specific agencies or, indeed, how these programmes will be co-ordinated in line with a whole-system approach. Evaluation of the effectiveness of obesity programmes was not defined and, therefore, success will be assumed to be measured through changes in the JSNA indicators. This approach to evaluation will not identify the strengths and weaknesses of any individual intervention. This illustrates that, although local policy development can follow the theoretical model, the focus has been on problem identification and the development of strategies rather than evaluation for forecasting.

ACTIVITY 11.5

- Identify other lifestyle factors that have been addressed by health policy – for example, smoking. How do these differ from obesity policy development? Why?
- Reflect on what you have read. Identify where improvements could be made in the causal pathway for lifestyle-related policy development. What barriers would there be to this? How could these barriers be addressed? Who are the stakeholders and how would you engage them?

Conclusion

In the 1970s perceptions about healthcare were nudged from that of a disease treatment service towards the suggestion that disease can be seen in a broader context of health and lifestyle. The development of lifestyle as a target for health policy can be traced through key documents over time. Since the recognition of lifestyle choice as a determinant of health in the 1970s, healthcare policy in England has gradually begun to recognise that focusing on lifestyle was a means by which to decrease the burden of disease within the population. Obesity, a consequence of lifestyle choice, was initially acknowledged as a risk factor for other diseases, such as heart disease and type 2 diabetes, that were also rapidly increasing in prevalence. Along with smoking cessation, good nutrition and increased physical activity became factors to be addressed in the prevention of specific chronic disease policies.

The 1992 *Health of the Nation* report (DoH, 1992) introduced the concept and need for inter-departmental working to reduce obesity rates in England. Throughout the development of obesity policies cross-departmental working has been continually highlighted as an area for improvement. The 2004 PSA (DoH, 2004d) and joint target setting between governmental departments aimed to create a holistic approach to enabling healthier lifestyle choices within the population. However, even after the introduction of this PSA, the need for cross-governmental action seemed to be a recurring theme suggestive of a failure of cohesive working.

The ethos of lifestyle policy related to obesity aimed to improve what is generally known as the obesogenic environment, i.e. reduced physical activity levels through an increasingly sedentary lifestyle and an abundance of energy-dense foods, and to address inequalities so as to enable people to make healthier choices. This concept originated with the Acheson Report in 1998 and has filtered throughout health-related policy since.

Personal responsibility is an important concept in encouraging populations to care for their health and improve compliance. However, throughout many reports there was an air of indifference in the ability of policy to impact upon lifestyle choice. Indeed, it is essential that people are enabled to be responsible for making informed choice regarding their behaviour. Interventions at local and national levels are highly dependent upon how clear and enforced a policy is. Without clear guidance and support, the obesogenic environment cannot be expected to show more than minimal change.

Chapter 11 summary

In using a theoretical model for policy development, it is possible to see that the reality of policy creation does not always fit with the theory of how it should be designed. The wider implications and outside influences from industry, and the political and personal ethos of policy makers will form the shape of a policy, particularly one related to individual lifestyle choice. The financial backdrop also affects the vigour with which lifestyle-related policy is used by government, both at a national and local level. Thus it is important in public health nutrition that the mechanisms and complexities of policy creation are understood by practitioners so that relevant policies can be constructed and promoted in a realistic and effective manner.

GOING FURTHER

Caroline Walker Trust (n.d.) *Improving Public Health Through Good Food.* Online at: www.cwt.org.uk/publications.html. *The CWT produces evidence-based reports that provide nutritional and practical guidelines to encourage eating well among specific vulnerable population groups.*

Kjærnes, U (2003) Food and nutrition policies of Nordic countries: how have they been developed and what evidence substantiates the development of these policies? *Proceedings of the Nutrition Society*, 62: 563–70. *This paper addresses the emergence and development of Nordic food and nutrition policies, with some reference to the types of nutrition policies characteristic of other north European countries.*

Macdiarmid, JI, Loe, J, Douglas, F, Ludbrook, A, Comerford, C and McNeill, G (2010) Developing a timeline for evaluating public health nutrition policy interventions. What are the outcomes and when should we expect to see them? *Public Health Nutrition*, August, 16: 1–1 (e-publication ahead of print). *This paper is about the methodology of developing a timeline for policy interventions so as to provide a realistic framework on which to base outcome evaluations.*

Weatherly, H, Drummond, M and Smith, D (2002) Using evidence in the development of local health policies. Some evidence from the United Kingdom. *International Journal of Technology Assessment in Health Care*, 18: 771–81. *This paper explores the use of evidence, focusing on economic evidence in particular, in the development of local health policies through an in-depth study of Health Improvement Programmes (HImPs) in England.*

chapter 12

Lifestyle Factors – Substance Use and Misuse: A UK Perspective

Lisa Luger

Meeting the Public Health Competences

Core area 3: Policy and strategy development and implementation to improve population health and wellbeing

This chapter will help you evidence the following competences for public health (Public Health Skills and Career Framework):

- Level 6(1): Contribute to the interpretation and application of policies and strategies in own area of work;
- Level 7(4): Contribute to the development of policies and strategies within own area of work;
- Level 7(5): Assess the actual or potential impact of policies and strategies on health and wellbeing;
- Level 9(1): Identify where new policies and strategies are needed to improve the population's health and wellbeing;
- Level 9(4): Influence the development of policies and strategies to improve the population's health and wellbeing.

This chapter will also assist you in demonstrating the following National Occupational Standard(s) for public health:

- PHS14: Assess the impact of policies and shape and influence them to improve health and wellbeing and reduce inequalities;
- PHP29: Work in partnership with others to develop and agree priorities and targets for improving health and wellbeing;
- PHP35: Advise how health improvement can be promoted in policy;
- PHP39: Present information and arguments to others on how policies affect health and wellbeing;
- DA AB 3: Contribute to the development of organisational policy and practice.

This chapter should also be useful in demonstrating Standard 10 of the Public Health Practitioner Standards:

Standard 10: Support the implementation of policies and strategies to improve health and wellbeing outcomes – demonstrating:

a. knowledge of the main public health policies and strategies relevant to own area of work and the organisations that are responsible for them;

b. how different policies, strategies and priorities affect own specific work and how to influence their development or implementation in own area of work;

c. critical reflection and constructive suggestions for how policies, strategies and priorities could be improved in terms of improving health and wellbeing and reducing health inequalities in own area of work.

Overview

This chapter will help you to identify and understand the relevant policies and strategies to address substance misuse. It will assist you in assessing these policies for their effectiveness and appropriateness, and to identify gaps. It will also help you to develop your thinking about how best to achieve the public health policy related to substance use and misuse, its development and implementation.

Introduction

A number of documentations endorsed the government's health policy commitment for the twenty-first century. The White Paper *Saving Lives: Our Healthier Nation* (DoH, 1999b) and the NHS plan (DoH, 2000) set the government's ambitious targets. 'Improving the health of the population' and 'reducing health inequality' are among the key themes of UK health policy. Both public health targets address issues that cut across the health field to the wider areas of society that influence the health of a population, and include environmental, social and economic factors. By setting these targets, the relationship between poverty and ill health is acknowledged, and it is recognised that, without tackling the underlying factors, such as lack of education, unemployment, poverty and social exclusion, the ill health of whole population groups will not be improved. It is also recognised that, in order to achieve these goals, partnership working and shared responsibility across government agencies, national and local government, community and industry was necessary.

Link between public health policy and drug policy

With the White Paper *Choosing Health: Making Healthier Choices Easier* (DoH, 2004b) the government took these key principles further, promising new policies that would reflect the reality of people's lives and respect freedom of individual choice in a diverse and open-minded modern society. The emphasis was for the NHS to support individuals in adopting, and maintaining, a healthy lifestyle. Behaviours such as smoking, obesity, alcohol and drug taking, sexually transmitted infections and unplanned pregnancies were identified as main targets. As not everyone would be able (or want) to adopt a healthy lifestyle, emphasis was given to training the NHS workforce to be able to provide trustworthy and credible information to enable informed choice, and advise individuals on how to improve their lifestyle and thereby their health. The policy endorsed that legislation may also be necessary (such as banning smoking in public places). This highlights the need to balance the right of individual freedom of choice with the right of others not to have their health damaged. Further, it is recognised that, in order to be effective in tackling health inequalities, support has to be tailored to the needs of individuals and communities – in particular the needs of those from deprived communities.

Public health policy to address substance use and misuse problems

The key targets of public health policy – 'improving the health of the population', 'reducing health inequality' and 'supporting individuals in making healthy lifestyle choices' – are also the key goals when working with people with drug and alcohol problems. This chapter examines the development of public health policies in tackling substance misuse, and discusses some of the challenges they face in the UK context. Drug policies are reviewed in terms of their effectiveness in achieving the public health goals and whether they are appropriate to the specific drug situation in the UK.

Drug policies usually cover illicit psychoactive substances, regulated by the Misuse of Drugs Act (1971) (Home Office, 2010; UK Statute Law Database, 2010b). Legal substances, such as alcohol and tobacco, are not covered by them. The focus of this chapter, therefore, will also mainly be on illicit drugs.

Contemporary drug policy usually operates at three different levels: prevention of drug use, drug treatment and supply control. Societal response to drug use, therefore, encompasses a range of programmes, including school drug prevention programmes to prevent or delay initiation to drug use; treatment of drug addiction with the aim of achieving abstinence, or reducing death or severe harm from the use of drugs; law-enforcement activities to control supply by arresting drug dealers or criminal sanctions such as penalties for drug possession (Babor, 2010). Public health approaches are important aspects of drug policy because of the effect the use of psychoactive drugs can have on the health of the population. However, they are only part of the strategy because many other aspects outside the health area affect drug use, or are affected by it and require action. The importance given to public health within the drug strategy depends on the priorities within the overall drug policy strategy adopted in a country at a given time. Drug policies differ greatly between countries, depending on the national context of how the drug problem affects a country, as well as the political structure and societal attitudes towards drug use. Some countries consider drugs mainly as a problem for law enforcement and trafficking; others place more emphasis either on education and prevention or on social and health policy by working with drug users to reduce their drug use or at least the harm from it.

The nature of the UK drug problem

Drug policies need to be developed in response to the reality of the national drug problem. When assessing drug policies it is therefore significant to have a knowledge and understanding of the nature and extent of the drug problem and the harm the use of psychoactive drugs can cause to the individual and society.

ACTIVITY 12.1 REFLECTING ON THE EXTENT OF PSYCHOACTIVE DRUG USE IN THE UK

Take a few moments to reflect on the questions below and write down your answers.

- Which psychoactive drug is used most?
- Who is using most drugs?
- Who is most vulnerable to drug use?

Comment

Some key facts from a recent report by the UK Drug Policy Commission are summarised below. Compare your answers with this information. Do your views match the evidence provided in the report?

- The UK has the highest level of dependent drug use and the highest levels of recreational drug use in Europe.
- About one-quarter of those born between 1976 and 1980 have used a Class A drug at least once. The percentage of young people who have used cannabis is about 45 per cent. However, most people use illegal drugs only for a short period of time.
- Occasional drug use is not the main concern of Britain's drug problem. Most drug-related harm (deaths, illness, crime and other social problems) occurs among the small number of people who are dependent on Class A drugs, mostly heroin and cocaine.
- With 1,644 identified drug-related deaths in the UK in 2005, the UK has the second-highest rate of drug-related death in Europe. The prevalence of HIV among injecting drug users in the UK is much lower than in other European countries (1.6 per cent of injecting drug users), however it is estimated that about 42 per cent of injecting drug users in England are infected with hepatitis C.
- Some of the estimated 327,000 problem drug users in England commit crime to fund their drug use.
- Problematic drug use is disproportionately concentrated in socially deprived areas among the most disadvantaged.

Source: UK Drugs Policy Commission (2007)

Classification of psychoactive drugs according to their perceived harm

In order to be able to assess whether drug policies are appropriate to the reality of drug use in this country it is vital to reflect in more detail on the evidence of the harm that psychoactive substances cause.

ACTIVITY 12.2 HOW HARMFUL ARE PSYCHOACTIVE DRUGS?

Take a few moments to reflect on your own views on the questions below.

- Which drugs are most harmful?
- What is the harm associated with the use of a particular drug?

Using the sources below, review the evidence from research and reflect on your answers. Do your views match the evidence provided in the literature?

Nutt, DJ and ACMD (2009) MDMA (Ecstasy): A Review of its Harms and Classification under the Misuse of Drugs Act 1971. Online at: www.drugs.homeoffice. gov.uk/publication-search/acmd/acmd-MDMA-report-2009.

Nutt, DJ et al. (2007) Development of a rational scale to assess the harm of drugs of potential misuse. The Lancet, March, 369(9566): 1047–53.

Rawlins, M et al. (2008) Cannabis: Classification and Public Health (Home Office online publication). Online at: www.drugs.homeoffice.gov.uk/publication-search/acmd/acmd-cannabis-report-2008.

Psychoactive drugs are regulated depending on their perceived harm, and divided into various groups, either as illegal according to the Misuse of Drugs Act, legally available when prescribed by a physician, regulated by the Medicines Act 1968 (UK Statute Law Database, 2010a) or sold over the counter by a pharmacist. The Misuse of Drugs Act (1971) (UK Statute Law Database, 2010b) regulates the different kinds of drugs into different classes (A, B and C) according to their alleged harmfulness. The different classes carry different levels of penalty for possession and dealing. Class A drugs are considered to cause most harm.

Table 12.1 The Misuse of Drugs Act: penalties for possession and dealing

		Possession	*Dealing*
Class A	Ecstasy, LSD, heroin, cocaine, crack, magic mushrooms, amphetamines (if prepared for injection)	Up to seven years in prison or an unlimited fine, or both	Up to life in prison or an unlimited fine, or both
Class B	Amphetamines, cannabis, methylphenidate (Ritalin), pholcodine	Up to five years in prison or an unlimited fine, or both	Up to 14 years in prison or an unlimited fine, or both
Class C	Tranquilisers, some painkillers, gamma hydroxybutyrate (GHB), ketamine	Up to two years in prison or an unlimited fine, or both	Up to 14 years in prison or an unlimited fine, or both

Source: Home Office (2010)

A number of psychoactive substances that are widely used and cause harm to the individual and society are not listed under these categories. For example, alcohol, tobacco and coffee are the most popular and common everyday drugs used by many people. They are easily available, apart from an age limit and time restrictions to buy and some restrictions on places where to consume. The recent public debate on the harm of smoking, and passive smoking, has resulted in a smoking ban in certain areas; reports on the increasing levels of alcohol-related morbidity and mortality have resulted in calls for stronger control of drinking. Yet, both tobacco and alcohol are heavily taxed by the government, and therefore, supposedly, contributing towards the cost of the harm they cause to the national healthcare system.

The classification of psychoactive drugs is based on a perception of what harm they are likely to cause to individuals and society. The Advisory Council for the Misuse of Drugs (ACMD), a committee of renowned experts, advises the government in this task by providing scientific evidence of the effects of drugs, as well as social and economic knowledge of the context of drugs. Recent debates – for example, the smoking ban in public areas or the reclassification of cannabis from Class C to B – have raised concerns as to whether the classification of drugs reflects the extent of their harmfulness. Concerns have been raised as to whether decisions on drug classifications are based on research evidence, public opinion or the moral views of politicians. Current debates inspired by new research by Nutt *et al.* (2007) have called for a reclassification of drugs to reflect the harm they cause to the individual and society.

Case Study: 30 October 2009: government drug adviser David Nutt sacked

Professor David Nutt, the government's chief drug adviser and chairman of the ACMD was sacked by then Home Secretary Alan Johnson after his claims that alcohol and tobacco were more harmful than many illegal drugs, including LSD, ecstasy and cannabis. In February 2009, Nutt had clashed with then Home Secretary Jacqui Smith, when he compared in an article in the *Journal of Psychopharmacology* the dangers of taking ecstasy to those of horse riding. Nutt had criticised politicians for distorting and ignoring research evidence in the debate over the classification of illicit drugs. In January 2009, the Home Office had cannabis reclassified from Class C to B, against the explicit wishes of the advisory council.

This incident raises questions as to the role of an expert advisory committee when its recommendations are rejected. It also raises concerns as to whether UK drug policy is based on scientific evidence, economic interests or moral positioning, particularly at times of elections.

The classification of drugs is a political decision and the government thereby seeks advice from a range of agencies and individuals. These include the ACMD, public consultations, UN policy on drugs, pressure groups and general public perception. The process of drug classification has become complex and highly politicised.

ACTIVITY 12.3 POLICY FORMULATION FOR THE CATEGORISATION OF PSYCHOACTIVE DRUGS

Consider the various players that have an input into policy formulation regarding the categorisation of psychoactive drugs. Reflect upon, and compare and contrast their possible interests and views.

Possible players are:

- the ACMD;
- the UN and other international partners;
- public consultation;
- pressure groups;
- the media;
- the public.

Comment

Refer to Nutt (2009), which discusses the complex task of estimating the harm of recreational drugs and the public perception of drugs. The author provides scientific research evidence on the harmfulness of drugs such as cannabis or ecstasy, and presents the results of public opinion polls on classification and penalties for cannabis users.

Why is the evidence base for classification so important? The classification determines penalties for possession and supply, whereby those considered most harmful carry the highest penalties. Public perception of the harmfulness of drugs appears confused. Many consider illicit drugs harmful because they are illegal, believing that the categorisation of drugs is based on evidence of their dangerousness. According to a MORI survey on public opinion (Rawlins *et al.*, 2008), on behalf of the ACMD, most people (32 per cent) wanted cannabis to be a Class A drug. At the same time, most respondents (41 per cent) rated that the penalty for possession should be two years only (as for a Class C drug), and 27 per cent wanted penalties to be abolished. This demonstrates a strong public opinion that drug laws should be used as a deterrent to scare but not to punish.

UK policy response to drug issues

In the UK the NHS response to drug misuse is characterised by a harm-reduction approach to reduce the harmful consequences of illicit drug use and other risk behaviours, alongside other approaches to reduce the supply and demand of illicit drugs. The concept of harm reduction is based on the realistic assumption that people who use drugs are unable or unwilling to stop using them at a particular time. Harm reduction is a pragmatic approach to treatment to reduce the harmful consequences of psychoactive drug use. Harm reduction argues that interventions need to be in place to reduce the harm from such use, but not necessarily reduce drug use itself. Staff in treatment services have to accept the fact that drug use will continue and they have to provide interventions that are acceptable to the drug user in order to engage them in treatment. Central to a harm-reduction approach for opiate users are the provision of clean injecting equipment and prescription of substitute drugs such as methadone.

Harm reduction

The harm-reduction approach to drugs is based on a strong commitment to public health and human rights. It refers to policies, programmes and practices that aim primarily to reduce the harmful health, social and economic consequences of the use of legal and illegal psychoactive drugs, without necessarily reducing their use. Harm reduction benefits people who use drugs, as well as their families and the community. Harm reduction complements approaches that aim to prevent or reduce the overall level of drug consumption. It is based on the pragmatic view that many people continue to use psychoactive drugs despite the strongest efforts to prevent the onset or continued use of psychoactive drugs. Harm reduction accepts that many people who use drugs are unable or unwilling to stop using drugs at this particular moment in time. Access to good-quality treatment is important, but many people with drug problems are unable or unwilling to get treatment. The majority of people who use drugs do not need treatment. However, there is a need for action to help minimise risks from continuing to use drugs, and reduce the harm for themselves or others. Harm-reduction interventions are vital to help keep people safe and healthy. Allowing people to suffer or die from preventable causes is not an option (International Harm Reduction Association (IHRA), 2009).

The concept of harm reduction, or risk reduction, is closely related to the concept of public health. The core ideas of public health, of improving health and reducing inequality, include risk management and reducing harm. However, harm reduction is not without challenges. Approaches to reduce the harm from illicit drug use often face criticism. Critics believe that, by adopting a harm-reduction approach, societal traditional values and norms would be lost and drug control measures would be undermined by initiatives that focus on reducing harm rather than eliminating drug use. Critics often accuse harm reduction of colluding with or condoning drug use and sending out an incorrect message to the community. In contrast, interventions based on abstinence and a punitive approach to illegal drug use are regarded as the morally correct response to drug use. However, proponents of harm reduction argue that drug laws would criminalise people and prevent them from taking up services.

The public health principles of improving health and reducing inequalities also need to apply to drug users. Equally, one should bear in mind that harm reduction is not a new concept. Initiatives such as charities providing food and shelter for people who have an alcohol problem, or drink driving laws, have widely been accepted as humanitarian. However, when it comes to the treatment of illicit drug use, emotions run high and risky behaviours are often condemned on moral grounds.

Case Study: The 'British System'

Britain has had a long-standing relationship between public health and drug policy, with collective efforts to improve the health of populations and control and manage diseases. Harm reduction is not a new approach in Britain. From early 1920s onwards medical doctors prescribed opiates to their addicted patients. This differed greatly from the drug policy of other countries, such as the USA where drug users were mostly considered as deviant and criminals. The Rolleston Committee (named after its chairman Sir Henry Rolleston) was set up to review the existing practice of the treatment of addiction. In 1926, the Rolleston Report verified the existing practice that confirmed the right of medical doctors to prescribe substitute treatment to their drug-addicted patients. This practice became known as the 'British System' and resulted in a policy towards addiction that was driven by health concerns rather than by drug control efforts. It considered addiction as a disease and the drug addict as a patient rather than a criminal. This practice continued until the 1960s, when incited by concerns of irresponsible prescribing practices by some doctors, a review (Second Brain Report, published in 1965) resulted in a significant change in drug treatment. The right to prescribe opiates became limited to specialist doctors in drug treatment centres.

Source: Drummond and Strang (2001)

The development of harm-reduction drug policy in the UK

The harm-reduction approach in the UK developed as a response to the emerging threat of HIV infection in the mid-1980s. The threat of the spread of HIV infection among injecting drug users, and towards the wider population, in the mid-1980s required radical approaches and helped to prepare the way for measures to reduce the harm from injecting drug use. The ACMD, encouraged by the positive results of harm-reduction measures in the Netherlands, recognised that HIV was a greater threat to individual and population health than drug use, and made the prevention of HIV a priority over the prevention of drug use (ACMD, 1988). A number of activities were introduced to prevent the spread of HIV among injecting drug users. The most important were needle exchange schemes and substitute prescription with methadone, as well as the provision of condoms to encourage safer sex, and outreach work to get in touch with hard-to-reach drug users. In order to engage drug users in drug treatment services, it was vital to establish a relationship of trust with them. This required a new ethos of working, in that staff in services and drug users needed to work together to address drug-related health problems. A non-judgemental attitude of staff towards drug users, and accepting the fact that people may not be willing, or able, to stop using drugs, was needed.

This new and pragmatic harm-reduction strategy was guided by the principles of public health approaches, and transformed drug policy and drug treatment in terms of safer drug use rather than abstinence. Although the concept of harm reduction accepts that abstinence may not be the immediate goal of the drug user, it may be their end goal in a long process. In the meantime, it is most important to get the drug user into treatment so they can use drugs more safely. The concept of safer drug use involves various steps, and ranges from safer use (not sharing injecting equipment, preventing abscesses when injecting by disinfecting injecting sites), safer modes of drug use (move from injecting to smoking) and reducing drug use (frequency and quantity), to stopping drug use altogether.

ACTIVITY 12.4 ANALYSING THE IMPACT OF KEY STAKEHOLDERS IN THE DEVELOPMENT OF HARM-REDUCTION POLICY IN THE 1980S

In order to understand the concepts of power, interests and ideology in the development of contemporary drug policy, it is helpful to reflect in more detail on the development of harm-reduction policies in the light of the threat of an HIV epidemic.

- What were the key drivers?
- Who were key players?
- What were their different views and interests?

Spend a few minutes thinking about these questions and then read the following key papers:

Stimson, GV (1995) Aids and injecting drug use in the United Kingdom, 1987–1993: the policy response and the prevention of the epidemic. *Social Science and Medicine*, 41(5): 699–716.
Stimson, GV (1998) Harm reduction in action: putting theory into practice. *International Journal of Drug Policy*, 9(6): 401–9.

How has government drug policy developed and changed over time?

The development of drug policy in the UK was not without tensions between the proponents of and opponents to harm reduction. The concept of harm reduction remains controversial. Despite the fact that, since 1986, the Department of Health has allocated funding for drug treatment services, fears prevailed that the existing harm-reduction practice would be replaced by an American-style drug policy based on abstinence, and that initiatives such as needle exchange schemes and methadone maintenance would be ended. Drug treatment services were under pressure to provide evidence of effectiveness. As a result, all harm-reduction initiatives were closely researched and evaluated. The government was particularly concerned about the cost-effectiveness of drug treatment, and especially the cost of treatment with methadone. An extensive taskforce was established to provide comprehensive reviews of existing treatment services. Key outcome indicators included:

- abstinence from drugs;
- reduction in drug use and risk-taking behaviour;
- improvement in physical health and psychological wellbeing;
- improved social functioning;
- reduction in criminal activity.

The effectiveness review concluded that treatment worked and was cost-effective (Gossop *et al.*, 1995). It was claimed that, for every £1 spent on treatment, at least £9.50 was saved on crime and health costs.

A vital policy document was the government's (HM Government, 1995) *Tackling Drugs Together* (TDT), in which it recognised drug misuse as a chronic relapsing condition, which may require a number of treatment attempts in order for an individual to become drug free. The emphasis of the three-year drug policy strategy was on working to reduce the health risks of drug use through effective treatment and rehabilitation. The strategy tackled the controversy on harm reduction by stating that, while abstinence was the aim, steps were needed to reduce the risk of spread of HIV and other communicable diseases and to save lives. Thus, harm reduction was considered a means towards the ultimate goal: abstinence. Based on the evidence and in line with the taskforce's recommendations, the Department of Health provided more funding for drug treatment services.

The three key areas of the drug policy, once considered equally important, gradually became more influenced by the crime-control agenda:

1. crime;
2. young people;
3. public health.

With the TDT strategy the British drug policy made a fundamental shift away from the harm-reduction approach to prevent the spread of HIV, towards an agenda based on crime, law enforcement and a greater involvement of the criminal justice system in drug-related issues. The drug–crime link became the driving force behind policy development. The goals were to reduce the incidence of drug-related crime and reduce the public's fear of drug-related crime.

From 1997 onwards, the Labour government built on the policy and achievements of the previous government. The ten-year drug strategy (1998–2008) *Tackling Drugs to Build a Better Britain* (HM Government, 1998) continued the harm-reduction approach with a promise to reach out to young people, women and minority ethnic groups, and to create safer communities. In 2002, the National Treatment Agency (NTA) was set up to oversee drug treatment within the NHS. The NTA published guidelines for drug treatment and developed standards of care for workers in the drug treatment sector.

In 2008, the NTA conducted a review of drug treatment services, collecting evidence of good practice in harm reduction, and concluded that harm reduction works (NTA, 2008). The new ten-year drug strategy (2008–18) (HM Government, 2008) emphasised the need to protect families and strengthen communities, and respective programmes were developed. However, at the same time, the Labour drug policy continued with its emphasis on crime reduction. Under the premise of protecting communities from drug-related antisocial behaviour, efforts were undertaken to reduce the level of repeat offending among drug users, and to try to break the vicious cycle of drugs and crime by investing in treatment services within the criminal justice system.

Based on the evidence that drug treatment works and is cost effective, a range of treatment interventions in the criminal justice system were introduced, assuming that coerced treatment is just as effective as voluntary treatment. Drug testing was introduced in prisons, with the aim of identifying people with drug problems and ensuring that they complied with treatment. Interventions, such as arrest referral schemes, drug testing and treatment orders (DTTOs), and drug intervention programmes (DIPs), were developed and funding was directed towards interventions within the criminal justice system to disrupt the cycle of drugs and crime.

While still balancing harm reduction and crime reduction, over time the overriding aim of drug policy was in danger of becoming that of crime reduction. This was based on an assumption that most drug users are committing crimes to pay for their drug habit, and that the drug problem would be solved by investing in treatment interventions within the criminal justice system. However, this new emphasis occurred at the expense of the many other drug users who were in need of treatment but did not commit crimes.

ACTIVITY 12.5 CRITICAL REFLECTION ON THE IMPACT OF KEY STAKEHOLDERS IN THE DEVELOPMENT OF UK HARM-REDUCTION POLICY SINCE 1995

Critically reflect on the developments since the introduction of the drug strategy *Tackling Drugs Together* (HM Government, 1995) up until the present day.

- What were the key drivers?
- Who were the key players?
- What were their different views and interests?
- What has changed since the introduction of the harm-reduction policy in the 1980s?

Spend a few minutes thinking about your answers to these questions, then compare your findings from this activity with those from Activity 12.4 (when facing the threat of an HIV epidemic). Identify similarities and differences.

Comment

The following may be useful sources.

Duke, K (2006) Out of crime and into treatment? The criminalization of contemporary drug policy since *Tackling Drugs Together. Drugs: Education, Prevention and Policy,* 13(5): 409–15.
MacGregor, S (2006) *Tackling Drugs Together: ten years on. Drugs: Education, Prevention and Policy,* 13(5): 393–8.
Stimson, GV (2010) Harm reduction: moving through the third decade. *International Journal of Drug Policy,* 21(2): 91–3.

The global picture of drug policy response

During the twentieth century there was no coherent international drug policy. Depending on a country's approach, drug policy was either driven by drug control measures and efforts to protect the moral values, or by public health concerns. Harm reduction was developed as a response to the failures of international drug policies that were unsuccessful in reducing the drug problem, whose focus was on prevention and supply control, resulting in the criminalisation of drug users.

The WHO recognised the increasing health problems resulting from a rise in the use of illicit drugs and, in 1973, called for the development of strategies that would give priority to public health over drug-control policies. Only with the onset of HIV/AIDS in the mid-1980s did the adoption of harm-reduction measures become possible within some countries' drug policies. Those countries with an established history of public health, such as the UK and the Netherlands, were able to respond quickly to the need to reduce the harm to the health of drug-using individuals, their families and communities. An international harm-reduction network was established, enabling support and the sharing of experiences among its members. In 2001, the UN encouraged the availability of harm-reduction measures to drug users by setting targets for countries. In 2003, all 192 WHO member states endorsed the Global Health Sector Strategy for HIV/AIDS, which included harm reduction as a core element. In 2005, UNAIDS included harm reduction as one of its essential actions for HIV prevention.

Analysis of the global response to harm reduction demonstrates that, in many countries, harm reduction has been successful and has been adopted as a response to the drug problem. Yet, despite comprehensive evidence of effectiveness many countries still have not adopted harm-reduction policies. As a result many injecting drug users have no access to needle exchange and opioid substitute programmes. Drug treatment programmes are grossly underfunded and the benefits of harm-reduction methods balanced against public health gains are not widely recognised. Harm reduction had its biggest success with the prevention of HIV infection in opioid users. Yet, harm reduction is also relevant to other psychoactive drugs, including alcohol and tobacco, focusing on harm prevention rather than stopping their use.

ACTIVITY 12.6 THE INFLUENCE OF THE HARM-REDUCTION APPROACH ON LEGAL SUBSTANCES

Using alcohol and tobacco as examples, examine drink-driving legislation and the availability of non-smokeable nicotine products. Explore how these policies have been influenced by the harm-reduction agenda.

Comment

The following may be useful sources.

Ball, A (2007) HIV, injecting drug use and harm reduction: a public health response. *Addiction*, 102(5): 684–90.
Rhodes, T and Hedrich, D (eds) (2010) Harm reduction evidence, impacts and challenges. *EMCDDA Monographs*. EMCDDA.

Analysis of UK drug policy

How successful has the UK policy approach been in tackling drug use and has it been able to meet the public health goals of improving the health of the population and reducing health inequalities?

With its public health approach of harm reduction, the UK government was able, to a certain extent, to reduce the moral arguments regarding treatment of users of illicit drugs. Harm reduction has proved to be successful in preventing a major HIV epidemic and getting people with drug problems into treatment rather than criminalising them. Yet the emphasis of drug policy changed over time. It gradually shifted from reducing harm to reducing crime. As a result, the public health aims of improving the health of the population and reducing health inequalities – all key elements of harm reduction – seem to have lost their significance at the expense of a policy that appears now focused on the link between drugs and crime, and upon criminalising drug users. The following section explores whether UK drug policy still has at its heart the public health goals 'improving the health of the population' and 'reducing health inequality'.

Is drug policy based on evidence or on moral views?

The recent debates regarding the classification of drugs to reflect the factual harm they cause raised concerns as to the basis on which such classifications are being made – whether they are based on scientific evidence or on moral views. As mentioned above, assessing the harm associated with the use of psychoactive drugs has important implications for drug policy. Drug policy needs to take into account that psychoactive drugs vary in the harm they cause to the individual and society. Some drugs, such as opioids and cocaine, may be more harmful to the health of individuals than other drugs, such as ecstasy or cannabis, although more people use the latter. On the other hand, some substances that are legal, such as alcohol and tobacco, can cause great harm. The risks to health also vary, depending on the amount taken, frequency of drug use and the how the drug is taken – be it orally, smoked or injected.

Classifying a drug as Class A does not seem to work as a deterrent. For example, ecstasy is ranked in the same category as heroin and cocaine, but many people use ecstasy on a regular basis without any problems. The most harm they suffer may be a criminal conviction and/or imprisonment, if caught in possession or dealing. Messages on the harmfulness of drugs may not be taken seriously and other, more dangerous, Class A drugs, such as heroin or cocaine, may be taken without much concern for the consequences. The harm alcohol and tobacco can cause is often underestimated because they are classified as legal. This should not be the intention of a drug policy based on the principle of reducing harm from drug use and the public health goal of improving the health of the population. For this reason, drug policy and the classification of drugs need to be based on contemporary scientific evidence, and need to be flexible if this evidence changes. If a drug policy wants to be successful, and its message trustworthy, it needs to reflect public perception and research evidence. Recent polls, which revealed increasing support for the legal regulation of cannabis and ecstasy, demonstrated that the public is ready for a mature debate on drug reclassification. Perhaps, politicians may even no longer have to be concerned about possible repercussions for their re-election if this debate is opened?

Furthermore, policy makers need to be aware of the fact that, in many cases, the harmful consequences are not necessarily due to the effects of the drug itself, but deeply entrenched within the social environment in which drug use is taking place. There needs to be an understanding of the reasons why people are using drugs, and of the underlying factors and context of their use. Issues such as education, environment, housing and family greatly influence the effect of drugs and problems related to their use. All these need to be addressed in order to break the cycle of drug use.

Improving the health of the population

Despite the increasing numbers of drug users in treatment, in particular within the criminal justice system, there is little evidence on the effectiveness of treatment for the individual, their family and the overall picture of problematic drug use in the UK (UKDCP, 2007). The prevailing goal of a drug policy based on crime reduction, to get offenders out of crime and into treatment, assumes a direct link between drugs and crime, and that the drug problem would be resolved by investing in treatment within the criminal justice system. However, such an approach does not take into account that coercive treatment may not be very successful. There is substantial evidence that a drug user's motivation to change their drug using behaviour is likely to lead to better treatment outcomes (Beckett et al., 2004).

Moreover, an emphasis on interventions within the criminal justice system, with its coercive treatment and drug testing, clashes with the spirit of harm reduction and public health policy, which seek to address inequalities of health by tackling social issues such as homelessness, poverty and unemployment. Although such issues are explored in the current drug policy, critics have argued that the emphasis is on their possible link with criminal behaviour rather than on social causes. Considering that harm reduction was developed in response to other approaches that considered drug users as criminals, this shift in policy is worrying as it departs from the very principles of harm reduction and public health. The current fixation on the link between drug use and crime has neglected the need of the many drug users who have not committed a crime but simply require treatment.

The focus on crime reduction with compulsory treatment within the criminal justice system has not had a significant long-term impact on drug use and drug-related crime. Healthcare professionals involved in the treatment of problematic drug use strongly argue that punishment is not the appropriate response to treating drug problems – indeed imprisonment can be counterproductive, whereas treatment and care that meet the many health and social needs of people with drug-related problems would facilitate the voluntary uptake of treatment and prevent drug-related crime. The United Nations Office on Drugs and Crime (UNDOC, 2010) also endorsed the need for treatment of drug problems through healthcare rather than punishment, and questioned the benefit of coercive treatment. The UNDOC's treatment approach entailed a wider view of improving the health of drug users that goes beyond the psychosocial or pharmacological treatment of the drug problem, and includes measures to facilitate social reintegration and reduce isolation and social exclusion. This strongly suggests that, for drug policy to be effective, the drug problem must, once again, be regarded as a health and social care problem rather than a criminal problem.

Addressing inequalities

An emphasis on crime reduction does not take into account the underlying factors of problematic drug use and the social context in which drug use occurs. People from all backgrounds take drugs for many reasons, including pleasure, to relieve boredom, ease physical or emotional pain, or to tackle stress or anxieties. Most of them will not develop any problems whatsoever. However, those most at risk of developing problems are those who are socially and economically marginalised. Their social context may be characterised by being disadvantaged, having limited perspectives in life, or a lack of education and resources. Social stress, poor social networks, low self-esteem, high rates of depression, anxiety and a lack of control have important impacts on life experiences. Drugs may be used for their psychosocial effects to counter such stresses and anxieties.

There is evidence of strong links between poverty, deprivation, inequalities and problematic drug use, and the relationship is complex (Scottish Drugs Forum, 2007; Hoare and Moon, 2010). Some population groups are disproportionately affected by poverty. While deprivation and poverty do not cause drug problems, they weaken protective factors and strengthen the risk factors. However, not everyone in a poor neighbourhood will take drugs and/or develop problems with their drug use. The causes of deprivation and social exclusion are social, but they are experienced individually. However, it is not always poverty and deprivation that cause drug use – drug use can also lead to poverty and deprivation.

Experts have long argued that drug policy can work only if more emphasis is placed on eliminating the causal factors of problematic drug use by addressing inequalities. This requires a complex and multi-faceted programme of action and working in partnership with a range of government agencies to ease the social stresses and improve the perspectives and qualities of people's lives. More emphasis needs to be given, for example, to the quality of education, programme of social inclusion and the development of young people, to raise their self-confidence and the level of control over their lives. Excellent experiences have been reported in other areas. For example, concerted programmes of education and support to reduce teenage pregnancy in the London borough of Hackney led to a 28 per cent fall in teenage pregnancy from 1998 to 2008 (Team Hackney, 2010). Tackling drugs would certainly benefit from such programmes, which are also core elements of public health approaches. A drug policy that criminalises problem drug users will not be effective, no matter how much money is put into the criminal justice sector.

With the new coalition government in office since May 2010 it is uncertain what shape its drug policy will take. So far, the new government has endorsed its commitment to improving the population's health and to tackling health inequalities (HM Government, 2010). Also, a public consultation on the new drug strategy is under way and a new drug policy has been promised for early 2011. This provides an excellent opportunity for collaborative working and the development of programmes and interventions to target those at risk of social exclusion and substance misuse problems. Public health, with its experience of multi-faceted collaborative working, would be best placed to provide interventions to those vulnerable groups to break the cycle of deprivation and drug use.

It will be very interesting to see where the emphasis will be – either towards public health and harm reduction or law enforcement – whether the body of evidence of the effectiveness of harm-reduction treatment will be taken into account, and whether the public health goals will be adhered to, as promised in the coalition document. While it is unclear as yet what form the new drug policy is likely to take, what is clear is that budget cuts will have a serious impact on the extent and effectiveness of future drug policy. Then again, policy makers need to recognise that investment in programmes that tackle social exclusion and deprivation is cost effective in the long term, and very likely to be the best way to tackle problematic drug use.

Conclusion

Harm reduction emerged directly from a crisis, in order to prevent an epidemic of HIV infection. Harm reduction demonstrated a strong commitment to the principles of public health and health promotion using public health interventions to reduce the harm to population groups. As such, harm reduction could be seen as a model for a successful public health intervention. Important aspects of harm reduction, such as creating a supportive environment, strengthening action within communities, developing healthy public policy and reorientating services towards the needs of disadvantaged population groups are also part of good public health practice.

Unfortunately, recent UK drug policy has gradually moved away from the public health and harm reduction-orientated approach. Evidence suggests that its focus on the link between substance use and crime achieved only limited success. Tackling drugs, therefore, should become once again a health rather than a crime issue. The treatment of people with drug problems should adopt a health approach in the widest sense, by also addressing issues of social exclusion, deprivation and personal development. Public health thereby has an important role to play.

Finally, one needs to be aware that tackling drugs is a difficult enterprise and there will always be people who use drugs. Even if a policy does work it cannot entirely eliminate drug problems, but it can reduce their negative impact on individuals and society.

Chapter 12 summary

This chapter began by identifying the main features of a public health policy related to substance use and misuse, its development and implementation. The main focus of the chapter was to develop an understanding of the different stages in the development and implementation of drug policy. The chapter highlighted how the diverse interests of the key players have impacted on the development of policy, and resulted in a shift away from a public health-orientated drug policy of harm reduction and towards an emphasis on crime reduction. Finally, based on an analysis of policy development, the chapter has provided some recommendations for policy development that may assist in successfully tackling the drug problem.

GOING FURTHER

Duke, K (2006) Out of crime and into treatment? The criminalization of contemporary drug policy since *Tackling Drugs Together. Drugs: Education, Prevention and Policy*, 13(5): 409–15. *This article examines the increasing interconnections between drugs, crime, punishment and treatment since the publication of the 1995 national drugs strategy*, Tackling Drugs Together.

Home Office: drugs and alcohol, online at: www.homeoffice.gov.uk/drugs. *Various topics related to this subject.*

Nutt, DJ *et al.* (2007) Development of a rational scale to assess the harm of drugs of potential misuse. *The Lancet*, March, 369(9566): 1047–53. *This article explores the problems for policy making of the current classification systems for harmful drugs.*

Stimson, GV (2010) Harm reduction: moving through the third decade. *International Journal of Drug Policy*, 21(2): 91–3. *This is the official journal of the International Harm Reduction Association.*

References

Aberdeen City Council (2009) *Middlefield Neighbourhood Community Action Plan Summary 2009/10*. Online at: www.communityplanningaberdeen.org.uk/web/FILES/NCAPNorth/Middlefield_-_2009-10_NCAP_28_July_2009.pdf, accessed 27 January 2011.

Acheson, D (1998) *Independent Inquiry into Inequalities in Health Report*. London: HMSO. Online at: www.archive.official-documents.co.uk/document/doh/ih/ih.htm, accessed 27 January 2011.

Adelman, L, Middleton, S and Ashworth, K (2003) *Britain's Poorest Children: Severe and Persistent Poverty and Social Exclusion*. London: Save the Children.

Advisory Council on the Misuse of Drugs (ACMD) (1988) *AIDS and Drug Misuse: Part One*. London: Department of Health and Social Security.

Aitchison, J and Carter, H (2004) *Spreading the Word: The Welsh Language 2001*. Talybon: Y Lolfa.

Alcock, P (2006) *Understanding Poverty* (3rd edn). Basingstoke: Palgrave Macmillan.

Alcock, P (2008) *Social Policy in Britain* (3rd edn). Basingstoke: Palgrave Macmillan.

Allsop, J (1995) *Health Policy and the NHS Towards 2000* (2nd edn). London: Longman.

Alvarez-Rosete, A, Bevan, G and Mays, N (2005) Information in practice: effect of diverging policy across the NHS. *British Medical Journal*, 331: 946–50.

Ambrose, P (2002) *Second Best Value: The Central Stepney SRB – How Non-joined-up Government Policies Undermine Cost-effectiveness in Regeneration*. University of Brighton: Health and Social Policy Research Centre.

Ambrose, P (2008) Defining moment. *Roof*, 29 September. London: Shelter.

Ambrose, P and Farrell, B (2009) *Housing our Future*. London: London Citizens.

Ambrose, P and Macdonald, D (2001) *For Richer, for Poorer? Counting the Costs of Regeneration in Stepney*. University of Brighton: Health and Social Policy Research Centre.

Ambrose, P and Stone, J (2010) *Happiness, Heaven and Hell in Paddington: A Comparative Study of the Empowering Housing Management Practices of WECH (Walterton and Elgin Community Homes)*. London: WECH.

American Journal of Public Health (AJPH) (2003) Special Issue: *Built Environment and Health,* 93: 9.

Anderson, JE (1975) *Public Policy-making.* New York: Holt, Praeger.

Appleby, J (2005) *Independent Review of Health and Social Care Services in Northern Ireland.* Online at: www.dhsspsni.gov.uk/publications/2005/appleby/appleby-report.pdf, accessed 27 January 2011.

Appleby, J, Crawford, R and Emmerson, C (2009) *How Cold Will it Be? Prospects for NHS Funding 2011–17.* London: King's Fund and Institute for Fiscal Studies.

Area Children and Young People's Committees (ACYPC) (2008) *Northern Ireland Children's Services Plan 2008–2011.* Belfast: ACYPC.

Assembly for Wales (n.d.) Online at: www.assemblywales.org.uk, accessed 14 November 2010.

Association for Public Health Observatories (2010) *Health Profiles 2010.* Online at: www.apho.org.uk/resource/view.aspx?QN=P_HEALTH_PROFILES, accessed 14 November 2010.

Babor, TF (2010) Drug policy and the public good: a summary of the book. *Addiction,* 105(7): 1137–45.

Baggott, R (2000) *Public Health Policy and Politics.* Basingstoke: Palgrave Macmillan.

Baggott, R (2007) *Understanding Health Policy.* Bristol: Policy Press.

Baggott, R (2010) *Public Health Policy and Politics* (2nd edn). Oxford: Wiley Blackwell.

Ball, A (2007) HIV, injecting drug use and harm reduction: a public health response. *Addiction,* 102(5): 684–90.

Bardach, E (1977) *The Implementation Game.* Cambridge, MA: MIT Press.

Barlow, J, Singh, D, Bayer, S and Curry, R (2007) A systematic review of the benefits of home telecare for frail elderly people and those with long term conditions. *Journal of telemedicine and Telecare,* 13: 172–9.

Barrett, S and Fudge, C (eds) (1981) *Policy and Action: Essays on the Implementation of Public Policy.* London: Methuen.

Beaumont, K, Douglas, J and Heller, T (2007) From an original chapter by Jones, L (2002) Making and changing healthy public policy, in Lloyd, C, Handsley, S, Douglas, J, Earle, S and Spurr, S (2007) *Policy and Practice in Promoting Public Health.* London, Sage.

Beck, U (1992) *Risk Society: Towards a New Modernity.* London: Sage.

Beck, U, Giddens, A and Lash, S (1994) *Reflexive Modernization: Politics, Tradition and Aesthetics in the Modern Social Order.* Cambridge: Polity Press.

Beckett, H, Heap, J, McArdle, P, Gilvarry, E, Christian, J, Bloor, R, Crome, I and Frischer, M (2004) Understanding problem drug use among young people accessing drug services: a multivariate approach using statistical modelling techniques. Home Office Online Report 15/04. Online at: rds.homeoffice.gov. uk/rds/pdfs04/rdsolr1504.pdf, accessed 30 November 2010.

Belfast Healthy Cities (2004) *Community Profile, Community Health Impact Assessment Developing a Community Profile*. Online at: www.belfasthealthycities. com, accessed 14 November 2010.

Bell, D (1960) *The End of Ideology: On the Exhaustion of Political Ideas in the Fifties*. New York: The Free Press.

Bernstein, H, Cosford, P and Williams, A (2010) *Enabling Effective Delivery of Health and Wellbeing*. London: Department of Health.

Beveridge Report (1942) *Social Insurance and Allied Services*. Cmd 6404. London: HMSO. Online at: www.sochealth.co.uk/history/beveridge.htm, accessed 27 January 2011.

Birkland, T (1997) *After Disaster: Agenda Setting, Public Policy and Focusing Events*. Washington: Georgetown University Press.

Birrell, D (2009) *The Impact of Devolution on Social Policy*. Bristol: Policy Press.

Black, D (1980) *Inequalities in Health* (The Black Report). London: Department of Health and Social Services/Penguin. Online at: www.sochealth.co.uk/Black/ black.htm.

Black, N (2001) Evidence based policy – proceed with care. *British Medical Journal*, 323(7307): 275.

Blackman, T and Harvey, J (2001) Housing renewal and mental health: a case study. *Journal of Mental Health*, 10(5): 571–83.

Blair, T (1999) Beveridge lecture, 18 March, Toynbee Hall, London.

Boyle, D and Harris, M (2009) *The Challenge of Co-Production – How Equal Partnerships Between Professionals and the Public are Crucial to Improving Public Services*. London: NESTA.

Braubach, M (2010) *The Health Relevance of the Immediate Housing Environment in Housing and Health in Europe: The WHO LARES Project*. London: Routledge.

Braybrooke, D and Lindblom, C (1963) *A Strategy of Decision: Policy Evaluation as a Social Process*. New York: Free Press of Glencoe.

Brereton, L and Vasoodaven, V (2010) *The Impact of the NHS Market*. London: CIVITAS: Institute for the Study of Civil Society.

British Medical Association (BMA) (2003) *Housing and Health: Building for the Future*. London: BMA.

British Medical Association (BMA) (2007) *Devolution and Health Policy: A Map of Divergence Within the NHS*. London: BMA Health Policy & Research Unit.

British Medical Association (BMA) (2010) *Devolution and Health Policy: A Map of Divergence*. London: BMA Health Policy & Research Unit.

British Medical Association (BMA) Board of Science (2005) *Preventing Childhood Obesity*. London: BMA Publications Unit. Online at: www.bma.org.uk/images/PreventingObesityfinal_tcm41-20659.pdf.

British Medical Association (BMA) Board of Science (2007) *Breaking the Cycle of Children's Exposure to Tobacco Smoke*. London: BMA.

Bullock, H, Mountford, J and Stanley, R (2001) *Better Policy Making*. London: Cabinet Office Centre for Management and Policy Studies. Online at: www.civilservant.org.uk/betterpolicymaking.pdf, accessed 14 November 2010.

Burridge, R and Ormandy, D (1993) *Unhealthy Housing: Research, Remedies and Reform*. London: E&FN Spon.

Buse, K, Mays, N and Walt, G (2005) *Making Health Policy*. Berkshire: Open University Press, McGraw-Hill Education.

Cabinet Office (1999) *Modernising Government*. London: HMSO.

Capon, C (2008) *Understanding Strategic Management*. Harlow: Prentice Hall.

Caroline Walker Trust (n.d.) Improving public health through good food. Online at: www.cwt.org.uk/publications.html.

Cattan, M and Tilford, S (2006) *Mental Health Promotion*. Berkshire: Open University Press.

Cawson, B (1982) *Corporatism and Welfare*. London: Heinemann Educational Books.

Chief Medical Officer (2009) *On the State of the Public Health: Annual Report of the Chief Medical Officer 2008*. London: HMSO.

Cm 289 (1988) *Public Health in England*. London: HMSO.

Cm 1986 (1992) *The Health of the Nation: A Strategy for Health in England*. London: HMSO.

Cm 3807 (1997) *The New NHS: Modern, Dependable*. London: HMSO.

Cm 4386 (1999) *Saving Lives: Our Healthier Nation*. London: HMSO.

Cm 4818 (2000) *The NHS Plan: A Plan for Investment, A Plan for Reform*. London: HMSO.

Cm 6374 (2004) *Choosing Health: Making Healthy Choices Easier*. London: HMSO.

Cm 7881 (2010) *Equity and Excellence: Liberating the NHS*. London: HMSO.

Cm 7985 (2010) *Healthy Lives, Healthy People: Our Strategy for Public Health in England*. London: HMSO.

Coffman, J (2007) Evaluation based on theories of the policy process. *The Evaluation Exchange,* XIII(1). Online at: www.hfrp.org/evaluation/the-evaluation-exchange/issue-archive/advocacy-and-policy-change/evaluation-based-on-theories-of-the-policy-process, accessed 14 November 2010.

Colebatch, HK (1998) *Policy.* Buckingham: Open University Press.

Colebatch, HK (2002) *Policy* (2nd edn). Buckingham: Open University Press.

Colebatch, HK (2006) What work makes policy? *Policy Sciences,* 39(4): 309–21.

Colebatch, HK (2009) *Policy* (3rd edn). Maidenhead: Open University Press.

Communities and Local Government (CLG) (2010) *A Review of Health and Safety Risk Drivers.* London: Department for Communities and Local Government.

Concordia (2007) *Childcare that Works.* Dungannon: Concordia.

Cowley, S (ed.) (2008) *Community Public Health in Policy and Practice. A Source-book* (2nd edn). Edinburgh: Bailliere Tindall Elsevier.

Cox, SJ and O'Sullivan, EFO (eds) (1995) *Building Regulation and Safety.* Watford: Building Research Establishment.

Cox, Y and Fenech, A (2010) *Public Service Adaptation* (unpublished model). University of Southampton: Faculty of Health Sciences.

Cox, Y and Rawlinson, M (2008) *Strategic Leadership for Health and Wellbeing,* in Coles, L and Porter, E (eds) *Public Health Skills: A Practical Guide for Nurses and Public Health Practitioners.* Oxford: Blackwell Publishing.

Crinson, I (2009) *Health Policy: A Critical Perspective.* London: Sage.

Crisis (2002) *Critical Condition: Homeless People's Access to GPs.* London: Crisis.

Curtice, J (2006) A stronger or weaker union? Public reactions to asymmetric devolution in the United Kingdom. *Publius: The Journal of Federalism,* 36(1): 95–113.

Dahrendorf, RG (1969) The nature and types of social inequality, in Beteille, A (ed.) *Social Inequality.* Middlesex: Penguin Books: 21.

Dailly, J and Barr, A (2008) *Understanding a Community Led Approach to Health Improvement. Health Communities.* Edinburgh: Scottish Government.

Dalziel, Y (2000) Community development as a strategy for public health, in Craig, P and Lindsay, G (eds) *Nursing for Public Health.* Edinburgh: Churchill Livingstone.

Davidson, M (2010) *Perceptions of Safety and Fear of Crime in Housing and Health in Europe: The WHO LARES Project.* London: Routledge.

Davies, J (2007) *A History of Wales.* Harmondsworth: Penguin.

Davies, J (2010) What are we doing to tackle the issue of obesity in Southampton? Online at: www.southampton.gov.uk/modernGov/mgConvert2PDF.aspx?ID=1530.

Day, G (2002) *Making Sense of Wales: A Sociological Perspective*. Cardiff: University of Wales Press.

Day, G, Dunkerley, D and Thompson, A (eds) (2006*) Civil Society in Wales: Policy, Politics and People: Policy, Politics and People* (Politics and Society in Wales Series). University of Wales Press.

Democratic Dialogue (2003) *Bare Necessities Poverty and Social Exclusion in Northern Ireland – Key Findings*. Belfast: Democratic Dialogue.

Department for Communities and Local Government (DCLG) (2007) *Homes for the Future: More Affordable, More Sustainable*. London: Department for Communities and Local Government.

Department of the Environment (DoE) (1996) *Private Sector Renewal: A Strategic Approach* (Circular 17/96). London: Department of the Environment.

Department of Environment, Food and Rural Affairs (DEFRA) (2000) *Warm Front*. London: Department for Environment, Food and Rural Affairs. Online at: ww2.defra.gov.uk/environment (accessed 1 September 2006).

Department of the Environment, Transport and the Regions (DETR) (1996) *Private Sector Renewal: a Strategic Approach* (Circular 17/96). London: Department of the Environment.

Department of the Environment, Transport and the Regions (DETR) (1998) *English House Condition Survey 1996*. London: Department of the Environment, Transport and the Regions.

Department of Health (DoH) (1992) *The Health of the Nation*. London: HMSO.

Department of Health (DoH) (1995a) *Tackling Drugs Together: A Strategy for England 1995–1998*. London: HMSO.

Department of Health (DoH) (1995b) *Variations in Health: What can the Department of Health and the NHS do*? London: Department of Health.

Department of Health (DoH) (1998) *Tackling Drugs to Build a Better Britain: The Government's Ten Year Strategy for Tackling Drugs Misuse*. London: HMSO.

Department of Health (DoH) (with the University of Leeds, University of Glamorgan, London School of Hygiene and Tropical Medicine) (1998) *The Health of the Nation – A Policy Assessed*. London: Department of Health. Online at: www.dh.gov.uk/prod_consum_dh/groups/dh_digitalassets/@dh/@en/documents/digitalasset/dh_4011788.pdf.

Department of Health (DoH) (1999a) *National Service Framework for Mental Health*. London: HMSO.

Department of Health (DoH) (1999b) *Saving Lives: Our Healthier Nation*. London: HMSO.

Department of Health (DoH) (1999c) *Smoking Kills: A White Paper on Tobacco* (CM 4177). London: HMSO.

Department of Health (DoH) (1999d) *Reducing Inequalities: An Action Report*. London: Department of Health. Online at: www.dh.gov.uk/prod_consum_dh/groups/dh_digitalassets/@dh/@en/documents/digitalasset/dh_4042496.pdf.

Department of Health (DoH) (2000) *The NHS Plan: A Plan for Investment, a Plan for Reform*. London: HMSO.

Department of Health (DoH) (2001) *Devolution Concordat on Health and Social Care; UK Department of Health, Cabinet of the National Assembly for Wales and Department of Health, Social Services and Public Safety*. London: Department of Health.

Department of Health (DoH) (2002) *Delivering the NHS Plan – Next Steps on Investment; Next Steps in Reform* and *Annual Report of the Chief Medical Officer: Health Check on the State of the Public Health*. London: Department of Health Publications. Online at: www.dh.gov.uk/prod_consum_dh/groups/dh_digita-lassets/@dh/@en/documents/digitalasset/dh_4081860.pdf.

Department of Health (DoH) (2003) *Tackling Health Inequalities: A Programme For Action*. London: Department of Health Publications.

Department of Health (DoH) (2004a) *Choosing Health? A Consultation on Action to Improve People's Health. Consultation Analysis Final Report*. London: HMSO. Online at: webarchive.nationalarchives.gov.uk/+/www.dh.gov.uk/en/Consultations/Responsestoconsultations/DH_4106017, accessed 14 November 2010.

Department of Health (DoH) (2004b) *Choosing Health: Making Healthy Choices Easier*. London: HMSO. Online at: webarchive.nationalarchives.gov.uk/+/www.dh.gov.uk/en/Publicationsandstatistics/Publications/PublicationsPolicyAndGuidance/Browsable/DH_4097491.

Department of Health (DoH) (2004c) *NHS Improvement Plan*. www.dh.gov.uk/en/Publicationsandstatistics/Publications/PublicationsPolicyAndGuidance/DH_4086057, accessed 14 November 2010.

Department of Health (DoH) (2004d) Spending Review. Online at: www.dh.gov.uk/en/Aboutus/HowDHworks/Servicestandardsandcommitments/DHPublicServiceAgreement/DH_4106188.

Department of Health (DoH) (2004e) *The NHS Knowledge and Skills Framework (NHS KSF) and the Development Review Process*. London: Department of Health. Online at: www.dh.gov.uk/en/Publicationsandstatistics/Publications/PublicationsPolicyAndGuidance/DH_4090843, accessed 14 November 2010.

Department of Health (DoH) (2005a) *Choosing a Better Diet: A Food and Health Action Plan*. London: Department of Health Publications. Online at: www.dh.gov.uk/prod_consum_dh/groups/dh_digitalassets/@dh/@en/docu-ments/digitalasset/dh_4105709.pdf.

Department of Health (DoH) (2005b) *Choosing Activity: A Physical Activity Action Plan*. Online at: www.dh.gov.uk/prod_consum_dh/groups/dh_digitalassets/@dh/@en/documents/digitalasset/dh_4105710.pdf.

Department of Health (DoH) (2005c) *Practice Based Commissioning*. Online at: www.library.nhs.uk/HealthManagement/ViewResource.aspx?resID=122205&tabID=288, accessed 14 November 2010.

Department of Health (DoH) (2006a) *Devolution Concordat on Health and Social Care: UK Department of Health and the Scottish Executive*. London: HMSO.

Department of Health (DoH) (2006b) *Our Health, Our Care, Our Say: A New Direction for Community Services*. Online at: www.dh.gov.uk/en/Publications andstatistics/Publications/PublicationsPolicyAndGuidance/DH_4136930, accessed 14 November 2010.

Department of Health (DoH) (2008a) *Drugs: Protecting Families and Communities. The 2008 Drug Strategy*. London: HMSO.

Department of Health (DoH) (2008b) *Healthy Weight, Healthy Lives: A Cross Government Strategy for England*. London: Department of Health Publications. Online at: www.dh.gov.uk/prod_consum_dh/groups/dh_digitalassets/documents/digitalasset/dh_084024.pdf.

Department of Health (DoH) (2008c) *High Quality Care For All: NHS Next Stage Review Final Report*. London: HMSO. Online at: www.dh.gov.uk/en/Publicationsandstatistics/Publications/PublicationsPolicyAndGuidance/DH_085825, accessed 14 November 2010.

Department of Health (DoH) (2008d) *Improving Access to Psychological Therapies*. London: HMSO.

Department of Health (DoH) (2009) *Tackling Health Inequalities: 2006–08 Policy and Data Update for the 2010 National Target*. London: HMSO.

Department of Health (DoH) (2010a) *Equity and Excellence: Liberating the NHS*. Online at: www.dh.gov.uk/en/Publicationsandstatistics/Publications/PublicationsPolicyAndGuidance/DH_117353, accessed 14 November 2010.

Department of Health (DoH) (2010b) *The NHS Constitution*. London: HMSO.

Department of Health (DoH) (2010c) *Healthy Lives, Healthy People: Our Strategy for Public Health in England*. London: HMSO.

Department of Health, Social Services & Public Safety Northern Ireland (DHSSPSNI) (2002) *Investing for Health Strategy*. Online at: www.dhsspsni.gov.uk/show_publications?txtid=10415, accessed 27 January 2011.

Department of Health, Social Services & Public Safety Northern Ireland (DHSSPSNI) (2005) *Independent Review of Health and Social Care Services in Northern Ireland*. Online at: www.dhsspsni.gov.uk/show_publications?txtid=13 662, accessed 27 January 2011.

Department of Health, Social Services & Public Safety Northern Ireland (DHSSPSNI) (2008) *Health Improvement Plan*. Online at: www.dhsspsni.gov.uk/index.htm, accessed 27 January 2011.

Department of Health & Social Security (DHSS) (1980) *Inequalities in Health: Report of a Research Working Party* (The Black Report). London: HMSO.

Department of Health and Social Services and Public Safety (DHSSPS) (1999) *Children First*. Belfast: DHSSPS.

Dignam, T (2003) *Low-Income Households 1990–2002: Methodology and Statistics Tables*. Belfast: OFMDFM.

Drummond, DC and Strang, J (2001) *British System of Drug-Addiction Treatment. Encyclopaedia of Drugs, Alcohol and Addictive Behaviour*. Online at: www.encyclopedia.com, accessed 20 September 2009.

Duke, K (2006) Out of crime and into treatment? The criminalization of contemporary drug policy since *Tackling Drugs Together*. *Drugs: Education, Prevention and Policy*, 13(5): 409–15.

Easton, D (1953) *The Political System*. New York: Alfred A Knopf.

Easton, D (1965) *A Systems Analysis of Political Life*. New York: Wiley.

Economic and Research Council (2004) *Findings from the Economic and Research Council's Research Programme on Devolution and Constitutional Change: What's Distinctive About Wales? Findings from a Comparison of Wales with Brittany*, Briefing No. 10, June. Online at: www.devolution.ac.uk/pdfdata/Cole_briefing_10.pdf, accessed 27 January 2011.

Economic and Social Data Service (2010) *Social Capital: Introductory User Guide*. Office of National Statistics. Online at: www.esds.ac.uk, accessed 27 January 2011.

Edwards, B (2007) *An Independent NHS: A Review of the Options*. London: Nuffield Trust.

Edwards, VK and Newcombe, LM (2003) *Evaluation of the Efficiency and Effectiveness of the Twf Project, Which Encourages Parents to Transmit the Language to their Children*. University of Reading. Online at: www.ncll.org.uk/50_research/10_research_projects/Twf_evaluation.pdf, accessed 27 January 2011.

Elementa Leadership (2010) Online at: www.elementaleadership.co.uk, accessed 27 January 2011.

Elmore, R (1979) Backward mapping, *Political Science Quarterly*, 94: 601–16. Reprinted in Williams, W (ed.) *Studying Implementation*. Chatham, NJ: Chatham House.

ESRC (2005) *Poverty and Income Distribution in Northern Ireland, ESRC Seminar Series, Mapping the Public Policy Landscape*. London: ESRC.

Etzioni, A (1967) Mixed scanning: a 'third' approach to decision making. *Public Administration Review*, 27(5): 385–92.

European Union (2010) *Determine*. Online at: www.health-inequalities.eu, accessed 27 January 2011.

Evans, D (2003) Hierarchy of evidence: a framework for ranking evidence evaluating healthcare interventions. *Journal of Clinical Nursing*, 12: 77–84.

Exworthy, M, Stuart, M, Blane, D and Marmot, M (2003) *Tackling Health Inequalities Since the Acheson Inquiry 2003*. Online at: www.jrf.org.uk/sites/files/jrf/jr140-health-inequalities-acheson.pdf.

Faculty of Public Health of the Royal College of Physicians of the United Kingdom (2007) *Public Health Training Curriculum 2007*. London: Faculty of Public Health. Online at: www.fph.org.uk/training_e-portfolio#post2007.

Fawcett, L (2009) Childcare matters. *Research Update*, 59. Online at: www.ark.ac.uk/publications/updates/update59.pdf.

Fitzpatrick, S, Kemp, P and Klinker, S (2000) *Research on Single Homelessness in Britain*. London: Joseph Rowntree Foundation.

Foresight (2007) *Tackling Obesities: Future Choices* (Project Report). London: HMSO. Online at: www.bis.gov.uk/assets/bispartners/foresight/docs/obesity/obesity_final_part1.pdf.

Friedman, MA (1962) *Freedom and Capitalism*. Chicago: University of Chicago Press.

General Register Office (2009) Online at: www.gro-scotland.gov.uk, accessed 27 January 2011.

George, V and Wilding, P (1994) *Welfare and Ideology*. Hemel Hempstead: Harvester Wheatsheaf.

Gilchrist, A (2007) Community development and networking for health, in Orme J, Powell, J, Taylor, M and Gray, M (eds) *Public Health for the 21st Century: New Perspectives on Policy, Participation, and Practice*. Buckingham: Open University.

Gillespie, A (2007) *Foundations of Economics, Additional Chapter on Business Strategy*. Oxford: Oxford University Press. Online at: www.oup.com/uk/orc/bin/9780199296378/01student/additional, accessed June 2010.

Gossop, M, Marsden, J, Edwards, C, Wilson, A, Segar, G and Steward, D (1995) *The National Treatment Outcome Research Study: A Report for the Task-force*. London: Department of Health.

Government of Wales Act (GOWA) (1998) (c. 38). Online at: www.opsi.gov.uk/acts/acts1998/ukpga_19980038_en_1, accessed 27 January 2011.

Government of Wales Act (GOWA) (2006) Statutory Instrument 1999, No. 672, National Assembly for Wales (Transfer of Functions) Order 1999. Online at: www.uklaws.org/statutory/instruments_21/doc21479.htm, accessed 27 January 2011.

Grayson, L and Gomersall, A (2003) *A Difficult Business: Finding the Evidence for Social Science Reviews*. ESRC UK Centre for Evidence Based Policy and Practice

Working Paper No. 19. London: Queen Mary, University of London. Online at: www.evidencenetwork.org, accessed 27 January 2011.

Green, DS (1987) *The New Right: The Counter Revolution in Political Economic and Social Thought*. Brighton: Wheatsheaf.

Green, J (1995) School sex education policies: a qualitative analysis of the process of policy development. *Journal of the Institute of Health Education*, 32(4): 106–11.

Green, J and Tones, K (2010) *Health Promotion Planning and Strategies*. London: Sage Publications.

Greer, S (2004a) *Four Way Bet: How Devolution has Led to Four Different Models for the NHS*. London: UCL.

Greer, SL (2004b) *Territorial Politics and Health Policy*. Manchester: Manchester University Press.

Greer, S (2008) Devolution and public health politics in the United Kingdom, in Dawson, S and Slote Morris, Z (eds) *Future Public Health: Burdens, Challenges and Opportunities*. Basingstoke: Palgrave Macmillan.

Griffiths, S, Jewell, T and Donnelly, P (2005) Public health in practice: the three domains of public health. *Public Health*, 119(10): 907–13.

Griffiths Report (1983) *NHS Management Inquiry*. London: HMSO.

Gunn, L (1978) Why is implementation so difficult? *Management Services in Government*, 33: 169–76.

Hall, P, Land, H, Parker, R and Webb, A (1975) C*hange, Choice and Conflict in Social Policy*. London: Heinemann.

Ham, C (1999) *Health Policy in Britain* (4th edn). Basingstoke: Palgrave.

Ham, C (2004) *Health Policy in Britain* (5th edn). Basingstoke: Palgrave.

Ham, C (2009) *Health Policy in Britain* (6th edn). Basingstoke: Palgrave Macmillan.

Ham, C and Hill, M (1993) *The Policy Process in the Modern Capitalist State*. Hemel Hempstead: Harvester Wheatsheaf.

Hancock, T (1992) The healthy cities: utopias and realities, in Ashton, J (ed.) *Healthy Cities*. Milton Keynes: Open University Press.

Handy, C (1985) *Understanding Organizations* (3rd edn). Harmondsworth: Penguin.

Hanley, L (2007) *Estates: An Intimate History*. London: Granta.

Harker, L (2006) *Chance of a Lifetime: The Impact of Bad Housing on Children's Lives*. London: Shelter.

Harkins, C (2010) The Portman Group. When it comes to alcohol awareness, is the government under the influence of the drinks industry? *British Medical Journal*, 340: 187.

Harrison, S and McDonald, R (2008) *The Politics of Healthcare in Britain*. London: Sage.

Hastings, GSM, McDermott, L, Forsyth, A, MacKintosh, AM, Rayner, M, Godfrey, C, Caraher, M and Angus, K (2003) *Review of Research on the Effects of Food Promotion to Children*. University of Strathclyde: Centre for Social Marketing. Online at: www.food.gov.uk/multimedia/pdfs/foodpromotionto-children1.pdf.

Hayek, FA (1944) *The Road to Serfdom*. Chicago: University of Chicago Press.

Hill, M (1997) *The Public Policy Process* (4th edn). Harlow: Pearson Longman.

Hill, M (2005) *The Public Policy Process* (4th edn). Harlow: Pearson Education Ltd.

Hirsch, D (2008) *What is Needed to End Child Poverty in 2020?* York: Joseph Rowntree Foundation.

HM Government (1995) *Tackling Drugs Together: A Strategy for England 1995–1998*. London: HMSO.

HM Government (1998) *Tackling Drugs to Build a Better Britain: The Government's Ten Year Strategy for Tackling Drugs Misuse*. London: HMSO.

HM Government (2008) *Drugs: Protecting Families and Communities. The 2008 Drug Strategy*. London: HMSO.

HM Government (2010) *The Coalition: Our Programme for Government*. London: Cabinet Office. Online at: www.cabinetoffice.gov.uk/media/409088/pfg_coalition.pdf.

HM Treasury (2002) *Securing our Future Taking a Long-term View – the Wanless Report*. London: HM Treasury. Online at: webarchive.nationalarchives.gov.uk/+/http://www.hm-treasury.gov.uk/consult_wanless_final.htm.

Hoare, J and Moon, D (eds) (2010) *Drug Misuse Declared: Findings from the 2009/10 British Crime Survey England and Wales*. British Crime Survey. Online at: rds.homeoffice.gov.uk/rds/pdfs10/hosb1310.pdf, accessed 27 January 2011.

Hodgson, S and Irving, Z (eds) (2007) *Policy Reconsidered: Meanings, Politics and Practices*. Bristol: Policy Press.

Hogwood, BW and Gunn, LA (1984) *Policy Analysis for the Real World*. Oxford: Oxford University Press.

Home Office (2010) *The Misuse of Drugs Act (1971)*. Online at: www.homeoffice.gov.uk/drugs/drug-law, accessed 25 November 2010.

Horgan, G and Monteith, M (2009) *What Can We Do to Tackle Child Poverty in Northern Ireland?* York: Joseph Rowntree Foundation.

House of Commons Committee of Public Accounts (2007) *Tackling Child Obesity*

– *First Steps: Eighth Report of Session 2006–07*. London: HMSO. Online at: www.publications.parliament.uk/pa/cm200607/cmselect/cmpubacc/157/157.pdf.

House of Commons Health Committee (2004) *Third Report on Session 2003–2004*. Online at: www.parliament.the-stationery-office.co.uk/pa/cm200304/cmselect/cmhealth/23/2302.htm.

House of Commons – Health Committee (2009) *Third Report on Health Inequalities*. Online at: www.publications.parliament.uk/pa/cm200809/cmselect/cmhealth/286/286.pdf, accessed 27 January 2011.

House of Commons Health Select Committee (2010) *Alcohol, First Report of Session 1*. London: HMSO. Online at: www.publications.parliament.uk/pa/cm200910/cmselect/cmhealth/151/15102.htm, accessed 27 January 2011.

Housing Act (1988) London: HMSO. Online at: http://www.legislation.gov.uk/ukpga/1988/50/contents, accessed 27 January 2011.

Housing Act (2004) London: HMSO. Online at: www.legislation.gov.uk/ukpga/2004/34/data.pdf, accessed 27 January 2011.

Housing Corporation (2006) *Good Housing and Good Health? A Review and Recommendations for Housing and Health Practitioners. Part 5*. Online at: http://www.hiaconnect.edu.au/files/Good_housing_and_good_health.pdf, accessed 27 January 2011.

Howden-Chapman, P and Carroll, P (2004) *Housing and Health: Research, Policy and Innovation*. Wellington, New Zealand: Steele Roberts.

Howden-Chapman, P, Matheson, A, Crane, J, Viggers, H, Cunninghan, M, Blakely, T, Cunninighan, C, Woodward, A, Woodward, A, Saville-Smith, K, O'Dea, D, Kennedy, M, Baker, M, Wainara, N, Chapman, R and Davie, G (2007) Effect of insulating existing houses on health inequality: cluster randomised study in the community. *British Medical Journal*, 334: 460.

Hunter, DJ (2003) *Public Health Policy*. Cambridge: Polity Press.

Hunter, S and Ritchie, P (2008) Co-production and personalization in social care: changing relationships in the provision of social care, in *Research Highlights in Social Work 49*. Gateshead: Althenaeum Press.

Independent Inquiry into Inequalities in Health (1998) *Report* (Acheson Report). London: HMSO.

Ineichen, B (1993) *Homes and Health: How Housing and Health Interact*. London: E&FN Spon.

International Harm Reduction Association (IHRA) (2009) *What is Harm Reduction? A Position Statement from the IHRA*. London: IHRA.

Ison, E (2002) *Rapid Appraisal Tool for Health Impact Assessment: A Task-based Approach*. Oxford: Institute of Health Sciences. Online at: www.fph.org.uk/uploads/Intro.pdf, accessed 27 January 2011.

Jenkins, M and Ambrosini, A (2002) *Strategic Management: A Multi-perspective Approach*. Basingstoke: Palgrave.

Jenkins, R (2002) The meaning of policy/policy as meaning, in Hodgson, S and Irving, Z (eds) *Policy Reconsidered: Meanings, Politics and Practices*. Bristol: Policy Press.

Jervis, P (2008) *Devolution and Health*. London. Nuffield Trust.

Jervis, P and Plowden, W (2003) *The Impact of Political Devolution on the UK's Health Services*. London: Nuffield Trust.

Jochelson, K (2005) *Nanny or Steward? The Role of Government in Public Health*. London: King's Fund.

John, P (1998) *Analysing Public Policy*. London: Creswell.

Johnson, G, Scholes, K and Whittington, R (2006) *Exploring Corporate Strategy*. Harlow: Prentice Hall.

Joseph Rowntree Foundation (1994) The health of single homeless people. *Housing Research*, 128.

Joseph Rowntree Foundation (2009) *Monitoring Poverty and Social Exclusion in Northern Ireland*, September, ref. 2392. York: JRF.

Journal of Public Health Management and Practice (2010) Volume 16, September/October, E-Supplement 5. Online at: journals.lww.com/jphmp/toc/2010/09001#-1750774083, accessed 27 January 2011.

Kenway, P, MacInnes, T, Kelly, A and Palmer, G (2006) *Monitoring Poverty and Social Exclusion in Northern Ireland*. York: JRF.

Kickbush, I (2010) Health in all policies: where to from here? *Health Promotion International*, 25(3): 261–4.

Kingdon, J (1984) *Agendas, Alternatives and Public Policies*. Boston: Little Brown.

Kingdon, J (2003) *Agendas, Alternatives and Public Policies*. New York: Longman.

Kjærnes, U (2003) Food and nutrition policies of Nordic countries: how have they been developed and what evidence substantiates the development of these policies? *Proceedings of the Nutrition Society*, 62: 563–70.

Klein, R (2005) Transforming the NHS: the story in 2004, in Powell, M, Bauld, L and Clarke, K (eds) *Social Policy Review 17: Analysis and Debate in Social Policy*. Bristol: Policy Press.

Labour Party (1997) *New Labour: Because Britain Deserves Better*. London: Labour Party.

Lalonde, M (1974) *A New Perspective on the Health of Canadians: A Working Document*. Ottawa: Minister of Supply and Services Canada. Online at: www.hc-sc.gc.ca/hcs-sss/pubs/system-regime/1974-lalonde/index-eng.php.

Lalonde, M (1977) The physician and health promotion. *Canadian Medical Association*, 116.

Laverack, G (2009) *Public Health. Power, Empowerment and Professional Practice.* Basingstoke: Palgrave Macmillan.

Layard, Lord (2006) *The Depression Report. A New Deal for Depression and Anxiety Disorders.* London School of Economics: The Centre for Economic Performance's, Mental Health Policy Group.

Leeke, M, Sear, C and Gay, O (2003) *An Introduction to Devolution in the UK, Research Paper 03/84.* Parliament and Constitution Centre: House of Commons Library. Online at: www.parliament.uk/documents/commons/lib/research/ rp2003/rp03-084.pdf, accessed 27 January 2011.

Leichter, H (1979) *A Comparative Approach to Policy Analysis: Health Care Policy in Four Nations.* Cambridge: Cambridge University Press.

Lewis, J and Flynn, R (1979) The implementation of urban and regional planning policies. *Policy and Politics*, 7: 123–42.

Leydon, KM (2003) Social capital and the built environment: the importance of walkable neighbourhoods. *American Journal of Public Health*, September, 93(9): 1546–51.

Liddell, C (2008) *The Impact of Fuel Poverty on Children. Policy Briefing.* Online at: www.savethechildren.org.uk/northernireland, accessed 27 January 2011.

Lifelong Learning UK. (2009) *National Occupational Standards for Community Development.* London: Lifelong Learning UK. Online at: www.fcdl.org.uk/ NOS_Consultation/Documents/NOS_CD_Eng_v2finalartworkedversion.pdf, accessed 27 January 2011.

Lindblom, C (1959) The science of muddling through. *Public Administration Review*, 19: 78–88.

Lipsky, M (1971) Street-level bureaucracy and the analysis of urban reform. *Urban Affairs Quarterly*, 6: 391–409.

Lipsky, M (1980) *Street Level Bureaucracy: Dilemmas of the Individuals in Public Services.* New York: Russell Sage Foundation.

Lister, R (2010) *Understanding Theories and Concepts in Social Policy.* Bristol: Policy Press.

Lloyd, C, Handsley, S, Douglas, J, Earle, S and Spurr, S (2007) *Policy and Practice in Promoting Public Health.* London: Sage.

Lloyd, C, Handsley, S, Douglas, J, Earle, S and Spurr, S (2009) *A Reader in Promoting Public Health* (2nd edn). Berkshire: Open University Press.

London Citizens Team (2008) *A Better Housed London.* Online at: www.londoncitizens.org.uk, accessed 27 January 2011.

Lukes, S (2004) *Power: A Radical View* (2nd edn). London: Palgrave.

Macdiarmid, JI, Loe, J, Douglas, F, Ludbrook, A, Comerford, C and McNeill, G (2010) Developing a timeline for evaluating public health nutrition policy interventions. What are the outcomes and when should we expect to see them? *Public Health Nutrition*, August, 16: 1.

Macdowell, W, Bonell, C and Davies, M (2006) *Health Promotion Practice*. Maidenhead: Open University Press.

MacGregor, S (2006) *Tackling Drugs Together: ten years on. Drugs: Education, Prevention and Policy*, 13(5): 393–8.

Mackenbach, JP (2006) Socio-economic inequalities in health in Western Europe, in Siegrist, J and Marmot, M (eds) *Social Inequalities in Health*. Oxford: Oxford University Press.

Mannion, R (2010) Eclipsing the clan culture in the NHS. *Health Service Journal*, 22 July: 20–1.

Mant, D and Muir Gray, JA (1986) *Building Regulation and Health*. Watford: Building Research Establishment.

Marmot Review (2010) *Fair Society, Healthy Lives. Strategic Review of Health Inequalities in England Post-2010* (Marmot Review). London: University College. Online at: www.marmotreview.org, accessed 27 January 2011.

Maryon-Davis, A and Jolley, R (2010) *Healthy Nudges – When the Public Wants Change and Politicians Don't Know It*. London: Faculty of Public Health.

Maslin-Prothero, S, Masterton, A and Jones, K (2008) Four parts or one whole: the National Health Service (NHS) post-devolution. *Journal of Nursing Management*, 16: 662–72.

Maslow, JH (1943) Theory of human motivation. *Psychological Review*, 50(4): 370–96.

Meerding, WJ, Mulder, S and Van Beeck, EF (2006) Incidence and costs of injuries in the Netherlands. *European Journal of Public Health*, 16(3): 217–77.

Meier, GM (1991) Policy lessons and policy formation, in Meier, GM (ed.) *Policy and Policy Making in Developing Countries. Perspectives on the New Political Economy*. San Francisco: ICS Press.

Mental Health Foundation (2010) Primary care and mental health. Online at: www.mentalhealth.org.uk/our-work/policy/primary-care/?locale=en.

Michael, P and Tanner, D (2007) Values vs policy in NHS Wales, in Greer, S and Rowand, D (eds) *Devolving Policy, Diverging Values? The Values of the United Kingdom's National Health Service*. London, Nuffield Trust.

Milio, N (1986) Multi-sectoral policy and health promotion: where to begin? *Health Promotion*, 1(2): 129–132. Also in Abel-Smith, B (1994) *Introduction to Health Policy, Planning and Financing*. London: Longman.

Monaghan, S, Huws, D and Navarro, M (2003) *The Case for a New UK Health of the People Act*. London: Nuffield Trust.

Montanari, JR and Bracker, JS (1986) The strategic management process at the public planning unit level, in Johnson, G, Scholes, K and Whittington, R (2006) *Exploring Corporate Strategy*. Harlow: FT Prentice Hall.

Monteith, M and McLaughlin, E (2004) *The Bottom Line: Children and Severe Poverty in Northern Ireland*, Belfast: Save the Children.

Monteith, M, Lloyd, K and McKee, P (2008) Persistent Child Poverty in Northern Ireland. Online at: www.savethechildren.org.uk/northernireland, accessed 27 January 2011.

Moore, A (2009) Are we drifting apart? *Nursing Standard*, 23: 3422–4.

Moore, R (2003) Personal communication (with permission).

Moran, M, Rein, M and Goodin, RE (2006) *The Oxford Handbook of Public Policy*. Oxford: Oxford University Press.

Morgan, G (1986) *Images of Organization*. Newbury Park, CA: Sage.

Morgan, R (2002) Clear red water. Speech to the University of Wales, Swansea, 11 December, National Centre for Public Policy Third Anniversary Lecture. Online at: www.sochealth.co.uk/Regions/Wales/redwater.htm, accessed 27 January 2011.

Morris, K, Barnes, M and Mason, P (2009) *Children, Families and Social Exclusion, New Approaches to Prevention*. Bristol: Policy Press.

Mulgan, G (2010) *Influencing Public Behaviour to Improve Health and Wellbeing*. London: Department of Health.

Naidoo, J and Wills, J (2005) *Public Health and Policy Promotion, Developing Practice* (2nd edn). Edinburgh: Bailliere Tindall: 67–85.

Naidoo, J and Wills, J (2009) *Foundations for Health Promotion* (3rd edn). Edinburgh: Bailliere Tindall Elsevier.

National Assembly of Wales (NAW) (2000) *Extending Entitlement*. Cardiff: NAW.

National Assembly of Wales (NAW) (2001) *Children and Adolescent Mental Health Services, Everybody's Business*. Cardiff: NAW. Online at: www.wales.nhs.uk/publications/men-health-e.pdf, accessed 27 January 2011.

National Audit Office (2001) *Tackling Obesity in England*. London: National Audit Office. Online at: www.nao.org.uk/publications/0001/tackling_obesity_in_england.aspx.

National Audit Office (2006) *Tackling Childhood Obesity – First Steps*. London: HMSO. Online at: www.nao.org.uk/publications/0506/tackling_child_obesity.aspx.

National Children's Bureau (2007) *The Day Care Needs of Disabled Young Children in Northern Ireland*. Belfast: NCB.

National Health Service (NHS) (2000) *The NHS Plan: A Plan for Investment, a Plan for Reform*. London: HMSO. Online at: www.dh.gov.uk/en/Publicationsand statistics/Publications/PublicationsPolicyAndGuidance/DH_4002960.

National Health Service (NHS) Information Centre (2009) *Health Survey for England – 2008 Trend Tables*. Online at: www.ic.nhs.uk/pubs/hse08trends.

National Health Service (NHS) Scotland and Scottish Executive Health Department (2007) *NHS Scotland eHealth Strategy – The Nursing, Midwifery and Allied Health Professions Contribution to Realising the Benefits of the National eHealth Programme*. Online at: www.ehealthnurses.org.uk/pdf/NMAHP%20eHealth%20 Action%20Plan.pdf, accessed 27 January 2011.

National Institute for Clinical Excellence (NICE) (2005) *Housing and Public Health: A Review of Reviews of Interventions for Improving Health*. Evidence Briefing Summary. London: NICE.

National Institute for Clinical Excellence (NICE) (2006) *Obesity Guidance on the Prevention, Identification, Assessment and Management of Overweight and Obesity in Adults and Children*. London: NICE. Online at: www.nice.org.uk/nicemedia/pdf/ CG43NICEGuideline.pdf.

National Institute for Clinical Excellence (NICE) (2009) *Nice Clinical Guideline CG90 on Depression*. Online at: www.nice.org.uk/usingguidance/commission-ingguides/cognitivebehaviouraltherapyservice/steppedcaremodels.jsp.

National Obesity Observatory (2010a) *Health Risks of Adult Obesity*. Online at: www.noo.org.uk/NOO_about_obesity/obesity_and_health/health_risk_adult.

National Obesity Observatory (2010b) *Health Risks of Childhood Obesity*. Online at: www.noo.org.uk/NOO_about_obesity/obesity_and_health/health_risk_ child.

National Treatment Agency (NTA) (2008) *Good Practice in Harm Reduction*. National Treatment Agency for Substance Misuse.

Neave, J (1999) in Masterton, A and Maslin-Prothero, S (eds) *Nursing and Politics: Power Through Practice*. London: Churchill Livingstone.

Needham, C and Carr, S (2009) *SCIE Research Briefing 31: Co-production: An Emerging Evidence Base for Adult Social Care Transformation*. London: Social Care Institute for Excellence.

Nettleton, S and Burrows, R (1998) Mortgage debt, insecure home ownership and health: an exploratory analysis. *Sociology of Health and Illness,* 20(5): 731–53.

NHS Management Inquiry (1983) *Report* (Chairman Mr ER Griffiths). London: Department of Health.

Nicol, S, Roys, M, Davidson, M, Ormandy, D and Ambrose, P (2010) *The Real Cost of Poor Housing*. Watford: BRE Press.

Northern Ireland Assembly (NIA) (2008a) *Comparing Child Poverty in Northern Ireland with Other Regions*, Briefing Note 23/08. Belfast: NIA.

Northern Ireland Assembly (NIA) (2008b) *Tackling Severe Childhood Poverty*, Briefing Note 09/08. Belfast: NIA.

Northern Ireland Assembly (NIA) (2008c) *Childcare Provision in the UK and the Republic of Ireland*, Research Paper 16/08. Belfast: NIA.

Northern Ireland Assembly (NIA) (2010) Child poverty and childcare strategy debates, 24 November. Online at: http://www.niassembly.gov.uk/record/committees2010/OFMDFM/101124_ChildPovertyChildcare.htm.

Northern Ireland Investing for Health Partnership (2008) Online at: www.dhssp-sni.gov.uk/61-north_down_and_ards_investing_for_health_partnership.pdf.

Northern Ireland Office (1998) *The Belfast Agreement*. Online at: www.nio.gov.uk/agreement.pdf, accessed 27 January 2011.

Northern Ireland Pre-School Association (NIPPA) (2006) *Response to the Draft Budget Statement by Peter Hain from NIPPA – The Early Years Organisation*. Belfast: NIPPA.

Northumbria University (2009) *PESTLE and SWOT Analysis*. Online at: www.jiscinfonet.ac.uk/tools/pestle-swot, accessed 17 June 2010.

Nuffield Council on Bioethics (2007) *Public Health: Ethical Issues*. Cambridge: Nuffield Council on Bioethics.

Nutt, DJ (2009) *Estimating Drug Harms: A Risky Business? Eve Saville Lecture*. Centre for Crime and Justice Studies, Briefing 10, October.

Nutt, DJ and Advisory Council on the Misuse of Drugs (ACMD) (2009) *MDMA (Ecstasy): A Review of its Harms and Classification Under the Misuse of Drugs Act 1971*. Online at: www.drugs.homeoffice.gov.uk/publication-search/acmd/acmd-MDMA-report-2009, accessed 27 January 2011.

Nutt, DJ, King, LA and Saulsbury, W (2007) Development of a rational scale to assess the harm of drugs of potential misuse. *The Lancet*, 369(9566): 1047–53, March.

OFCOM (2008) *Code on the Scheduling of Television Advertising*. London: OFCOM. Online at: stakeholders.ofcom.org.uk/binaries/broadcast/other-codes/tacode.pdf.

Office of the Deputy Prime Minister (ODPM) (2003a) *English House Condition Survey 2001*. London: Office of the Deputy Prime Minister.

Office of the Deputy Prime Minister (ODPM) (2003b) *Statistical Evidence to Support the Housing Health and Safety Rating System Vols I, II, and III*. London: Office of the Deputy Prime Minister.

Office of the Deputy Prime Minister (ODPM) (2004) *A Decent Home: The Definition and Guidance for Implementation*. London: Office of the Deputy Prime Minister.

Office of the Deputy Prime Minister (ODPM) (2005) *Public Sector Service Agreement Target 7*. London: Office of the Deputy Prime Minister. See also www. communities.gov.uk/index.asp?id=1152136, accessed 20 June 2006.

Office of the Deputy Prime Minister (ODPM) (2006a) *Housing Health and Safety Rating System: Operating Guidance*. London: Office of the Deputy Prime Minister.

Office of the Deputy Prime Minister (ODPM) (2006b) *English House Condition Survey 2003*. London: Office of the Deputy Prime Minister.

Office of the Deputy Prime Minister (ODPM) (2006c) *Minority Ethnic Issues in Social Exclusion and Neighbourhood Renewal*. London: Office of the Deputy Prime Minister, SEU REPORT: 101–2.

Office of the First Minister and Deputy First Minister (OFMDFM) (2006) *Our Children and Young People – Our Pledge: A Ten Year Strategy for Children and Young People in Northern Ireland 2006–2016*. Belfast: OFMDFM.

Office of the First Minister and Deputy First Minister (OFMDFM) (2010a) *Child Poverty Strategy, Consultation Document*, December. Belfast: OFMDFM.

Office of the First Minister and Deputy First Minister (OFMDFM) (2010b) *Lifetime Opportunities Monitoring Opportunities*. Baseline report, 14 October. Online at: www.ofmdfmni.gov.uk/annex_3_lifetime_opportunities_monitoring_framework_oct_2010_pdf.pdf.

Ordnance Survey (2010) Online at: www.ordnancesurvey.co.uk/oswebsite/business/sectors/health/docs/Bolton%20Health%20Inequality%20small.pdf, accessed 27 January 2011.

Ormandy, D (2009) *Housing and Health in Europe (Housing and Society Series): The WHO LARES Project*. London: Routledge.

Osborne, D and Gaebler, T (1992) *Reinventing Government: How the Entrepreneurial Spirit is Transforming the Public Sector*. Reading, MA: Addison-Wesley.

Parkes, A and Kearns, A (2004) *The Multi-dimensional Neighbourhood and Health. A Cross Sectional Analysis of the Scottish Household Survey, 2001*. ESRC Centre for Neighbourhood Research (CNR).

Parsons, W (1996) *Public Policy: An Introduction to the Theory and Practice of Policy Analysis*. Cheltenham: Edward Elgar.

Pencheon, D, Guest, C and Melzer, D (2001) *Oxford Handbook of Public Health Practice*. Oxford: Oxford University Press.

Pinker, R (2008) The Conservative tradition of social welfare, in Alcock, P, May, M and Rowlingson, K (eds) *The Student's Companion to Social Policy* (3rd edn). Oxford: Blackwell.

Plaid Cymru (2007) *One Wales*. Online at: www.plaidcymru.org/uploads/publications/281.pdf, accessed 27 January 2011.

Porter, ME (1980) *Competitive Strategy: Techniques for Analysing Industries and Competitors*. New York: Free Press.

Public Health Resource Unit and Skills for Health (2008) *Public Health Skills and Career Framework: Multidisciplinary/Multi-agency/Multi-professional*. Oxford: Public Health Resource Unit, Skills for Health. Online at: www.phru.nhs.uk/pages/PHD/publichealthcareer, accessed 27 January 2011.

Putnam, R, Leonardi, R and Nanetti, R (1993) *Making Democracy Work: Civic Traditions in Modern Italy*. New Jersey: Princeton University Press.

Quilgars, D, Johnsen, S and Pleace, N (2008) *Youth Homelessness in the UK*. London: Joseph Rowntree Foundation.

Ranson, R (1991) *Healthy Housing: A Practical Guide*. London: E&FN Spon.

Raw, GJ and Hamilton, RM (eds) (1995) *Building Regulations and Health*. Watford: Building Research Establishment.

Raw, GJ, Aizlewood, CE and Hamilton, RM (eds) (2001) *Building Regulation, Health and Safety*. Watford: Building Research Establishment.

Rawlins, M, Chairman and members of the Advisory Council on Misuse of Drugs (2008) *Cannabis: Classification and Public Health* (Home Office online publication). Online at: www.drugs.homeoffice.gov.uk/publication-search/acmd/acmd-cannabis-report-2008, accessed 27 January 2011.

Reeves, R (2010) *A Liberal Dose? Health and Wellbeing: The Role of the State*. London: Department of Health. Online at: www.dh.gov.uk/en/Publicationsand statistics/Publications/PublicationsPolicyAndGuidance/DH_111697, accessed 10 January 2011.

Rennie, D, Chen, Y and Lawson, J (2005) Differential effect of damp housing on respiratory health in women. *Journal of American Medical Women's Association*, Winter, 60(1): 46–51.

Reviews on Environmental Health (RenvH) (2004) Special Issue: *Housing, Health and Well-being*, 19: 3–4.

Rhodes, T and Hedrich, D (eds) (2010) *Harm Reduction Evidence, Impacts and Challenges*. EMCDDA Monographs. EMCDDA.

Ross, W and Tomaney, J (2001) Devolution and health policy in England. *Regional Studies*, 35(3): 265–70.

Rowe, J (2002) *Planning Public Health Strategies*, in Cowley, S (ed.) *Public Health in Policy and Practice: A Source Book for Health Visitors and Community Nurses*. Edinburgh: Bailliere Tindall.

Royal College of Physicians (1992) *Smoking and the Young*. London: RCP.

Royles, E (2007) *Revitalising Democracy: Devolution and Civil Society in Wales* (Politics and Society in Wales). University of Wales Press.

Sabatier, PA (1986) What can we learn from implementation research?, in Kaufman, FX *et al.* (eds) *Guidance, Control and Evaluation in the Public Sector.* New York: de Gruyter.

Sabatier, P and Jenkins-Smith, H (1993) *Policy Change and Learning.* Boulder, CO: Westview Press.

Save the Children (2008) *Children in Severe Poverty in Wales: An Agenda for Action.* Cardiff: The Wales Programme of Save the Children. Online at: www. savethechildren.org.uk/en/docs/wales_poverty_report_08_eng.pdf, accessed 27 January 2011.

Save the Children (2009) *A Child's Portion: An Analysis of Public Expenditure on Children in the UK.* Northern Ireland Briefing.

Save the Children (2010) *Measuring Severe Child Poverty in Northern Ireland.* Online at: www.savethechildren.org.uk, accessed 27 January 2011.

Scottish Drugs Forum (SDF) (2007) *Drugs and Poverty: A Literature Review.* Scottish Drugs Forum (SDF).

Scottish Executive (2003a) *Partnerships for Care. Scotland's Health White Paper.* Edinburgh: Scottish Executive.

Scottish Executive (2003b) *Improving Health in Scotland: The Challenge.* Edinburgh: Scottish Executive.

Scottish Executive (2004) *Community Health Partnerships. Statutory Guidance.* Edinburgh: Scottish Executive.

Scottish Executive (2005) *Delivering for Health.* Edinburgh: Scottish Executive.

Scottish Executive (2007) *Better Health, Better Care: Discussion Document.* Edinburgh: Scottish Executive.

Scottish Government (2005a) *Building a Health Service Fit for the Future* (Kerr Report). Online at: www.scotland.gov.uk/Publications/2005/05/23141307/13 348, accessed 27 January 2011.

Scottish Government (2005b) *Delivering for Health.* Online at: www.scotland. gov.uk/resource/Doc/76169/0018996.pdf, accessed 27 January 2011.

Scottish Government (2007a) *Better Health, Better Care: Discussion Document.* Online at: www.scotland.gov.uk/Publications/2007/08/13165824/0.

Scottish Government (2007b) *Better Health, Better Care: Action Plan.* Edinburgh: Scottish Government.

Scottish Government (2008a) *Delivering for Remote and Rural Health Care: What it Means to You.* Edinburgh: Scottish Government.

Scottish Government (2008b) *Equally Well: Report of the Ministerial Task Force on Health Inequalities*. Edinburgh: Scottish Government.

Scottish Government (2009a) *Scottish Community Empowerment Action Plan. Celebrating Success. Inspiring Change*. Edinburgh: Scottish Government.

Scottish Government (2009b) *Scottish Index of Multiple Deprivation*. Online at: www.scotland.gov.uk/Topics/Statistics/SIMD, accessed 15 November 2010.

Scottish Government (2010) *Official Gateway to Scotland*. Online at: www.scotland.org/facts/population, accessed 11 November 2010.

Scottish Office (1999) *Towards a Healthier Scotland: Opening the Door to a Healthier Scotland*. Edinburgh: Scottish Office.

Secretary of State for Health (1989) *Working for Patients*. London: HMSO.

Sergeant, E (2008) *Aberdeenshire Council Telecare Project*. Online at: www.aberdeenshire.gov.uk/about/departments/AberdeenshireTelecareProjectEvaluationReport.pdf, accessed 8 November 2010.

Sergrott, J, Holliday, J, Roberts, J, Phillips, C and Murphey, S (2009) *Evaluation of the Cooking Bus in Wales: Final Report*. Cardiff: Institute of Society, Health and Ethics.

Sheffield Hallam University (2010) *Analysing the Environment*. Online at: www.shu.ac.uk/ad/marriott/MSc%20Organisational%20Environment%20Module%20.pdf, accessed 17 June 2010.

Shelter (2009) *Eviction of Children and Families: The Impact and the Alternatives*. Scotland: Shelter.

Simon, H (1957) *Models of Man: Social and Rational*. London: John Wiley.

Sines, D, Saunders, M and Forbes-Burford, J (eds) (2009) *Community Health Care Nursing* (4th edn). Oxford: Wiley-Blackwell.

Skills for Health (2008) *Public Health Skills and Career Framework*. Oxford: Public Health Resource Unit.

Skills for Health (2009) *Public Health Skills and Career Framework*. Oxford: Public Health Resource Unit.

Smith, KE, Bambra, C, Joyce, KE, Perkins, N, Hunter, DJ and Blenkinsopp, EA (2009) 'Partners in Health?' A systematic review of the impact of organisations and partnerships on public health outcomes in England between 1997–2008. *Journal of Public Health*, 30 January: 1–12.

Smith, KR, Brown, BB, Yamada, I and Kowaleski-Jones, L (2008) Walkability and body mass index density, design, and new diversity measures. *American Journal of Preventative Medicine*, September, 35(3): 237–44.

Smith, T and Babbington, E (2006) *Devolution: A Map of Divergence in the NHS. Health Policy Review*. London: BMA Health Policy Research Unit, BMA House.

Southampton City (2008) *Fit-4-Life Strategy for Southampton 2008–13*. Online at: www.southampton-partnership.com/images/Fit%20For%20Life%20Strategy_tcm23-264617.pdf.

Southampton City NHS Primary Care Trust, Southampton City Council (2008) *Southampton's Joint Strategic Needs Assessment for Health and Well-being. 2008 to 2011*. Online at: http://www.southamptonhealth.nhs.uk/aboutus/publichealth/hi/public-health-data/jsna, accessed 27 January 2011.

Southampton City PCT and Southampton City Council (2003) *An Obesity Strategy for Southampton 2003–2008*. Online at: www.southamptonhealth.nhs.uk/publichealth/plans/obesity.

Southampton Partnership (2009) *Southampton's Health and Wellbeing Strategic Plan 2009/12*. Online at: www.southampton-partnership.com/images/2009.03.20%20Minutes_tcm23-224991.pdf.

South East England Health Strategy (2008) Online at: www.sepho.org.uk/Download/Public/11138/1/South%20East%20England%20Health%20Strategy%20(Feb-08).pdf.

Statistics for Wales (2009) *Wales's Population: A Demographic Overview 2009*. Cardiff: Welsh Assembly Government. Online at: wales.gov.uk/docs/statistics/2009/090326walespop09en.pdf, accessed 27 January 2011.

Statutory Instrument (1999) No. 672, The National Assembly for Wales (Transfer of Functions), Order 1999. Online at: www.opsi.gov.uk/si/si1999/19990672.htm, accessed 27 January 2011.

Stimson, GV (1995) AIDS and injecting drug use in the United Kingdom, 1987–1993: the policy response and the prevention of the epidemic. *Social Science and Medicine*, 41(5): 699–716.

Stimson, GV (1998) Harm reduction in action: putting theory into practice. *International Journal of Drug Policy*, 9(6): 401–9.

Stimson, GV (2010) Harm reduction: moving through the third decade. *International Journal of Drug Policy*, 21(2): 91–3.

Strategic Review of Health Inequalities in England Post-2010 (2010) *Fair Society, Healthy Lives* (Marmot Review). London: UCL.

Sullivan, A, Cara, O, Joshi, H, Sosthenes, K and Obolenskaya, P (2010) *The Consequences of Childhood Disadvantage in Northern Ireland at age 5*. London: Institute of Education.

Sustainable Development Commission (2006) *Stock Take: Delivering Improvements in Existing Housing*. Online at: www.sd-commission.org.uk/publications/downloads/Stock_Take.pdf, accessed 4th July 2010.

Sutcliffe, S and Court, J (2006) *A Toolkit for Progressive Policymakers in Developing Countries*. London: Overseas Development Institute.

Tawney, RH (1931) *Equality*. London: Allen & Unwin.

Team Hackney (2010) *Challenging Teenage Pregnancy in Hackney*. Online at: www.hackney.gov.uk/servapps/TeamHackneyProjectsPublic/PressReleasesView.aspx?PressReleaseID=14, accessed 27 January 2011.

Thaler, RH and Sunstein, CR (2008) *Nudge: Improving Decisions about Health, Wealth and Happiness*. New Haven and London: Yale University Press.

Thompson, JL (2001) *Strategic Management* (4th edn). London: Thompson Learning.

Titmuss, R (1970) *The Gift Relationship. From Human Blood to Social Policy*. New York: New Press.

Titmuss, R (1974) *Social Policy: An Introduction*. London: George Allen & Unwin.

Torjman, S (2005) *What is Policy?* Ottawa: Caledon Institute of Social Policy.

Tudor-Smith, C, Head of Health Improvement, Welsh Assembly Government, *Tackling Health Inequalities in Wales*. PowerPoint presentation. Online at: www.dur.ac.uk/resources/wolfson.institute/Neil_Riley.pdf, accessed 27 January 2011.

UK Drugs Policy Commission (UKDPC) (2007) *An Analysis of UK Drug Policy. UK Drugs Policy Commission*. Online at: www.ukdpc.org.uk/publications.shtml#Analysis_Drug_Policy, accessed 27 January 2011.

UK Statute Law Database (2010a) *Medicines Act 1968 (c. 67) OPSI, Office of Public Sector Information*. Online at: www.statutelaw.gov.uk/legResults.aspx?LegType=All+Legislation&title=Medicines+Act+1968&searchEnacted=0&extentMatchOnly=0&confersPower=0&blanketAmendment=0&TYPE=QS&NavFrom=0&activeTextDocId=1662209&PageNumber=1&SortAlpha=0, accessed 25 November 2010.

UK Statute Law Database (2010b) *Misuse of Drugs Act 1971 (c. 38) OPSI, Office of Public Sector Information*. Online at: www.statutelaw.gov.uk/content.aspx?LegType=All+Legislation&title=Misuse+of+Drugs+Act+1971&searchEnacted=0&extentMatchOnly=0&confersPower=0&blanketAmendment=0&sortAlpha=0&TYPE=QS&PageNumber=1&NavFrom=0&parentActiveTextDocId=1367412&ActiveTextDocId=1367412&filesize=260094, accessed 25 November 2010.

UNICEF (2009) *The State of the World's Children: Celebrating 20 Years of the Convention on the Rights of the Child Statistical Tables*. New York: UNICEF. Online at: www.unicef.org/publications/files/SOWC_Spec_Ed_CRC_Statistical_Tables_EN_111809.pdf, accessed 27 January 2011.

United Kingdom Public Health Association (UKPHA) (2010) *Housing and Health Framework*. Online at: www.ukpha.org.uk, accessed 27 January 2011.

United Nations General Assembly (1989) *Convention on the Rights of the Child. Resolution 25 Session 44*. Geneva: United Nations. Online at: http://www.un.org/documents/ga/res/44/a44r025.htm, accessed 27 January 2011.

United Nations Office on Drugs and Crime (UNDOC) (2010) *From Coercion to Cohesion: Treating Drug Dependence through Health Care, Not Punishment. Discussion Paper Based on a Scientific Workshop*. Vienna: UNDOC.

Van Kamp, I, Ruysbroek, A and Stellato, R (2010) *Residential Environmental Quality and Quality of Life, in Housing and Health in Europe: The WHO LARES Project*. London: Routledge.

Vostanis, P (2002) Mental health of homeless children and their families. *Advances in Psychiatric Treatment*, 8: 463–9.

Wales Centre for Health (2009) *Public Health Practitioner's Public Engagement Toolkit*. Online at: www.wales.nhs.uk/sitesplus/documents/888/Public%5FHeal th%5FPractitioner%27s%5FPublic%5FEngagement%5FToolkit1.pdf, accessed 27 January 2011.

Walt, G (1994) *Health Policy: An Introduction to Process and Power*. London: Zed Books.

Walt, G and Gilson, L (1994) Reforming the health sector in developing countries: the central role of policy and analysis. *Health Policy and Planning*, 9: 353–70.

Walt, G, Shiffman, J, Schneider, H, Murray, SF and Brugha, R (2008) Doing health policy analysis: methodological and conceptual reflections and challenges. *Health Policy and Planning*, 23: 308–17.

Wanless, D (2002) *Securing our Future Health: Taking a Long-term View* (final report). London: HM Treasury. Online at: http://www.dh.gov.uk/en/Publicati onsandstatistics/Publications/PublicationsPolicyAndGuidance/DH_4009293, accessed 27 January 2011.

Wanless, D (2003) *The Review of Health and Social Care in Wales, Welsh Assembly Government*. Online at: www.wales.gov.uk/topics/health/publications/health/ reports/wanless/?lang=en. accessed 27 January 2011.

Wanless, D (2004) *Securing Good Health for the Whole Population: Final Report Summary*. London: HMSO. Online at: www.dh.gov.uk/en/Publicationsandstatis tics/Publications/PublicationsPolicyAndGuidance/DH_4074426.

Weatherly, H, Drummond, M and Smith, D (2002) Using evidence in the development of local health policies. Some evidence from the United Kingdom. *International Journal of Technology Assessment in Health Care*, 18: 771–81.

Weber, M (1947) *The Theory of Social and Economic Organisation* (trans. Henderson, AM and Parsons, T). Glencoe: Free Press.

Wells, P (2007) New Labour and evidence based policy making: 1997–2007. *People, Place and Policy Online*, 1(1): 22–9. Online at: extra.shu.ac.uk/ppp-online/issue_1_220507/documents/new_labour_evidence_base_1997–2007. pdf, accessed 27 January 2011.

Welsh Assembly Government (WAG) (2000) *Promoting Health and Wellbeing:*

Implementing the National Health Promotion Strategy (2000). Online at: www.wales.nhs.uk/publications/prom-health-e.pdf, accessed 27 January 2011.

Welsh Assembly Government (WAG) (2001a) *Improving Health in Wales: A Plan for the NHS with its Partners (2001)*. Online at: http://www.wales.nhs.uk/publications/NHSStrategydoc.pdf, accessed 27 January 2011.

Welsh Assembly Government (WAG) (2001b) *Targeting Poor Health*. Online at: www.wales.nhs.uk/publications/TargetingPoorhealth_ENGLISH.pdf, accessed 27 January 2011.

Welsh Assembly Government (WAG) (2002) *Well Being in Wales*. Online at: www.healthcarealliances.co.uk/Public/documents/AM0212WBW.pdf, accessed 27 January 2011.

Welsh Assembly Government (WAG) (2004a) *About Health Challenge Wales*. Cardiff: Welsh Assembly Government. Online at: wales.gov.uk/docs/health-challenge/publications/organisation/090202organisationen.pdf, accessed 27 January 2011.

Welsh Assembly Government (WAG) (2004b) *Children and Young People: Rights to Action*. Online at: www.assemblywales.org/N00000000000000000000000000016990.pdf, accessed 27 January 2011.

Welsh Assembly Government (WAG) (2005a) *Committee on the Better Governance for Wales White Paper*. Cardiff: Welsh Assembly Government.

Welsh Assembly Government (WAG) (2005b) *Designed for Life*. Online at: www.wales.nhs.uk/documents/designed-for-life-e.pdf, accessed 27 January 2011.

Welsh Assembly Government (WAG) (2005c) *Inequalities in Health: The Welsh Dimension 2002–2005*. Online at: wales.gov.uk/dhss/publications/health/reports/inequalitieshealth/inequalitieshealthe.pdf;jsessionid=Xh4HMVTF311ryZFKc51v1d3FZ4fbLMcRCwxb22pxK53TRG0JhV2K!-42672990?lang=en, accessed 27 January 2011.

Welsh Assembly Government (WAG) (2007a) *One Wales: A Progressive Agenda for the Government of Wales*. Cardiff: WAG.

Welsh Assembly Government (WAG) (2007b) *One Wales: A Progressive Agenda for the Government of Wales. An Agreement between the Labour and Plaid Cymru Groups in the National Assembly* Cardiff: WAG. Online at: www.wales.gov.uk/strategy/strategies/onewales/onewalese.pdf?lang=en, accessed 18 November 2010.

Welsh Assembly Government (WAG) (2007c) *Children in Wales: A Wales Fit for Children and Young People*. Cardiff: WAG.

Welsh Assembly Government (WAG) (2007d) *Food and Fitness Policy*. Cardiff: WAG. Online at: www.healtheschool.org.uk/teachers/school-food-fitness-policy-e.pdf, accessed 18 November 2010.

Welsh Assembly Government (WAG) (2008a) *Guidance for Working with*

Schools at Each Phase of the Programme: Welsh Network of Healthy Schools Network (WNHSN). Cardiff: WAG.

Welsh Assembly Government (WAG) (2008b) *Making a Difference: Good Practice Communities First*. Cardiff: WAG. Online at: www.wales.gov.uk/dsjlg/publications/communityregendevelop/making/guide.pdf?lang=en, accessed 18 November 2010.

Welsh Assembly Government (WAG) (2008c) *Primary School Free Breakfast Initiative*. Cardiff: WAG. Online at: http://wales.gov.uk/publications/circular/circulars2006/1552917/?lang=en, accessed 18 November 2010.

Welsh Assembly Government (WAG) (2009) *Services for Children and Young People with Emotional Needs.* Cardiff: WAG. Online at: www.wao.gov.uk/assets/englishdocuments/CAMHS_eng.pdf, accessed 18 November 2010.

Welsh Assembly Government (WAG) (2010a) *Eco Schools Wales*. Online at: www.eco-schoolswales.org/home.asp, accessed 11 December 2010.

Welsh Assembly Government (WAG) (2010b) *Doing Well, Doing Better*. Online at: http://wales.gov.uk/topics/health/publications/health/ministerial/health-servicesstandards/;jsessionid=CJKLMKnJQ2bTFJpLVvJFxBhJk9L2F5cJ32Nmvl5hjrtPGLxdT12h!82924164?lang=en, accessed 18 November 2010.

Welsh Assembly Government (WAG) (2010c) *Free Swimming for Children and Young People*. Cardiff: WAG. Online at: http://wales.gov.uk/newsroom/cultureandsport/2010/100608swimming/?lang=en, accessed 11 December 2010.

Welsh Assembly Government (WAG) (2010d) *Proposals for a Rights of Children and Young Persons (Wales) Measure*. Cardiff: WAG. Online at: http://wales.gov.uk/consultations/childrenandyoungpeople/righsofchildrenyoung/?lang=en, accessed 18 November 2010.

Welsh Assembly Government (WAG) (2010e) *Setting the Direction*. Online at: www.wales.nhs.uk/sitesplus/867/opendoc/157072?uuid=4E4F17BD-1143-E756-5C1BCD843D069AE5, accessed 18 November 2010.

Welsh Assembly Government (WAG) (2010f) *The Foundation Phase*. Online at: http://wales.gov.uk/topics/educationandskills/earlyyearshome/foundation_phase/?lang=en, accessed 11 December 2010.

Welsh Assembly Government (WAG) (2010g) *Welsh Language Policy and Legislation*. Online at: http://wales.gov.uk/topics/welshlanguage/legislation/updates/3842878/;jsessionid=vlvLN2nYj1Jw6JCbThy1Jn5jzXdDJN9pvYVXmrd2LN0lYjTvV52m!-547148533?lang=en.

Welsh Language Act 1993 (c. 38) *Put Welsh and English on an Equal Basis in Public Life in Wales*. Online at: www.byig-wlb.org.uk/English/publications/Publications/523.pdf-, accessed 18 November 2010.

Welsh Office (1998a) *Better Health, Better Wales*. Online at: http://www.wales.nhs.uk/publications/greenpaper98_e.pdf, accessed 18 November 2010.

Welsh Office (1998b) *Putting Patients First*. Online at: http://www.wales.nhs.uk/publications/whitepaper98_e.pdf, accessed 18 November 2010.

Wilkinson, R and Pickett, K (2010) *The Spirit Level: Why Equality is Better for Everyone*. London: Penguin.

Williams, C (ed.) (2007) *Social Policy for Social Welfare Practice in a Devolved Wales*. Birmingham: Venture Press, the Wales Planning Policy Development Programme. Online at: www.cymru.gov.uk/topics/planning/planningresearch/?lang=en, accessed 18 November 2010.

Wills, J (2009) Community development in public health and primary care, in Sines, D, Saunders, M and Forbes-Burford, J (eds) (2009) *Community Health Care Nursing* (4th edn). Oxford: Wiley-Blackwell.

World Health Organization (WHO) (1986) *The Ottawa Charter for Health Promotion. Health Promotion Action Means: Build a Healthy Public Policy*. Ottawa: World Health Organization. Online at: www.who.int/healthpromotion/conferences/previous/ottawa/en/index1.html.

World Health Organization (WHO) (1999) *Charter on Transport, Environment and Health*. EUR/CP/EHCO 02 02 05/9 (rev. 4th edn). Copenhagen: WHO. Online at: www.euro.who.int/_data/assets/pdf_file/0006/88575/E69044.pdf.

World Health Organization (WHO) (2003) *The Social Determinants of Health: The Solid Facts* (ed. Wilkinson, R and Marmot, M). Online at: www.euro.who.int/__data/assets/pdf_file/0005/98438/e81384.pdf, accessed 18 November 2010.

World Health Organization (WHO) (2005a) *Commission on Social Determinants of Health (CSDH)*. Online at: www.who.int/social_determinants/en/, accessed 18 November 2010.

World Health Organization (WHO) (2005b) *Health Service Planning and Policy-making: A Toolkit for Nurses and Midwives. Module 4: Policy Development Process*. Manila: WHO, Western Pacific Regional Publications. Online at: whqlibdoc.who.int/wpro/2005/9290611863_eng.pdf.

World Health Organization (WHO) MIND Project (2010) Online at: www.who.int/mentalhealth/policy/en, accessed 18 November 2010.

World Health Organization (WHO) and World Organization of Family Doctors (WONCA) (2008) *Integrating Mental Health into Primary Care: A Global Perspective*. Online at: www.who.int/mental_health/policy/Integratingmhintoprimarycare2008_lastversion.pdf, accessed 18 November 2010.

YouTube (2008) *NHS at 60. A Look at Bevan and Tredegar* (BBC, 2008). Online at: www.youtube.com/watch?v=2lLBRs-sT6o&feature=related, accessed 18 November 2010.

Zacchaeus 2000 Trust (2005) *Memorandum to the Prime Minister on Unaffordable Housing*. London: Z2K Trust.

Index